BARBARA O'NEILL COMPLETE COLLECTION

Over 400 Pages About Natural Solutions and Herbal Remedies for Everyday Ailments and Lasting Wellbeing

Janet Moore

Table of Contents

BOOK 1: DR. BARBARA O'NEILL'S MUST-HAVE HERBAL ENCYCLOPEDIA

BOOK 2: THE LOST BOOK OF HERBAL SOLUTIONS

BOOK 3: THE ESSENTIAL BARBARA O'NEILL COOKBOOK

CHAPTER 15: HEALING BEVERAGES 364

PART III: IMPLEMENTING WELLNESS INTO EVERYDAY LIFE 374

Thank you so much for purchasing my book! I'm thrilled to have you as part of my reading family.

If you could take a moment to scan the QR code below and leave your honest review on Amazon, I would be deeply grateful.

If you are reading the ebook version, please click on this link:

https://www.amazon.com/review/create-review?&ASIN=B0CWMCM7BK

Your feedback is incredibly important to me—it helps me grow as a writer and makes our community stronger. I genuinely love hearing from you and value your thoughts immensely!

DR. BARBARA O'NEILL'S
MUST-HAVE
HERBAL
ENCYCLOPEDIA

Everything You Need to Know About Natural Solutions for Everyday Ailments and Lasting Wellbeing

Janet Moore

Introduction to Dr. Barbara O'Neill's Philosophy

Barbara O'Neill, as a natural health educator and advocate for the use of herbal remedies, promotes a philosophy centered around the healing power of nature and the body's inherent ability to heal itself given the right conditions. Her approach to health and wellness is holistic, emphasizing the importance of natural foods, herbal remedies, and lifestyle changes to achieve optimal health.

O'Neill believes strongly in the effectiveness of natural remedies, including herbs, to prevent and treat various health conditions. She advocates for using plants and natural substances as medicines, which have been used for centuries across different cultures and civilizations.

Her philosophy encompasses a holistic view of health, considering the physical, mental, emotional, and spiritual aspects of an individual. She emphasizes that true healing involves addressing all these components rather than just treating symptoms.

O'Neill is dedicated to educating people about health and nutrition, empowering them to take control of their health through informed choices. She provides resources, workshops, and lectures to disseminate her knowledge on natural healing and healthy living.

A core aspect of her philosophy is the emphasis on prevention of disease through a healthy lifestyle, including diet, exercise, and stress management. She advocates for proactive measures to maintain health rather than reactive measures to treat diseases.

Diet and nutrition play a central role in her approach to health and wellness. O'Neill promotes a diet rich in whole, plant-based foods and minimizes processed foods, believing that such a diet can support the body's healing processes and maintain vitality.

She also speaks to the importance of detoxification and cleansing as methods to rid the body of toxins and support overall health. Herbal remedies, along with other natural practices, are often recommended as part of detoxification protocols.

Barbara O'Neill's philosophy on herbal remedies and natural health is comprehensive, emphasizing education, prevention, and the use of natural methods to achieve and maintain optimal health. For those interested in her teachings, it would be beneficial to look into her published works, online resources, or attend her workshops for more detailed insights.

Chapter 1: Who is Dr. Barbara O'Neill?

Background: From Hippie to Health Educator

Dr. Barbara O'Neill, often referred to in the context of natural health and wellness, has a background that traces from an early interest in natural living and holistic health to becoming a recognized educator and advocate for natural healing practices. While there might be some confusion due to the existence of multiple professionals with a similar name, the Barbara O'Neill referred to here is best known for her contributions to natural health education. This profile outlines her journey from a lifestyle initially inspired by holistic and 'hippie' values to her role as a health educator and speaker.

Dr. Barbara O'Neill's journey into the world of natural health often begins with a narrative of personal discovery and passion for understanding the body's natural healing abilities. Inspired by the holistic health movement that gained prominence in the 1960s and 1970s, which was closely tied to the 'hippie' culture of that era, she embraced the principles of natural living, organic eating, and the therapeutic use of herbs and natural remedies. This early interest laid the foundation for her future career.

Driven by her passion for health and wellness, O'Neill pursued formal education in the field of natural health. She has been described as obtaining qualifications in naturopathy, nutrition, herbal medicine, and health education. Her academic and professional journey equipped her with a broad understanding of holistic health principles and practices, allowing her to blend traditional knowledge with scientific research in her teachings.

As a health educator, Dr. Barbara O'Neill has dedicated much of her career to teaching others about the benefits of natural health practices. She is known for conducting seminars, workshops, and lectures where she shares her knowledge on nutrition, detoxification, natural remedies, and the body's ability to heal itself. Her approach is often characterized by a focus on preventative health measures and the adoption of a holistic lifestyle.

O'Neill has authored several books and produced a variety of educational materials, including videos and online courses, to reach a broader audience. Her work often emphasizes practical advice on how to incorporate natural health strategies into everyday life, aiming to make holistic health accessible to everyone.

It's important to note that while O'Neill's teachings have been influential for many seeking alternative health solutions, she has also faced criticism and controversy. Some of her views, particularly those skeptical of conventional medicine and vaccination, have sparked debate within the medical and health communities. Despite the controversies, Dr. Barbara O'Neill's impact on the field of natural health education is undeniable. Her journey from a 'hippie' inspired by the holistic health movement to a respected health educator underscores the importance she places on natural, preventative health measures and the body's healing capabilities. Her work continues to inspire those interested in natural health practices and holistic wellness.

Embracing a Life Aligned with Nature

Barbara O'Neill, as a natural health educator, embodies the philosophy of embracing a life aligned with nature through her teachings and personal practices. Her approach to health and wellness is deeply rooted in the belief that the body can heal itself if given the right natural conditions and support.

Here's how Dr. O'Neill's philosophies and teachings reflect the principles of living in harmony with nature:

- Holistic Approach to Health: O'Neill advocates for a comprehensive view of health that includes physical, emotional, mental, and spiritual well-being. She emphasizes the importance of addressing all aspects of an individual's life to achieve true health.
- Nature as a Healing Space: Dr. O'Neill encourages spending time in nature to support healing and well-being. She believes that direct contact with the earth, fresh air, and natural light are essential for health.
- Learning from Nature: She often highlights how observations of the natural world can inform healthier living practices, stressing the importance of living in a way that is respectful and mindful of the natural environment.
- Sustainable Practices: In her teachings, O'Neill promotes sustainable living habits, such as reducing waste, choosing organic and locally sourced foods, and minimizing one's ecological footprint.
- Ethical Considerations: She also touches upon the ethical dimensions of living in harmony with nature, including animal welfare and the equitable distribution of resources.
- Herbal Medicine: A significant aspect of Dr. O'Neill's approach includes the use of herbal remedies and natural supplements to support health and treat illness, emphasizing the healing power of plants.
- Plant-Based Nutrition: She advocates for a diet that is rich in plant-based foods, minimally processed items, and organic produce, suggesting that such a diet is not only healthier for the individual but also less harmful to the environment.
- Empowering Through Knowledge: O'Neill is dedicated to educating individuals on how to take control of their health through natural means. She provides resources, workshops, and lectures that empower people to make informed decisions about their health.
- Self-Care Practices: She teaches self-care practices that individuals can incorporate into their daily lives, advocating for proactive health measures that align with natural principles.
- Mindfulness and Meditation: Emphasizing the importance of mental and spiritual well-being, O'Neill encourages practices like meditation and mindfulness to foster a sense of peace, balance, and connection with the self and nature.

Chapter 2: Understanding Your Body

The Body's Innate Ability to Heal

Dr. Barbara O'Neill, with her background in natural health education, emphasizes the body's innate ability to heal itself. This belief is central to her teachings and practices, reflecting a fundamental principle of naturopathy and holistic medicine. According to O'Neill, when provided with the right environment, nutrition, and care, the body can often rectify imbalances and recover from illness without the need for invasive treatments.

Let's delve deeper into how Dr. O'Neill applies these principles in her teachings:

Fundamental Beliefs

- Whole Person Health: O'Neill's approach goes beyond addressing isolated symptoms; it involves assessing the whole person. This includes not only physical health but also emotional well-being, mental health, social connections, and spiritual life.
- Prevention is Primary: Emphasizing preventive care to avoid the onset of illness is a key part of her philosophy. This involves educating individuals on how to live healthily and make choices that promote long-term wellness.

The healing power of nature

- Vis Medicatrix Naturae: O'Neill often refers to the concept of "Vis Medicatrix Naturae," or the healing power of nature, which suggests that the body inherently knows how to heal itself, given the right conditions. This principle is foundational to her approach to health and wellness. Central to the idea of Vis Medicatrix Naturae is the understanding that the body is not just a collection of parts to be fixed but is a complex, dynamic system capable of self-regulation and self-healing. O'Neill emphasizes that the body strives to maintain equilibrium and health, and when provided with the right conditions, it can often initiate healing processes without external interventions.
- Natural Surroundings: O'Neill advocates for spending time in natural environments to support health and healing. Nature is seen as a source of healing energy and a means to reduce stress and promote physical activity.
- Reduced Exposure to Toxins: Limiting exposure to environmental toxins, including chemicals in food, water, and personal care products, is considered important for allowing the body to heal.

Nutrition and Detoxification

- Nutritional Support: A cornerstone of Dr. O'Neill's teachings is the role of nutrition in supporting the body's healing processes. She advocates for a diet rich in whole, plant-based foods, which provide the nutrients necessary for repair and maintenance of health.
- Detoxification: O'Neill emphasizes the importance of detoxification in facilitating healing. She advocates for practices and diets that support the body's natural detoxification processes, helping to eliminate toxins that can impede health.

Lifestyle and Environmental Factors

- Holistic Lifestyle: The adoption of a lifestyle that reduces stress, incorporates physical activity, ensures adequate rest, and fosters positive relationships is essential in O'Neill's philosophy. She believes such a lifestyle supports the body's natural healing mechanisms.
- Healthy Environment: Creating an environment that supports health, including clean air, water, and a toxin-free living space, is also seen as crucial to enabling the body's innate ability to heal.

The Role of Mind and Spirit

- Mental and Emotional Well-being: Dr. O'Neill teaches that mental and emotional health is deeply connected to physical health. Stress management techniques, positive thinking, and emotional healing practices are recommended to support the body's healing capacity.
- Spiritual Health: She also highlights the importance of spiritual wellness, suggesting that a sense of purpose and connection can significantly impact one's ability to heal and maintain health.

Education and Empowerment

- Self-Care: Dr. O'Neill empowers individuals to take an active role in their health journey. She educates her audience on how to listen to their bodies and apply natural health principles to support healing.
- Informed Decision-Making: She advocates for individuals to become informed about their health options and to make decisions that align with the body's natural healing processes.

Key Functions and How They Support Health

Dr. Barbara O'Neill, with her background in natural health education, emphasizes several key bodily functions as vital to maintaining health and supporting the body's innate healing abilities. Her teachings focus on understanding and supporting these functions through natural means, such as diet, lifestyle changes, and natural therapies. Here's an overview of some key functions according to her perspective and how they support health:

Digestion and Nutrient Absorption

- Role in Health: Proper digestion and the efficient absorption of nutrients are essential for health, as they ensure the body receives the necessary building blocks for repair, growth, and energy production.
- Support Strategies: Dr. O'Neill advocates for a diet rich in whole, plant-based foods, minimizing processed foods to enhance digestive health. She also emphasizes the importance of proper meal timing and chewing food thoroughly to aid digestion.

Detoxification

- Role in Health: The body's ability to detoxify, primarily through the liver, kidneys, skin, and lungs, is crucial for removing toxins and waste products. Efficient detoxification prevents the accumulation of harmful substances that can lead to illness.
- Support Strategies: O'Neill recommends practices such as fasting, consuming detoxifying foods (like leafy greens and cruciferous vegetables), staying hydrated, and using saunas to support the body's natural detoxification processes.

Immune Function

- Role in Health: A robust immune system protects the body from infections and disease. It identifies and neutralizes pathogens like bacteria, viruses, and other foreign bodies.
- Support Strategies: To support immune function, O'Neill emphasizes the importance of a nutrient-dense diet, adequate sleep, stress reduction, and regular physical activity. She may also recommend specific herbs and supplements known to support immune health.

Hormonal Balance

- Role in Health: Hormones regulate numerous bodily functions, including metabolism, growth and development, and mood. Maintaining hormonal balance is essential for overall health and well-being.
- Support Strategies: O'Neill suggests managing stress, avoiding endocrine disruptors found in some plastics and pesticides, and consuming foods that support hormonal health, such as those rich in omega-3 fatty acids and phytoestrogens.

Circulation and Cardiovascular Health

- Role in Health: Efficient circulation ensures that oxygen, nutrients, and hormones are delivered to the cells, and waste products are removed. Good cardiovascular health supports this process and prevents disease.
- Support Strategies: Regular exercise, a diet low in saturated fats and high in fruits, vegetables, and whole grains, and avoiding smoking are key recommendations for supporting circulatory and cardiovascular health.

Nervous System Function

- Role in Health: The nervous system controls body movements, responds to sensory information, and regulates body functions. Its health is critical for overall well-being and quality of life.
- Support Strategies: O'Neill promotes stress management techniques, adequate sleep, and nutrients that support nervous system health, such as B vitamins, omega-3 fatty acids, and magnesium.

Mental and Emotional Well-being

- Role in Health: Mental and emotional health significantly impact physical health. Stress, anxiety, and depression can lead to physical health issues and vice versa.
- Support Strategies: Practices such as meditation, mindfulness, physical activity, and connecting with nature are recommended to enhance mental and emotional well-being.

Chapter 3: Foundations of Health

Importance of Water and Hydration

Dr. Barbara O'Neill, with her expertise in natural health education, places a significant emphasis on the importance of water and hydration for maintaining health and supporting the body's natural healing processes. Water is fundamental to life and plays a critical role in virtually every function of the body, including digestion, detoxification, circulation, and nutrient absorption. Here are some of the key points Dr. O'Neill might highlight regarding the importance of water and hydration:

- Cell Function: Every cell in the body requires water to function properly. Water participates in the biochemical reactions within cells, helps maintain cell structure, and facilitates the transport of nutrients and removal of waste.
- Elimination of Toxins: Water is crucial for the body's natural detoxification processes. It aids the kidneys in filtering waste from the blood and helps remove toxins through urine. Adequate hydration also supports liver function, another key organ in detoxification.
- Digestive Health: Water is essential for healthy digestion. It helps dissolve nutrients so that they can be absorbed by the intestines and supports the movement of food through the gastrointestinal tract, preventing constipation.
- Thermoregulation: Through the process of perspiration and evaporation, water helps regulate the body's temperature. Staying hydrated is especially important during physical activity and in hot environments to prevent overheating.
- Physical Activity: Hydration affects muscle function and endurance. Dehydration can lead to fatigue, reduced coordination, and muscle cramps, thereby impacting physical performance.
- Blood Volume and Pressure: Adequate hydration is important for maintaining proper blood volume, which affects blood pressure and heart rate. Water helps ensure that the heart can efficiently pump blood throughout the body.
- Skin Health: Water contributes to skin hydration, which affects its elasticity, appearance, and ability to act as a barrier against pathogens and environmental pollutants.
- Mental Health: Hydration has a significant impact on brain function, including concentration, memory, and mood. Dehydration can lead to headaches, cognitive impairment, and mood swings.

Dr. O'Neill typically recommends drinking pure, clean water as the best source of hydration. She may also emphasize the importance of listening to your body's signals, such as thirst, and adjusting your water intake based on activity level, climate, and individual health needs. She often suggests avoiding or minimizing beverages that can lead to dehydration, such as those high in caffeine or sugar.

Furthermore, Dr. O'Neill might highlight the role of foods in hydration, pointing out that fruits and vegetables with high water content can contribute significantly to daily water intake.

Overall, Dr. Barbara O'Neill's teachings underscore water's vital role in health and healing, advocating for regular, adequate hydration as a cornerstone of a healthy lifestyle and natural wellness.

The Role of Air and Breathing

Dr. Barbara O'Neill, with her focus on natural health practices, emphasizes the critical role of air quality and proper breathing techniques in maintaining health and enhancing the body's innate healing capabilities. Understanding that the act of breathing is not just about oxygen intake but also about detoxification and energy distribution, she highlights several key aspects of how air and breathing support health:

Oxygenation of the Body

- Essential for Life: Breathing is the process by which the body takes in oxygen from the air and expels carbon dioxide. Oxygen is essential for cellular respiration, the process by which cells produce energy.
- Enhanced Cellular Function: Proper oxygenation ensures that every cell in the body functions optimally, supporting overall health and vitality.

Detoxification

- Removal of Waste: Breathing is a major route for the body to expel toxins, with carbon dioxide being a primary waste product of metabolism. Deep, effective breathing can enhance this detoxification process.
- Supports Lymphatic System: Proper breathing supports the lymphatic system, which helps to remove toxins from the body. The lymphatic system relies on muscle movement and breathing to pump lymph fluid through the body.

Stress Reduction

- Calming Effect: Deep, mindful breathing has a calming effect on the nervous system. It can reduce stress and anxiety by activating the parasympathetic nervous system, which induces a state of relaxation.
- Improves Mental Clarity: Regular practice of deep breathing techniques can improve mental clarity, concentration, and emotional stability.

Supports Immune Function

Enhanced Immune Response: Adequate oxygenation and the removal of toxins through breathing are essential for a strong immune system. Proper breathing can help to fend off infections and promote healing.

Energy Levels

Increased Energy: Effective breathing techniques can increase energy levels by ensuring that the body's cells receive the oxygen they need for efficient energy production.

Breathing Techniques and Exercises

- Deep Breathing: Encourages full oxygen exchange and stimulates the body's relaxation response.
- Diaphragmatic Breathing: Focuses on engaging the diaphragm during breathing, which is more efficient than shallow chest breathing.
- Breath Awareness: Involves being mindful of the breath, which can enhance emotional well-being and reduce stress.

The Importance of Clean Air

Environmental Health: Dr. O'Neill also highlights the importance of breathing clean, unpolluted air. She may advocate for spending time in natural, green environments, using air purifiers indoors, and avoiding exposure to airborne toxins and pollutants.

Sunshine: Nature's Healer

Dr. Barbara O'Neill underscores the vital role of sunshine in maintaining health and supporting the body's natural healing processes. Recognized as "Nature's Healer," sunlight provides numerous health benefits, central to which is the production of Vitamin D, a critical nutrient for overall health. Here's how Dr. O'Neill might articulate the healing properties of sunshine and practical ways to harness its benefits:

Vitamin D Synthesis

- Critical for Bone Health: Vitamin D, produced by the skin in response to sunlight, is essential for calcium absorption, making it crucial for maintaining healthy bones and preventing conditions such as osteoporosis.
- Supports Immune Function: Vitamin D plays a significant role in modulating the immune system, enhancing the body's ability to fight off infections and reduce inflammation.

Mood Enhancement

Fights Depression: Exposure to sunlight can improve mood and energy levels, partly through the production of serotonin, a neurotransmitter associated with a feeling of well-being and happiness. This is particularly beneficial in combating seasonal affective disorder (SAD) and other forms of depression.

Circadian Rhythm Regulation

Improves Sleep Quality: Sunlight exposure, especially in the morning, can help regulate the body's circadian rhythm, leading to improved sleep patterns and quality. This regulation is vital for overall health, affecting everything from hormone production to cognitive function.

Skin Conditions

Therapeutic Effects: Controlled sun exposure can have therapeutic effects on certain skin conditions, such as psoriasis, eczema, and acne, through anti-inflammatory properties and promoting healing.

Practical Advice for Safe Sun Exposure

Dr. O'Neill emphasizes the importance of balancing sun exposure to harness its benefits while minimizing risks such as skin damage and increased risk of skin cancer:
- Timing: She might recommend getting sunlight exposure during the safer times of the day, typically in the morning or late afternoon, when the sun's rays are less intense.
- Duration: For Vitamin D synthesis, short daily exposure (about 10 to 15 minutes for lighter skin and slightly longer for darker skin tones) is often sufficient, depending on the individual's skin type, geographic location, and time of year.
- Protection: When exposure exceeds these brief periods, she advises using protective measures such as wearing hats, sunglasses, and applying broad-spectrum sunscreen to exposed skin to prevent overexposure and damage.
- Diet and Supplements: In regions with limited sunlight or during the winter months, Dr. O'Neill might suggest Vitamin D-rich foods or supplements to ensure adequate levels.

Recognizing the interconnectedness of all aspects of health, Dr. O'Neill likely advocates for a holistic approach to sun exposure, considering individual needs and environmental factors. She would stress the importance of listening to one's body and respecting its signals, encouraging a mindful approach to sunbathing that seeks to balance the benefits of sunlight with the need for skin protection.

Chapter 4: Nutrition for Healing

Plant-Based Diet: Benefits and How to Transition

D r. Barbara O'Neill strongly advocates for the benefits of a plant-based diet. Emphasizing whole, minimally processed foods derived from plants, this diet aligns with her holistic approach to health, highlighting the interconnectedness of diet, bodily health, and the natural world.

A plant-based diet centers around foods derived from plants, including vegetables, fruits, grains, nuts, seeds, and legumes, with few or no animal products. It's not necessarily vegetarian or vegan but focuses on consuming more plant-derived foods in their whole, minimally processed forms. The idea is to maximize the intake of nutrient-dense plant foods while minimizing processed foods, meats, and dairy products.

Here are the key components and principles of a plant-based diet:
- Vegetables and Fruits. These are the cornerstone of a plant-based diet, providing essential vitamins, minerals, fiber, and antioxidants that support overall health and help prevent chronic diseases.
- Grains. Whole grains like brown rice, quinoa, barley, and whole wheat products are preferred over refined grains because they retain their fiber and nutrient content.
- Nuts and Seeds. Nuts and seeds are excellent sources of healthy fats, proteins, vitamins, and minerals. Including a variety of them ensures a good intake of essential nutrients.
- Legumes. Beans, lentils, and peas are important plant-based protein sources, offering fiber, iron, and B vitamins, making them great alternatives to meat.
- Healthy Fats. A focus on healthy fats from avocados, nuts, seeds, and olive oil, rather than saturated fats found in animal products and certain oils.
- Limited Processed Foods. Emphasis is placed on whole, minimally processed foods, reducing intake of highly processed snacks, sweets, and fast foods, which are often high in unhealthy fats, sugars, and sodium.
- Sustainability. A plant-based diet is also recognized for its environmental benefits, as plant-based food production generally requires less energy, land, and water, and produces fewer greenhouse gases compared to animal-based food production.

Adopting a plant-based diet offers a multitude of health, environmental, and ethical benefits. Here's a detailed look at some of these advantages:

Health Benefits
1. Heart Health: A plant-based diet is linked to a lower risk of heart disease. It typically includes high amounts of fruits, vegetables, whole grains, nuts, and seeds, which are known to reduce blood pressure and improve cholesterol levels.
2. Weight Management: People following a plant-based diet often find it easier to maintain a healthy weight because plant-based foods are generally lower in calories and fat than animal products, and higher in fiber, which can help you feel full longer.
3. Diabetes Prevention and Management: Eating a diet rich in whole, plant-based foods can improve insulin sensitivity and reduce the risk of type 2 diabetes. For those already diagnosed, it may help in managing blood sugar levels.
4. Cancer Risk Reduction: Certain plant-based diet components, like fruits, vegetables, and whole grains, contain antioxidants and phytochemicals that could lower the risk of certain cancers.
5. Improved Digestive Health: The high fiber content in a plant-based diet supports gut health by promoting regular bowel movements, preventing constipation, and reducing the risk of gastrointestinal diseases.

6. Longevity: Some research suggests that a plant-based diet could be associated with a longer lifespan, likely due to its impact on risk factors for chronic diseases.

Environmental Benefits
1. Lower Carbon Footprint: Plant-based diets generally require less energy, land, and water to produce than diets rich in animal products, resulting in a lower carbon footprint and less strain on the environment.
2. Reduced Greenhouse Gas Emissions: The production of plant-based foods typically generates fewer greenhouse gas emissions compared to raising livestock for meat, dairy, and eggs.
3. Conservation of Resources: Adopting plant-based eating habits can contribute to water conservation and reduced deforestation, as agriculture is a major driver of water usage and forest conversion to farmland, especially for livestock.

Ethical Benefits
1. Animal Welfare: Choosing plant-based foods can reduce the demand for animal farming, thereby potentially leading to higher welfare standards for animals.
2. Promoting Food Security: Plant-based diets can be more sustainable and efficient in terms of calorie production per acre, which could contribute to global food security by making more food available for human consumption rather than being used to feed livestock.

Nutritional Benefits
1. Nutrient-Rich: Plant-based diets are rich in vitamins, minerals, antioxidants, and phytonutrients that support overall health.
2. Healthy Fats: They encourage the consumption of healthy fats from sources like avocados, nuts, and seeds, which support heart health and cognitive function.

Transitioning to a plant-based diet in a gradual, flexible manner can make the shift more sustainable and enjoyable, reducing the likelihood of feeling overwhelmed by drastic changes. Here's a deeper look into practical steps and considerations for gradually adopting a plant-based lifestyle:

- Incorporate More of What You Already Eat: Begin by increasing portions of plant-based foods you already enjoy, such as adding extra vegetables to dishes, expanding the variety of fruits for snacks, and incorporating more whole grains into your meals.
- Plant-Based Alternatives: Experiment with plant-based substitutes for familiar animal products. Try almond or oat milk instead of cow's milk, use lentils or beans in place of ground meat in recipes, and explore cheese alternatives made from nuts.
- Expand Your Recipe Repertoire: Explore plant-based recipes online, in cookbooks, or through cooking classes. Learning to cook a variety of tasty plant-based meals can keep your diet interesting and satisfying.
- Meal Planning: Planning your meals can help ensure you're including a variety of nutrients in your diet and can make the transition smoother. Start by planning a few plant-based meals each week and gradually increase as you feel comfortable.
- Understand Nutritional Needs: Educating yourself about the nutritional aspects of a plant-based diet is important to ensure you're getting all the nutrients your body needs. Pay particular attention to nutrients that may require more attention in a plant-based diet, such as vitamin B12, iron, calcium, and omega-3 fatty acids.
- Diverse Protein Sources: Familiarize yourself with plant-based protein sources like beans, lentils, tofu, tempeh, and seitan. These can be great substitutes for meat in many recipes and offer a variety of textures and flavors.
- Reduce Animal Products Gradually: If you currently eat a lot of meat, dairy, or eggs, consider reducing your consumption gradually. You might designate certain days of the week as plant-based or start with one plant-based meal a day.
- Adjust According to Your Needs: Pay attention to how your body responds to dietary changes. You may need to adjust your food choices based on energy levels, digestion, and overall well-being.

- Seek Support: Connecting with others who are interested in plant-based eating can provide support, inspiration, and practical advice. Look for online communities, local meetups, or plant-based cooking classes.
- Flexibility is Key: Remember that transitioning to a plant-based diet is a journey. There may be setbacks or challenges, but each plant-based choice is a step toward your goals. Be patient and allow yourself the flexibility to enjoy the process.

By taking these gradual steps, you're not only moving toward a healthier diet but also contributing to a more sustainable and ethical world. The key is to find joy and satisfaction in exploring new foods and discovering the benefits of a plant-based lifestyle.

Understanding Fats and Sugars

Dr. Barbara O'Neill places a significant emphasis on understanding the roles of fats and sugars in our diet, advocating for informed choices that support overall health. Her teachings likely emphasize the complexity of these macronutrients, debunking common misconceptions and highlighting their impact on bodily functions. Here's how she might approach the topic:

Understanding Fats

Fats have often been misunderstood and wrongly vilified in the diet. Dr. O'Neill might stress the importance of distinguishing between different types of fats, understanding their roles in the body, and recognizing which sources of fats are healthiest.

Healthy Fats:
- Essential Fatty Acids: Omega-3 and omega-6 fatty acids are essential for heart health, brain function, and reducing inflammation. Sources include flaxseeds, chia seeds, hemp seeds, walnuts, and fatty fish (for those who include fish in their diet).
- Monounsaturated Fats: Found in olive oil, avocados, and nuts, these fats are beneficial for heart health and can help lower bad cholesterol levels.

Unhealthy Fats:
- Saturated Fats: While not all saturated fats are inherently bad, excessive intake, especially from processed meats and dairy products, can increase the risk of heart disease.
- Trans Fats: Virtually all health experts agree that trans fats, found in many processed foods, should be avoided as they significantly raise the risk of heart disease and other health issues.

Understanding Sugars

Sugar, particularly added sugar, is a major concern in modern diets. Dr. O'Neill would likely highlight the difference between natural sugars found in fruits and vegetables and added sugars used in processed foods.

Natural Sugars:
- Whole Foods: Sugars found in whole fruits and vegetables come with fiber, vitamins, and minerals, which help regulate blood sugar levels and provide essential nutrients.

Added Sugars
- Health Risks: Excessive consumption of added sugars has been linked to obesity, type 2 diabetes, heart disease, and other metabolic disorders. Dr. O'Neill would advise minimizing foods with high levels of added sugars.

Practical Advice

For Fats
- Choose Healthy Sources: Incorporate healthy fats into your diet while minimizing the intake of unhealthy fats. Reading labels can help identify hidden sources of trans and saturated fats.
- Cooking with Healthy Fats: Use oils rich in monounsaturated and polyunsaturated fats for cooking and dressings.

For Sugars
- Read Labels: Be vigilant about reading food labels to identify added sugars, which can appear under many different names.
- Whole Foods First: Prioritize whole foods over processed ones to naturally reduce sugar intake and increase fiber, aiding in sugar metabolism.

Overall Approach
- Balance and Moderation: Understanding that fats and sugars are not inherently bad, but rather their sources and amounts consumed can lead to different health outcomes.
- Educational Empowerment: Empower yourself with knowledge about these macronutrients to make informed dietary choices that support health and well-being.

Dr. O'Neill's approach to fats and sugars would be grounded in the principle of balance and informed choice, advocating for a diet that supports the body's natural healing processes and promotes long-term health. Through education and practical guidance, she encourages a nuanced understanding of these critical dietary components.

The Role of Superfoods

Dr. Barbara O'Neill often emphasizes the importance of whole, nutrient-dense foods in supporting the body's natural healing processes and maintaining overall health. In this context, she might discuss the concept of "superfoods" and their role in a healthy diet. Superfoods are typically foods that are particularly rich in nutrients, antioxidants, vitamins, and minerals, offering significant health benefits beyond their nutritional content.

Superfoods don't have a strict scientific definition but are generally recognized as foods with a high nutrient density that may offer health benefits, such as reducing the risk of certain diseases or enhancing any number of bodily functions. Examples include berries, dark leafy greens, nuts and seeds, whole grains, and fatty fish (for those not following a strict plant-based diet), among others.

The Role of Superfoods According to Dr. O'Neill
- Nutrient Density. Dr. O'Neill would highlight that superfoods are packed with vitamins, minerals, antioxidants, and other phytonutrients essential for health and vitality. Incorporating a variety of these foods can help ensure a wide range of nutrients in the diet.
- Antioxidant Properties. Many superfoods contain high levels of antioxidants, which help combat oxidative stress and may reduce the risk of chronic diseases such as heart disease, cancer, and Alzheimer's disease. Foods like blueberries, spinach, and dark chocolate are noted for their antioxidant content.
- Support for Natural Healing. Dr. O'Neill might emphasize how superfoods support the body's innate healing abilities. For example, the anti-inflammatory properties of turmeric or the omega-3 fatty acids found in chia seeds and flaxseeds can support the body's natural healing processes.
- Enhancing Digestive Health. The fiber in many superfoods, such as legumes, whole grains, and fruits, supports digestive health, promoting regular bowel movements and a healthy gut microbiome.

- Energy and Vitality. Superfoods can contribute to sustained energy levels and overall vitality due to their complex carbohydrates, healthy fats, and protein content, along with vitamins and minerals that support metabolic processes.

Practical Tips for Incorporating Superfoods
1. Variety: Dr. O'Neill would likely recommend incorporating a wide range of superfoods to ensure a diverse intake of nutrients.
2. Whole Foods Over Supplements: While supplements can have their place, obtaining nutrients from whole foods ensures you benefit from the synergy of nutrients present in their natural form.
3. Seasonal and Local: Choosing seasonal and local superfoods can maximize their nutrient content and environmental sustainability.
4. Daily Diet: Incorporating superfoods into daily meals and snacks rather than viewing them as occasional additions can maximize their health benefits.

Dr. O'Neill would also caution against the perception that superfoods are a magic solution to health issues. She would stress the importance of a balanced diet, where superfoods are part of an overall healthy eating pattern rather than a cure-all. A holistic approach to health, considering not just diet but also lifestyle factors like stress management, physical activity, and sleep, is vital for achieving and maintaining optimal health.

Chapter 5: The Power of Exercise

Incorporating Movement into Daily Life

D r. Barbara O'Neill, with her holistic approach to health, emphasizes the importance of incorporating movement into daily life as a key component of overall well-being. Recognizing that modern lifestyles often lead to prolonged periods of sitting and inactivity, she advocates for finding ways to integrate more physical activity into our routines, regardless of fitness levels or age. Here are some principles and practical tips she might suggest for making movement a natural part of daily life:

Principles of Incorporating Movement:
- Consistency Over Intensity. Dr. O'Neill might stress that consistent, moderate activity is more beneficial in the long term than sporadic, intense exercise. The goal is to make movement a regular part of your lifestyle.
- Variety is Key. Incorporating different types of movement can prevent boredom, address various aspects of fitness (such as strength, flexibility, and endurance), and reduce the risk of injury by not overusing certain muscle groups.
- Listen to Your Body. It's important to choose forms of movement that feel good and don't cause pain. Dr. O'Neill would likely encourage listening to your body's signals and adjusting activities accordingly to avoid burnout and injuries.

Practical Tips for Daily Movement
1. Start Small. Begin with small, achievable goals, like a 10-minute walk each day, gradually increasing duration and intensity as your fitness improves.
2. Make It Convenient. Choose activities that fit easily into your daily routine. This might mean walking or cycling to work, taking stairs instead of elevators, or doing body-weight exercises at home.
3. Use Technology Wisely. Use fitness trackers or apps to set goals, track progress, and remind you to move if you've been inactive for too long. However, Dr. O'Neill would also advise against becoming too dependent on technology or letting it dictate your self-worth based on daily activity metrics.
4. Integrate Movement into Work and Leisure. For those with sedentary jobs, standing desks, walking meetings, or desk exercises can integrate movement into the workday. Leisure time can also include active hobbies like gardening, dancing, or playing sports.
5. Involve Family and Friends. Activities like hiking, biking, or playing games together can make exercise more enjoyable and provide motivation through social support.
6. Mindful Movement. Practices such as yoga, tai chi, or Pilates can offer both physical benefits and stress reduction, aligning with Dr. O'Neill's holistic view of health.
7. Be Flexible and Forgiving. Dr. O'Neill would remind us that there will be days when it's hard to find time or motivation for exercise. The key is to be flexible, forgiving, and to get back on track as soon as possible.

Dr. O'Neill's advice would likely go beyond just the physical benefits of movement, such as weight management and improved cardiovascular health. She would also emphasize the mental and emotional benefits, including stress relief, improved mood, and increased energy levels. Integrating movement into daily life is a holistic practice that supports not only physical health but also emotional and mental well-being, reflecting her comprehensive approach to health and wellness.

Exercise Regimens That Promote Healing

Dr. Barbara O'Neill likely advocates for exercise regimens that not only support physical fitness but also promote healing and overall well-being. Her recommendations would typically emphasize gentle, restorative activities that can be beneficial for individuals recovering from illness, managing chronic conditions, or simply seeking to enhance their health. Here are some exercise regimens she might suggest, emphasizing their healing properties:

Walking
- Healing Benefits: Walking is a low-impact exercise that can improve cardiovascular health, aid in weight management, and reduce stress. It's accessible to people of most fitness levels and can be easily incorporated into daily routines.
- Implementation: Start with short walks, gradually increasing the duration and intensity. Incorporating nature walks can also enhance mental well-being through exposure to fresh air and green spaces.

Yoga
- Healing Benefits: Yoga combines physical postures, controlled breathing, and meditation, making it effective for reducing stress, improving flexibility and balance, and enhancing mental clarity. Certain yoga practices can be particularly beneficial for healing, offering gentle stretching and strengthening without strain.
- Implementation: Seek out styles like Hatha, Yin, or Restorative yoga, which focus on gentle movements and stress relief. Classes designed for beginners or those with specific health concerns can provide a supportive environment.

Tai Chi and Qigong
- Healing Benefits: These ancient Chinese practices involve slow, deliberate movements and deep breathing, promoting relaxation, balance, and overall physical and mental well-being. They are particularly noted for improving joint health and reducing symptoms of stress and anxiety.
- Implementation: Join a class or find online tutorials that cater to beginners. Regular practice, even for short periods, can yield significant health benefits.

Swimming and Water Aerobics
- Healing Benefits: Water-based exercises are excellent for those with joint issues or recovering from injuries. The buoyancy of water reduces stress on the body, allowing for movement without the impact associated with many land-based exercises.
- Implementation: Look for local pools offering lap swimming or group water aerobics classes. Even gentle movement in the water can help build strength and flexibility.

Pilates
- Healing Benefits: Pilates focuses on core strength, flexibility, and mindful movement. It can be particularly beneficial for spinal health and posture, offering a foundation for physical balance and reducing the risk of injury.
- Implementation: Start with beginner classes or one-on-one sessions with a certified instructor who can modify exercises to accommodate any health issues or injuries.

Gentle Strength Training
- Healing Benefits: Strength training, when done gently and with proper form, can improve muscle tone, bone density, and metabolic rate. It can also play a crucial role in managing chronic conditions like arthritis and diabetes.
- Implementation: Begin with light weights or resistance bands, focusing on slow, controlled movements. Consulting with a fitness professional to ensure correct form can prevent injuries.

Cycling

- Healing Benefits: Stationary or outdoor cycling provides cardiovascular benefits without the high impact on joints found in some other forms of exercise. It can improve leg strength and endurance in a controlled, measured way.
- Implementation: For outdoor cycling, choose flat, safe routes and adjust the pace as needed. Stationary bikes offer the advantage of exercising in any weather and tailoring the difficulty level.

Dr. O'Neill would likely emphasize the importance of listening to one's body and choosing activities that feel rejuvenating rather than depleting. Integrating exercise into one's lifestyle should be a joyful and enriching experience, supporting not just physical healing but also fostering emotional and mental well-being. She would also remind individuals to consult with healthcare providers before starting any new exercise regimen, especially if recovering from illness or managing health conditions.

Chapter 6: Rest and Rejuvenation

The Critical Role of Sleep

D
r. Barbara O'Neill, with her holistic view on health, would place a strong emphasis on the critical role of sleep for rest and rejuvenation. Recognizing sleep as foundational to healing, well-being, and overall quality of life, she likely advocates for strategies that promote restorative sleep patterns. Here's how she might articulate the importance of sleep and provide guidance for enhancing sleep quality:

Physical Health
- Healing and Repair: Sleep is crucial for the body's repair processes, including muscle growth, tissue repair, and hormone production, particularly growth hormone, which is essential for growth and tissue repair.
- Immune Function: Adequate sleep supports the immune system, helping to fight off infections and illnesses.
- Metabolic Health: Sleep affects the body's hunger hormones, ghrelin and leptin, as well as insulin sensitivity, playing a significant role in weight management and risk reduction for metabolic disorders like type 2 diabetes.

Mental and Emotional Well-being
- Cognitive Function: Sleep is vital for cognitive processes including memory consolidation, learning, problem-solving, and decision-making.
- Emotional Regulation: Adequate sleep helps regulate mood, reducing the risk of stress, anxiety, and depression.

Strategies for Enhancing Sleep Quality
Dr. O'Neill might suggest a multifaceted approach to improving sleep, focusing on lifestyle adjustments, environment, and routines that promote relaxation and readiness for sleep.
1. Routine: Going to bed and waking up at the same time every day helps regulate the body's internal clock, improving sleep quality.
2. Comfort: Ensure your sleeping environment is conducive to rest, with a comfortable mattress and pillows, and a cool, quiet, and dark room.
3. Electronics: Minimize exposure to screens and electronic devices before bedtime, as the blue light emitted can interfere with the production of the sleep hormone melatonin.
4. Caffeine and Alcohol: Limit intake of caffeine and alcohol, especially in the hours leading up to bedtime, as they can disrupt sleep patterns.
5. Heavy Meals: Avoid heavy or large meals within a couple of hours of bedtime.
6. Wind-Down Routine: Engage in relaxing activities before bed, such as reading, taking a warm bath, or practicing relaxation exercises like deep breathing or meditation.
7. Limit Stimulating Activities: Avoid stimulating activities and stressful discussions before bedtime.
8. Regular Exercise: Regular, moderate exercise can help promote better sleep, but intense exercise should be avoided close to bedtime.
9. Daylight: Exposure to natural light during the day, especially in the morning, can help regulate sleep patterns and improve sleep quality.

Dr. O'Neill would likely remind individuals to listen to their bodies' signals for sleep and rest, acknowledging that sleep needs can vary by person and may change with age or lifestyle. She would also stress the importance of addressing any underlying health issues or sleep disorders with a healthcare professional.

Emphasizing sleep's integral role in a holistic approach to health, Dr. O'Neill would likely advocate for viewing sleep as a priority, not a luxury. Rest and rejuvenation through sleep are essential for maintaining balance, supporting the body's natural healing processes, and ensuring optimal function across all aspects of health.

Techniques for Relaxation and Stress Management

Dr. Barbara O'Neill likely emphasizes the importance of relaxation and effective stress management for maintaining optimal health. Understanding the negative impacts of chronic stress on the body, including its contribution to heart disease, obesity, diabetes, and mental health issues, she would advocate for incorporating various relaxation techniques into daily life. Here are some strategies she might suggest for managing stress and promoting relaxation:

Deep Breathing Exercises
- Technique: Dr. O'Neill might recommend deep breathing techniques as a foundational method for reducing stress. Techniques such as diaphragmatic breathing, where you focus on making the diaphragm expand and contract, can help activate the body's relaxation response.
- Practice: She would suggest setting aside specific times throughout the day for deep breathing exercises, especially during periods of high stress.

Progressive Muscle Relaxation (PMR)
- Technique: PMR involves tensing each muscle group in the body tightly, but not to the point of strain, and then slowly relaxing them. This process helps identify areas of tension and encourages relaxation throughout the body.
- Application: Dr. O'Neill might advise practicing PMR before bedtime or in situations where physical tension is noticeable.

Meditation and Mindfulness
- Mindfulness Meditation: Focusing on the present moment without judgment can help reduce stress and improve emotional well-being. She might recommend starting with short periods of meditation and gradually increasing the time as comfort with the practice grows.
- Guided Meditation: For beginners, guided meditations provided through apps or online resources can be a helpful way to get started.

Regular Physical Activity
- Exercise: Engaging in regular physical activity, such as walking, yoga, swimming, or cycling, can significantly reduce stress levels. Dr. O'Neill would likely stress finding an activity that is enjoyable and fits into one's lifestyle.
- Nature Walks: Incorporating walks in nature into one's routine can also offer the dual benefits of exercise and exposure to natural surroundings, which have been shown to lower stress levels.

Adequate Sleep and Rest
- Recognizing the cycle between stress and sleep, where stress can lead to poor sleep, and poor sleep can increase stress, Dr. O'Neill would emphasize the importance of prioritizing sleep as a critical component of stress management.

Healthy Diet
- Nutrition: Consuming a balanced diet rich in fruits, vegetables, whole grains, and lean proteins can support the body's ability to cope with stress. Dr. O'Neill might also highlight the importance of staying hydrated and limiting high-sugar and high-caffeine foods and beverages.

Time Management and Setting Boundaries
- Prioritizing Tasks: Effective time management, including prioritizing tasks and setting realistic deadlines, can help reduce stress. Dr. O'Neill would likely advise against overcommitting and recommend setting clear boundaries to maintain a work-life balance.

Seeking Social Support
- Connection: Maintaining a supportive network of friends and family can provide emotional support and reduce feelings of isolation, which is important for managing stress.

Engaging in Hobbies and Interests
- Leisure Activities: Pursuing hobbies and activities that bring joy can serve as an effective outlet for stress. Dr. O'Neill might suggest identifying activities that provide a sense of satisfaction and making time for them regularly.

Dr. O'Neill's approach to relaxation and stress management would be holistic, recognizing that effective stress reduction involves addressing both the mind and the body. By incorporating these techniques into daily routines, individuals can improve their resilience to stress and enhance their overall well-being.

Chapter 7: Detoxifying Your Life

Eliminating Toxins from Your Diet and Environment

Dr. Barbara O'Neill likely emphasizes the importance of minimizing exposure to toxins in both diet and environment as a way to support the body's natural healing processes and maintain optimal health. Toxins can come from various sources, including processed foods, pesticides, household chemicals, and pollutants, and can have a range of negative effects on health. Here are some strategies she might suggest for reducing toxin exposure:

Eliminating Toxins from Your Diet

- Choose Organic and Locally Sourced Foods: Opting for organic foods can reduce exposure to pesticides and chemicals used in conventional farming. Locally sourced foods are often fresher and have a lower environmental impact due to reduced transportation.
- Reduce Processed Foods: Processed foods can contain additives, preservatives, and artificial ingredients that may be harmful to health. Dr. O'Neill would likely advocate for a diet based on whole, minimally processed foods.
- Clean Produce Properly: Washing fruits and vegetables thoroughly can help remove surface pesticides and bacteria. Using a natural produce wash or a solution of vinegar and water can be effective.
- Be Cautious with Fish Consumption: Some fish may contain high levels of mercury and other contaminants. She might recommend choosing smaller, younger fish or species known to have lower mercury levels, such as sardines, salmon, and trout.
- Minimize Plastics: Plastic containers can leach chemicals into food and drinks, especially when heated. Dr. O'Neill might advise using glass, stainless steel, or BPA-free plastics and avoiding microwaving food in plastic containers.

Reducing Environmental Toxins

- Use Natural Cleaning Products: Many household cleaners contain harsh chemicals. Dr. O'Neill might suggest using natural cleaning alternatives like vinegar, baking soda, and essential oils, which are effective and less harmful.
- Improve Indoor Air Quality: Indoor air can be more polluted than outdoor air due to chemicals from paints, furniture, and cleaning products. She may recommend using air purifiers, keeping indoor plants, and ensuring good ventilation to improve air quality.
- Choose Natural Personal Care Products: Personal care products, including cosmetics, shampoos, and deodorants, can contain potentially harmful chemicals. Opting for products with natural ingredients or making homemade personal care items can reduce exposure.
- Be Mindful of Water Quality: Contaminants in tap water can vary depending on the location. Dr. O'Neill might suggest using water filters that remove contaminants specific to your area's water supply.
- Reduce Electronic Waste: Electronic devices can emit electromagnetic fields (EMFs) and contain toxic substances. Limiting unnecessary electronic devices and disposing of electronic waste properly can minimize exposure.
- Wear Natural Fibers: Synthetic fabrics can be treated with chemicals, while natural fibers like cotton, wool, and linen are less likely to be processed with harmful substances.

Dr. O'Neill's approach would likely extend beyond specific toxin reduction strategies to encompass holistic lifestyle changes that support overall health and well-being. This might include stress management techniques, regular physical activity, and ensuring adequate sleep, all of which can help the body detoxify naturally and strengthen its resilience against environmental toxins.

Emphasizing education and empowerment, Dr. O'Neill would likely encourage individuals to become informed consumers, making choices that not only benefit personal health but also contribute to a healthier planet.

Natural Detox Methods

Dr. Barbara O'Neill, with her expertise in natural health, emphasizes the body's inherent ability to detoxify itself through its liver, kidneys, digestive system, skin, and lungs. She advocates for supporting these natural processes with lifestyle and dietary choices rather than relying on extreme detox diets or commercial detox products. Here are some natural detox methods that Dr. O'Neill might recommend enhancing the body's detoxification capabilities:

Hydration

Hydration plays a central role in the body's natural detoxification process, with water serving as the primary vehicle for flushing toxins out of the body. By maintaining adequate hydration, individuals support their kidneys in efficiently filtering toxins from the bloodstream. Water also facilitates the digestive system's ability to eliminate waste, ensuring that toxins are promptly removed from the body through feces. Beyond its direct role in detoxification, water is essential for overall metabolic processes, including cellular hydration and nutrient transport, which are foundational for maintaining health and supporting the body's self-healing mechanisms.

In addition to plain water, certain herbal teas offer unique benefits that further support the body's detoxification efforts. For example, dandelion tea is praised for its diuretic properties, which can help the kidneys flush out excess toxins and water, enhancing the natural detoxification process. Green tea, rich in antioxidants, particularly catechins, supports liver function, a critical organ in the body's natural detoxification system. The liver works to neutralize and prepare toxins for elimination, and the antioxidants found in green tea may aid in protecting the liver from damage and supporting its detoxifying functions.

The inclusion of herbal teas as part of one's hydration strategy not only diversifies the sources of fluids but also introduces beneficial compounds that can aid in detoxification and overall health. Whether through increasing water intake or incorporating specific herbal teas, staying adequately hydrated is a simple yet effective strategy for supporting the body's natural ability to detoxify, highlighting the importance of hydration in maintaining health and facilitating the body's inherent healing processes.

Diet

Incorporating fiber-rich foods into one's diet is a cornerstone of supporting the body's natural detoxification processes. Foods that are high in fiber, such as vegetables, fruits, whole grains, and legumes, play a critical role in regulating the digestive system. Fiber aids in moving food through the digestive tract more efficiently, allowing for the timely elimination of waste and toxins through feces. This not only helps keep the colon clean but also reduces the likelihood of constipation, which can hinder the body's ability to rid itself of waste. Moreover, certain types of fiber act as prebiotics, feeding beneficial gut bacteria and promoting a healthy gut microbiome, which is essential for effective detoxification and overall health.

Choosing organic produce whenever possible is another strategy that can minimize the body's exposure to harmful pesticides and chemicals commonly used in conventional farming. These substances can accumulate in the body over time, contributing to the toxic load and potentially disrupting bodily functions. Organic foods are grown without synthetic pesticides or fertilizers, making them a cleaner choice that reduces the intake of these harmful chemicals. While organic foods can sometimes be more expensive or less accessible, prioritizing organic options for high-risk produce known to have higher pesticide residues, often referred to as the "Dirty Dozen," is a practical approach to reducing exposure.

Incorporating specific detoxifying foods into the diet further supports the body's natural detox mechanisms, particularly those of the liver and kidneys, which are central to processing and eliminating toxins. Foods like garlic, beets, and leafy greens are renowned for their detoxification benefits. Garlic contains sulfur compounds that aid in the liver's detoxification pathways, while beets contain antioxidants and nutrients that support liver health and promote increased bile production, aiding in the elimination of fat-soluble toxins. Leafy greens, rich in chlorophyll, help cleanse the blood and protect the liver. These foods, among others with detoxifying properties, offer natural ways to support and enhance the body's detoxification processes.

Emphasizing fiber-rich foods, organic produce, and detoxifying foods is not just about removing toxins from the body; it's about creating an internal environment that supports ongoing health and prevents disease. This approach aligns with the body's natural processes, ensuring that detoxification is a gentle, continuous process rather than an occasional intervention, thereby promoting long-term health and well-being.

Exercise

Regular physical activity is a vital component of maintaining health and enhancing the body's natural detoxification capabilities. Exercise serves multiple roles in this process, primarily through its ability to increase blood circulation and promote sweating. Improved circulation ensures that nutrients and oxygen are efficiently distributed throughout the body, while also facilitating the quicker removal of toxins and waste products from bodily systems. Sweating, on the other hand, not only helps regulate body temperature during physical exertion but also allows for the direct excretion of toxins through the skin, one of the body's primary detoxification pathways.

Moreover, engaging in regular physical activity contributes to enhanced respiratory function. As the intensity of exercise increases, so does the depth and rate of breathing. This deepened breathing allows for more substantial oxygen intake and helps in expelling carbon dioxide and other airborne toxins from the body more effectively. The combined effect of increased circulation and improved breathing during exercise significantly aids the body's efforts to detoxify and cleanse itself.

Yoga and stretching introduce a more targeted approach to supporting the body's detoxification processes. Certain yoga poses are specifically designed to aid in digestion and stimulate the lymphatic system, a critical component of the body's innate detoxification mechanism. The lymphatic system, which transports lymph, a fluid containing white blood cells and waste products, relies on muscle movement and body positions to facilitate fluid flow. Yoga and stretching exercises can effectively stimulate this system, helping to move toxins from tissues to the lymph nodes where they are neutralized or expelled from the body. Furthermore, yoga's emphasis on mindful breathing and relaxation can enhance the body's detoxification processes by reducing stress, which is known to impede the efficient functioning of detoxification organs like the liver.

Incorporating a mix of cardiovascular exercises, strength training, yoga, and stretching into a weekly routine can provide a holistic approach to exercise that not only supports physical fitness but also optimizes the body's natural detoxification processes. This holistic approach to physical activity ensures that the body is not only strong and healthy but also efficient in eliminating toxins, contributing to overall well-being and disease prevention.

Sauna and Steam Baths

The use of saunas and steam baths has long been recognized for its health benefits, particularly in cultures around the world that have integrated these practices into their wellness routines for centuries. The principle behind their detoxifying effect lies in the promotion of sweating, a natural mechanism through which the body regulates temperature and eliminates toxins. When the body is exposed to the high heat of a sauna or the humid warmth of a steam bath, it begins to produce sweat in an effort to cool down. This process not only helps rid the body of excess salt and other substances but also facilitates the removal of toxins absorbed from the environment and the products we consume.

The benefits of sweating in a controlled environment like a sauna or steam bath extend beyond simple detoxification. The heat can help relax muscles, soothe aches and pains in muscles and joints, and can have a profound relaxing effect on the mind. However, the key to harnessing these benefits safely lies in staying hydrated and being attuned to the body's signals. The intense heat can lead to rapid fluid loss through sweat, which is why replenishing lost fluids is crucial to prevent dehydration. Drinking water before, during, and after using a sauna or steam bath ensures that the body remains hydrated and the kidneys function properly, further aiding the detoxification process.

Moreover, listening to your body is essential to avoid overheating, which can lead to heat exhaustion or heat stroke, particularly in environments as intensely warm as saunas and steam baths. It's recommended to limit sessions to a duration that feels comfortable — typically between 15 to 20 minutes for most people — and to exit the environment if you begin to feel dizzy, nauseous, or overly fatigued. Gradually acclimating to the heat over several sessions can also help your body adjust more comfortably.

Integrating sauna or steam bath sessions into a holistic wellness routine can complement other detoxification methods like a balanced diet, regular exercise, and sufficient water intake. Together, these practices can enhance the body's natural ability to detoxify, contributing to improved health, increased energy, and a greater sense of well-being. As with any health practice, individuals with pre-existing health conditions or those who are pregnant should consult with a healthcare provider before incorporating sauna or steam baths into their wellness regimen to ensure it's appropriate and safe for their specific health circumstances.

Reduce Intake of Toxins

Reducing the intake of toxins through mindful consumption is a proactive approach to safeguarding health and supporting the body's inherent detoxification processes. This strategy involves a heightened awareness and scrutiny of the everyday products and foods we consume, recognizing that many can contain chemicals and substances potentially harmful to our health. The essence of mindful consumption lies in making informed choices, prioritizing products that are natural, minimally processed, and free from harmful additives.

When it comes to food, mindful consumption entails favoring organic produce where possible, as it's grown without the use of synthetic pesticides and fertilizers that can accumulate in the body over time. For items where organic options are not available or affordable, washing fruits and vegetables thoroughly or peeling them when appropriate can help reduce exposure to surface pesticides. Additionally, minimizing processed foods in the diet, which often contain artificial preservatives, colors, and flavors, further decreases the ingestion of unnatural substances.

Beyond diet, the principle of mindful consumption extends to personal care products and household cleaners, many of which contain a cocktail of chemicals. These can include endocrine disruptors, carcinogens, and skin irritants, among others. Opting for products with natural ingredients and fewer synthetic additives can significantly reduce the body's chemical burden. Reading labels becomes crucial in this context, as it allows consumers to identify and avoid harmful ingredients, opting instead for products with simpler, recognizable ingredient lists.

The environment we live in also plays a role in our overall exposure to toxins. Mindful consumption in this arena might involve choosing home furnishings, building materials, and clothing made from natural materials, thus avoiding the volatile organic compounds (VOCs) often found in synthetic materials. Additionally, reducing plastic use, especially in food storage and packaging, can decrease exposure to bisphenol A (BPA) and phthalates, which have been linked to various health issues.

Adopting a mindset of mindful consumption does not necessitate a radical lifestyle overhaul overnight but rather encourages gradual changes towards healthier choices. It's about doing the best one can within one's means to choose products that not only benefit personal health but also have a lesser impact on the environment. Over time, these choices can contribute to a significant reduction in the body's toxin load, facilitating better health and well-being. The journey towards mindful consumption is a personal one, shaped by individual priorities, health goals, and available resources, yet it's a powerful step anyone can take towards living a cleaner, healthier life.

Supportive Supplements and Herbs

Incorporating supportive supplements and herbs into one's wellness routine can play a significant role in enhancing the body's detoxification capabilities, particularly with respect to liver health, which is central to processing and eliminating toxins. Herbs like milk thistle, turmeric, and spirulina have been recognized for their potential to support these natural processes, each bringing unique properties that contribute to their efficacy.

Milk thistle is renowned for its silymarin content, a compound that has antioxidant and anti-inflammatory properties. It's thought to promote liver cell regeneration and protect the liver against toxins. This herb has been used traditionally to treat liver disorders, including hepatitis and cirrhosis, and to protect the liver from potential damage caused by toxins.

Turmeric, a staple in traditional medicine systems such as Ayurveda, contains curcumin, a component with potent anti-inflammatory and antioxidant effects. Curcumin is believed to aid in the detoxification process by stimulating bile production in the liver, which helps eliminate toxins. Additionally, its antioxidant action can help protect the liver from damage by free radicals and toxins.

Spirulina, a type of blue-green algae, is packed with nutrients including proteins, vitamins, minerals, and antioxidants. It has been shown to possess liver-protective effects, possibly due to its high antioxidant content, which can combat oxidative stress and aid the liver in processing and removing toxins from the body.

While the addition of these supplements and herbs can provide targeted support for detoxification and liver health, it's crucial to approach their use with care. The effects of supplements can vary greatly depending on the individual, and not all supplements are suitable for everyone. Factors such as existing health conditions, current medications, and overall health goals can influence whether a particular supplement is appropriate. For example, certain herbs might interact with medications, potentially leading to adverse effects or diminished efficacy of treatment.

Mindfulness and Stress Reduction

Mindfulness and stress reduction practices play a crucial role in supporting the body's natural detoxification processes, not only by contributing to the elimination of physical toxins but also by facilitating a mental and emotional detox. Engaging in meditation, deep breathing exercises, and mindfulness practices can significantly reduce stress levels, which is essential since chronic stress can impair the immune system and hamper the body's ability to detoxify efficiently.

Meditation, a practice with ancient roots across various cultures, involves sitting quietly and focusing the mind, which can lead to a deep state of relaxation and tranquility. Regular meditation has been shown to lower cortisol levels, the body's primary stress hormone, thereby enhancing immune function and enabling the body to dedicate more resources to detoxification and healing. Furthermore, meditation can improve sleep quality, which is another crucial factor in the body's natural detoxification cycle.

Deep breathing exercises are another powerful tool for reducing stress and supporting detoxification. By focusing on slow, deep breaths, these exercises stimulate the parasympathetic nervous system, the part of the autonomic nervous system responsible for the 'rest and digest' state. This not only helps alleviate immediate stress but also promotes better digestion and circulation, both of which are vital for effectively removing toxins from the body.

Mindfulness, the practice of being fully present and engaged in the moment without judgment, can be integrated into daily activities to help manage stress. Whether it's mindful eating, walking, or listening, mindfulness encourages a state of awareness and acceptance that can reduce stress-induced reactivity and impulsivity. This heightened state of awareness can also foster better choices regarding diet and lifestyle, indirectly supporting the body's detoxification efforts by minimizing the intake of new toxins.

The interconnectedness of mental, emotional, and physical health is central to the concept of a holistic detox. Chronic stress not only contributes to physical ailments but can also lead to emotional imbalances, creating a cycle that further impedes the body's natural healing capabilities. By adopting practices that reduce stress and promote mental and emotional well-being, individuals can enhance their body's resilience and capacity to detoxify.

Incorporating mindfulness and stress reduction practices into one's routine doesn't require significant time commitments or drastic lifestyle changes. Even a few minutes of meditation or deep breathing exercises daily can yield noticeable benefits. As these practices become more integrated into daily life, they can lead to profound changes in stress levels, overall health, and well-being, supporting the body's natural detoxification processes and contributing to a healthier, more balanced life.

Chapter 8: Emotional and Spiritual Wellness

The Connection Between Mind, Body, and Spirit

Dr. Barbara O'Neill emphasizes the profound and intricate connection between the mind, body, and spirit, viewing health as a holistic interplay of these components rather than isolated physical symptoms. This perspective reflects a core principle of holistic health, which posits that true wellness encompasses emotional, mental, spiritual, and physical well-being, with each aspect influencing the others.

Mind-Body Connection

The concept of the mind-body connection is foundational to understanding how integral our thoughts, emotions, and beliefs are to our physical health. This interplay suggests that our mental state is not just a reflection of our physical well-being but a determinant of it. Stress and anxiety, for example, are not merely psychological states; they manifest physically, affecting heart rate, blood pressure, and even the digestive system, demonstrating the direct impact of mental health on physical conditions. Similarly, physical health issues, such as chronic pain or nutritional deficiencies, can lead to significant mental health challenges, including depression and anxiety, further illustrating the cyclical nature of the mind-body relationship.

Practices like mindfulness and meditation are not merely exercises in mental discipline but are powerful tools for physical health. Through mindfulness, individuals learn to live in the present moment, reducing the stress that can exacerbate or lead to physical ailments. Meditation, by fostering a state of relaxation and calm, can lower stress levels, thereby potentially reducing the risk of stress-related physical disorders. These practices contribute to a more balanced state of mind, which in turn can lead to better physical health outcomes, including improved sleep quality and immune function.

Stress management techniques, which may include deep breathing exercises, yoga, or even engaging in hobbies and activities that bring joy, are also critical in the effort to harmonize the mind and body. By actively reducing stress, individuals can mitigate its harmful effects on the body, promoting healthier physiological functioning. The reduction of stress not only improves cardiovascular health and digestive function but can also enhance the body's immune response, making it more effective in fighting off illnesses.

Dr. O'Neill might advocate for these practices not just as therapeutic interventions but as integral components of daily life, emphasizing their potential to not only improve physical health outcomes but also to enhance overall quality of life. By recognizing and nurturing the connection between the mind and body, individuals can work towards achieving a state of health that encompasses both mental and physical well-being, illustrating the profound impact of our mental state on our physical health and vice versa.

Body-Spirit Connection

The body-spirit connection underscores the profound interplay between our physical form and our spiritual essence, revealing how each influence and enhances the other. This connection posits that the body is more than a collection of biological processes; it's a reflection of our spiritual state, serving as a bridge between the tangible world and the intangible aspects of our being. Spiritual practices, irrespective of their specific traditions or rituals, foster a deep sense of connection to something greater than oneself, whether that's a higher power, the natural world, or an inner sense of peace and purpose. These practices, by nurturing the spirit, can yield substantial benefits for physical health.

The benefits of a strong body-spirit connection extend to mental health, providing a sense of purpose and reducing feelings of isolation. This sense of belonging and purpose has been directly linked to improved physical health outcomes, such as enhanced immune function. When individuals feel connected to a larger purpose or community, it can bolster the immune system, making it more efficient in fighting off infections and diseases. Moreover, this connection can contribute to a more positive outlook on life, which in itself has been associated with better health outcomes, including increased longevity. People who maintain a positive spiritual practice tend to have a more hopeful perspective on life and its challenges, which can directly influence their physical health by encouraging healthier lifestyle choices and a proactive approach to managing health.

The body-spirit connection also emphasizes the importance of treating the body with respect and care, recognizing it as the vessel that enables our engagement with the world and our pursuit of spiritual fulfillment. Practices that honor the body, such as nutritious eating, regular physical activity, and adequate rest, are seen not just as acts of self-care but as expressions of gratitude and reverence for the life and health we've been granted. This holistic view encourages a lifestyle that supports both physical health and spiritual well-being, reinforcing the idea that caring for the body is intrinsically linked to nurturing the spirit.

In embracing the body-spirit connection, individuals are invited to explore practices that resonate with their personal beliefs and experiences, finding ways to integrate these into their daily lives. This integration not only enhances physical health but enriches the human experience, offering a pathway to a more balanced, healthy, and fulfilling life.

Integrating Mind, Body, and Spirit

Dr. O'Neill likely encourages an integrated approach to health that addresses the mind, body, and spirit to promote healing and wellness. This could involve:

- Nutrition: Adopting a diet rich in whole foods that nourishes the body and supports mental health.
- Exercise: Engaging in physical activity that not only improves physical health but also relieves stress and improves mental well-being.
- Rest and Sleep: Prioritizing quality sleep, which is crucial for physical repair, cognitive function, and emotional regulation.
- Nature: Spending time in nature to support spiritual health, reduce stress, and improve physical well-being.
- Community and Relationships: Fostering supportive relationships and community connections, which are vital for mental and spiritual health and can positively impact physical health.

By addressing health from this holistic perspective, Dr. O'Neill emphasizes that healing and wellness are multi-dimensional processes that require balance and harmony between the mind, body, and spirit. She advocates for personalized care strategies that reflect the unique needs and beliefs of the individual, encouraging practices that not only prevent and address physical ailments but also nurture the mental and spiritual aspects of health, leading to a more balanced and fulfilled life.

Practices for Mental Health and Emotional Balance

Dr. Barbara O'Neill, with her comprehensive understanding of natural health, likely emphasizes the importance of maintaining mental health and emotional balance as essential components of overall well-being. Recognizing that emotional and mental health are as crucial as physical health, she would advocate for a holistic approach that includes a variety of practices to support emotional balance and mental clarity. Here's how she might approach the subject:

Prioritizing Self-Care

Self-care is foundational to maintaining mental health and emotional balance. Dr. O'Neill would encourage individuals to identify activities that nourish and rejuvenate them, whether that's spending time in nature, engaging in creative pursuits, or simply taking moments of rest and reflection. Understanding that self-care is not selfish but necessary for well-being is key.

Establishing a Routine

A regular routine can provide a sense of stability and security, which is important for mental health. Dr. O'Neill might suggest establishing consistent habits related to sleep, nutrition, exercise, and relaxation to help create a balanced daily structure that supports mental and emotional well-being.

Mindfulness and Meditation

Mindfulness meditation is a powerful tool for cultivating mental clarity and emotional stability. Dr. O'Neill would likely advocate for the practice of mindfulness — paying attention to the present moment without judgment — as a way to reduce stress, enhance self-awareness, and promote a state of calm. She might recommend starting with short, daily sessions and gradually increasing the duration as comfort with the practice grows.

Physical Activity

Exercise is well-documented to have profound benefits for mental health, including reducing symptoms of depression and anxiety. Dr. O'Neill would encourage finding forms of physical activity that are enjoyable and sustainable, emphasizing that exercise doesn't have to be intense or time-consuming to be effective. Even regular walks or gentle yoga can significantly impact emotional balance.

Healthy Eating

Nutrition plays a critical role in mental health. Dr. O'Neill would stress the importance of a balanced diet rich in whole foods, which can support brain function and emotional health. She might highlight the importance of omega-3 fatty acids, antioxidants, and vitamins found in fruits, vegetables, nuts, and seeds.

Quality Sleep

Recognizing the strong link between sleep and mental health, Dr. O'Neill would emphasize the importance of good sleep hygiene practices. Ensuring adequate, restful sleep can help manage stress, improve mood, and enhance overall mental well-being.

Social Connections

Maintaining meaningful relationships and social connections can provide emotional support and reduce feelings of isolation, which are crucial for mental health. Dr. O'Neill might suggest actively nurturing relationships with family, friends, and community members as a way to maintain emotional balance.

Seeking Professional Help

Dr. O'Neill would also acknowledge the importance of seeking professional help when needed. Whether it's counseling, therapy, or exploring other mental health services, professional support can be invaluable for navigating life's challenges and maintaining emotional health.

By integrating these practices into daily life, individuals can foster resilience, improve mental health, and maintain emotional balance. Dr. O'Neill's approach would likely be one of compassion and empowerment, encouraging individuals to take proactive steps toward nurturing their mental and emotional well-being as part of a holistic view of health.

Chapter 9: The Comprehensive Guide to Over 150 Medicinal Herbs

Creating a comprehensive list of 150 medicinal herbs, inspired by the approaches often advocated by natural health practitioners like Dr. Barbara O'Neill, who focuses on holistic health and natural remedies, involves selecting herbs known for their healing properties across various cultures and traditions. The list below includes herbs that are recognized for their medicinal benefits, though it's essential to consult healthcare professionals before using them, especially to understand their proper usage, dosages, and potential interactions with other medications.

Abscess Root

Abscess root (Polemonium reptans), also known as Jacob's ladder, is a perennial plant native to North America, traditionally used in herbal medicine for its expectorant, anti-inflammatory, and astringent properties.

Properties	Expectorant: Helps in the expulsion of phlegm from the respiratory tract, beneficial for treating coughs and congestion. Anti-inflammatory: Can reduce inflammation, useful in treating conditions such as sore throat and fever. Astringent: The astringent properties of abscess root can help in tightening tissues and reducing secretions, useful in digestive disorders.
What disease it fights	Respiratory Conditions: Effective in treating symptoms of colds, flu, bronchitis, and other respiratory ailments by reducing cough and aiding in the clearance of mucus. Sore Throat: Its anti-inflammatory and astringent effects can soothe sore throats. Fever: May help reduce fever associated with colds and flu.
How it works	The healing effects of abscess root are attributed to its constituents, which include saponins, tannins, and flavonoids. These compounds work together to exert expectorant, anti-inflammatory, and astringent effects, thereby aiding in the relief of respiratory symptoms, reducing inflammation, and supporting the tightening of tissues.
How to use	Tea: Dried abscess root can be steeped in hot water to make a tea. This is the most common method of use, particularly for respiratory conditions and sore throat. Tincture: An alcohol extract of abscess root can be used for its concentrated properties.
Dosage	Tea: Use 1-2 teaspoons of dried herb per cup of boiling water, steeped for 10-15 minutes. Drink 2-3 times daily. Tincture: Follow the manufacturer's instructions, typically 1-2 ml three times a day
How long to use	Abscess root is generally used for the duration of acute symptoms, such as during a cold or respiratory infection, often not exceeding two weeks. Long-term use is not well documented and should be approached with caution, under the guidance of a healthcare professional, to monitor for potential side effects or interactions with other medications.

Acai

Acai (Euterpe oleracea) is a dark purple berry from the Amazon rainforest, celebrated for its antioxidant properties. It's become popular worldwide, particularly in the form of supplements, juices, and smoothie bowls.

Properties	Antioxidant: High in anthocyanins, which combat oxidative stress and may reduce the risk of chronic diseases. Anti-inflammatory: Contains anti-inflammatory compounds that may help reduce the risk of inflammatory diseases. Heart Health: The fatty acids found in acai, like those in olive oil, can support heart health. Digestive Health: A good source of fiber, aiding in digestive health and regularity.
What disease it fights	Chronic Diseases: Its antioxidant properties can help protect against various chronic diseases, including heart disease, diabetes, and cancer. Inflammation: May help reduce systemic inflammation, beneficial in managing conditions like arthritis. Oxidative Stress: Helps in reducing the cellular damage caused by oxidative stress, supporting overall health and aging.
How it works	The health benefits of acai berries are primarily attributed to their high antioxidant content, particularly anthocyanins, which help neutralize free radicals in the body. This action can reduce oxidative stress and inflammation, contributing to the prevention of several chronic diseases. The fiber in acai supports digestive health, while its healthy fats contribute to cardiovascular wellness.
How to use	Juice/Smoothies: Acai is commonly consumed in juice or smoothie form, often mixed with other fruits to enhance its nutritional value. Powder: Acai powder can be added to smoothies, yogurt, or oatmeal for an antioxidant boost. Capsules: Acai supplements are available for those who prefer a concentrated dose in capsule form.
Dosage	Juice/Smoothies: Typically, 100-200 ml of acai juice or 1-2 tablespoons of acai powder per day. Capsules: Follow the manufacturer's instructions, usually 1,000-2,000 mg per day.
How long to use	Acai can be incorporated into the daily diet as a regular part of a healthy eating plan. For those taking acai in supplement form, it's wise to follow the manufacturer's recommended duration or consult with a healthcare professional, especially if using acai supplements for specific health issues.

Alfalfa

Alfalfa (Medicago sativa), often referred to as the "Father of All Foods," is a nutrient-rich plant that has been used in traditional medicine for centuries. Its leaves, seeds, and sprouts are consumed for their health benefits.

Properties	Nutrient-Rich: Alfalfa is a good source of vitamins (A, C, E, and K4) and minerals (calcium, potassium, phosphorus, and iron), supporting overall nutritional status. Antioxidant: Contains antioxidants that help protect the body from oxidative stress and reduce the risk of chronic diseases. Estrogenic: Contains compounds that can mimic estrogen, potentially beneficial for menopausal symptoms. Detoxifying: Traditionally used for its diuretic and detoxifying effects, promoting kidney and urinary tract health. Cholesterol-Lowering: Some studies suggest alfalfa can help lower cholesterol levels by binding to cholesterol in the gut and preventing its absorption.
What disease it fights	High Cholesterol: Can aid in reducing cholesterol levels, supporting cardiovascular health. Menopausal Symptoms: Its estrogenic properties may help alleviate hot flashes and other symptoms associated with menopause. Digestive Issues: The high fiber content can promote digestive health and prevent constipation. Inflammatory Conditions: Anti-inflammatory properties may help with arthritis and other inflammatory diseases.
How it works	Alfalfa's health benefits stem from its rich nutritional profile, providing essential vitamins, minerals, and antioxidants that support overall health. The saponins found in alfalfa are believed to be responsible for its cholesterol-lowering effect, while its coumestans and isoflavones offer mild estrogenic effects, which can be beneficial for hormone balance.
How to use	Leaves and Seeds: Can be consumed in salads or as a green leafy vegetable. Sprouts: Alfalfa sprouts are commonly added to sandwiches, salads, and smoothies. Supplements: Available in capsules, tablets, or powders for those who prefer a concentrated form.
Dosage	Fresh Leaves/Sprouts: Can be consumed daily as part of a balanced diet. There's no specific dosage, but moderation is key due to its potent effects. Supplements: Typical dosages range from 500-1,000 mg per day for capsules or tablets. Follow the manufacturer's instructions for the correct dosage.
How long to use	Alfalfa can be included as part of a regular diet in moderate amounts over an extended period. When taking alfalfa supplements for specific health conditions like high cholesterol or menopausal symptoms, it might be used for several months, but it's wise to consult a healthcare professional for guidance on duration and monitoring for any potential side effects, especially due to its estrogenic activity.

Aloe vera

Aloe vera (scientific name: Aloe vera) is a succulent plant widely recognized for its health, beauty, and medicinal uses. Its leaves contain a gel-like substance rich in vitamins, minerals, enzymes, and amino acids. Aloe vera has been used historically to treat a wide range of conditions, both internally and externally.

Properties	Healing: Aloe vera is renowned for its wound-healing properties, especially for burns, cuts, and other skin injuries. Moisturizing: The gel is deeply hydrating, making it beneficial for dry skin conditions. Anti-inflammatory: Contains compounds that help reduce inflammation, useful in treating conditions like sunburn. Digestive Aid: When ingested, it can help soothe and heal the digestive tract, and promote regular bowel movements. Antimicrobial: Offers antimicrobial benefits, which can help prevent infection in wounds and improve skin health.
What disease it fights	Skin Conditions: Such as burns, acne, and psoriasis, thanks to its healing and anti-inflammatory properties. Digestive Issues: Including indigestion, constipation, and acid reflux. Aloe vera can help soothe the digestive tract lining. Oral Health: Can be used as a mouthwash to reduce dental plaque and combat gum inflammation.
How it works	The healing properties of aloe vera gel come from its complex mix of components. For skin application, it works by providing a protective barrier that helps keep moisture in and promotes collagen production, speeding up wound healing. For digestive health, its soothing properties help to calm irritation in the stomach and intestines, and it encourages healthy bowel movements.
How to use	Topical Application: Apply the gel directly to the skin for burns, wounds, or as a moisturizer. Oral Consumption: Drink aloe vera juice for digestive benefits. Ensure the juice is decolorized and purified for safe consumption. Dental Care: Use as a mouthwash by diluting aloe vera juice with water.
Dosage	Topically: As needed, depending on the condition being treated. There's generally no limit to the frequency of application for skin conditions. Orally: For aloe vera juice, recommended dosages vary, but a common guideline is about 2 to 4 ounces (60 to 120 milliliters) per day. Start with a smaller dose to assess tolerance. Dental Use: Rinse with a half-and-half mixture of aloe vera juice and water once or twice daily.
How long to use	Topical Use: Can be used as long as the skin condition persists, and improvement is seen. For moisturizing, it can be included in daily skincare routines indefinitely. Oral Use: For digestive health, some sources suggest using it for a few weeks, then taking a break or reducing frequency to prevent possible laxative dependency or other side effects. Continuous, long-term internal use is generally not recommended without consulting a healthcare professional.

Angelica

Angelica (Angelica archangelica), often referred to as wild celery, is a plant that has been used in traditional medicine across Europe, Asia, and North America. Its roots, seeds, and leaves are used for various medicinal purposes.

Properties	Digestive Aid: Angelica is known for its ability to stimulate digestion, relieve gas, and soothe stomach cramps. Expectorant: Helps to clear mucus from the respiratory tract, making it beneficial for coughs and colds. Anti-inflammatory: Contains compounds that may reduce inflammation, useful in treating arthritis and other inflammatory conditions. Circulatory Stimulant: Believed to improve circulation, which can benefit overall cardiovascular health. Antispasmodic: Can relieve muscle spasms, including those in the digestive tract.
What disease it fights	Digestive Disorders: Effective in treating indigestion, gas, and bloating. Respiratory Conditions: Used to alleviate symptoms of colds, such as coughs and congestion. Rheumatic Conditions: Its anti-inflammatory properties can help reduce pain and inflammation associated with arthritis. Menstrual Disorders: Can be used to ease menstrual cramps due to its antispasmodic properties.
How it works	Angelica's various health benefits are attributed to its active components, including volatile oils, coumarins, and flavonoids. These compounds work synergistically to stimulate digestive enzymes, improve blood flow, reduce inflammation, and expel mucus from the respiratory system.
How to use	Tea: Both the roots and leaves of angelica can be brewed into a tea to support digestive and respiratory health. Tincture: A concentrated form of angelica, useful for more specific therapeutic purposes such as menstrual pain or circulatory issues. Essential Oil: Used in aromatherapy for relaxation and improving digestion; should be diluted before topical application.
Dosage	Tea: Steep 1 teaspoon of dried root or leaves in boiling water for 5-10 minutes. Drink up to 3 times daily. Tincture: Typically, 1-2 ml three times daily, but it's important to follow specific product recommendations or consult with a healthcare provider. Essential Oil: For topical use, dilute with a carrier oil following a 2% dilution guideline (about 12 drops of essential oil per ounce of carrier oil).
How long to use	For acute conditions like digestive upset or a cold, angelica can be used until symptoms improve, typically for a few days up to two weeks. For chronic conditions or ongoing support, such as for circulatory health or menstrual pain, use under the guidance of a healthcare provider to determine the appropriate duration and monitor for any potential interactions or side effects.

Arnica

Arnica Montana, commonly known as Arnica, is an herbaceous plant in the sunflower family, renowned for its medicinal properties. It's traditionally used for its anti-inflammatory and pain-relieving effects, particularly for bruises, sprains, and muscle soreness. Arnica is popular in homeopathic medicine and is also applied topically in the form of creams, gels, ointments, or oils.

Properties	Anti-inflammatory: Helps reduce swelling and inflammation. Analgesic: Offers pain relief for various conditions, such as bruises, joint pain, and muscle aches. Anti bruising: Promotes the healing of bruises. Immunostimulant: Some components may stimulate the immune system.
What disease it fights	Bruises and Swelling: Applied topically to reduce the severity and duration of bruises. Muscle and Joint Pain: Used to alleviate pain and inflammation associated with arthritis, sprains, and muscle aches. Post-Surgical Recovery: Sometimes used to reduce pain and swelling after minor surgeries. Insect Bites: Can be applied to reduce itching and swelling.
How it works	Arnica contains several compounds, including sesquiterpene lactones (such as helenalin), flavonoids, and phenolic acids, which contribute to its anti-inflammatory and analgesic properties. These compounds are thought to inhibit the processes that lead to inflammation and pain at the site of injury.
How to use	Topically: Arnica is most commonly used in a gel, cream, ointment, or oil form applied directly to the skin over the affected area. It should not be applied to broken skin or open wounds. Homeopathic Preparations: These are available in oral form, such as pellets or drops, and are used for broader systemic effects, including pain and bruising.
Dosage	Topically: Apply to the affected area 2 to 3 times daily or as needed. Follow the specific product instructions for application. Homeopathic Arnica: The dosage can vary widely depending on the condition and the product's concentration. Common dosages include 30C potency, taken as directed on the product packaging or by a healthcare provider.
How long to use	For acute conditions like bruises, sprains, or muscle soreness, Arnica is generally used until symptoms improve, which is typically within a few days to a week. For chronic conditions, or when using homeopathic Arnica, its use might be longer-term, but it's important to evaluate its effectiveness regularly.

Ashwagandha

Ashwagandha (Withania somnifera) is a prominent herb in Ayurvedic medicine, revered for its adaptogenic properties. It helps the body manage stress, provides energy, and promotes overall health.

Properties	Adaptogenic: Helps the body manage stress and combat fatigue. Anti-inflammatory: Reduces inflammation, beneficial for arthritis and other inflammatory conditions. Antioxidant: Protects cells from oxidative stress and damage. Thyroid Modulating: Can help normalize thyroid function, particularly in cases of hypothyroidism. Anxiolytic and Antidepressant: Reduces anxiety and depression symptoms without causing drowsiness. Immune Boosting: Enhances the immune system's functioning.
What disease it fights	Stress and Anxiety: Helps reduce cortisol levels, mitigating the effects of stress on the body. Depression: Its adaptogenic effects contribute to mood stabilization. Chronic Fatigue: Provides energy and vitality, combatting fatigue. Inflammatory Conditions: Beneficial in managing conditions like arthritis. Thyroid Disorders: Assists in regulating thyroid hormone levels. Insomnia: Promotes restful sleep due to its stress-reducing properties.
How it works	Ashwagandha's adaptogenic properties are attributed to its bioactive compounds, including withanolides, which help modulate the body's stress response systems. It influences neurotransmitter systems to reduce anxiety and improve mood, and it can enhance endocrine function, including thyroid and adrenal health, for better hormonal balance.
How to use	Powder Form: Ashwagandha root powder can be mixed with water, milk, or honey and consumed. It can also be added to smoothies or other foods. Capsule/Tablet Form: For those who prefer not to taste the herb, capsules or tablets are convenient options. Tea: Ashwagandha tea, made from the powder or leaves, is another way to consume the herb.
Dosage	The dosage can vary depending on the form of Ashwagandha and the individual's health condition: Powder: 3–6 grams per day, typically divided into two or three doses. Capsules/Tablets: 300–500 mg of standardized extract twice daily.
How long to use	Ashwagandha is generally considered safe for long-term use, with many benefits observed over extended periods. However, it's often recommended to take breaks or evaluate its effects periodically. A common approach is to use it for 2–3 months, then take a break for a week or two.

Astragalus

Astragalus (Astragalus membranaceus) is a perennial plant whose roots have been used in Traditional Chinese Medicine for centuries, primarily to boost the immune system and help prevent respiratory infections. It's also recognized for its adaptogenic properties, aiding the body in handling stress.

Properties	Immunomodulatory: Enhances the immune system, potentially reducing the frequency of colds and other infections. Adaptogenic: Helps protect the body against various stresses, including physical, mental, or emotional stress. Antioxidant: Protects cells from oxidative damage by neutralizing free radicals. Anti-inflammatory: Reduces inflammation, which can help manage conditions related to chronic inflammation. Cardioprotective: Offers protective effects on the heart and vascular system, potentially improving heart health and function. Antiviral: Some studies suggest it can help fight against viruses, including those that cause respiratory infections.
What disease it fights	Common Colds and Respiratory Infections: By boosting the immune system, it can help reduce the incidence and severity of these conditions. Chronic Fatigue Syndrome: Its adaptogenic properties may help improve energy levels and overall well-being. Heart Disease: May help protect against heart disease by improving vascular health and reducing inflammation. Autoimmune Diseases: Astragalus has been used to regulate immune function, which can be beneficial in managing autoimmune conditions.
How it works	Astragalus works by stimulating and modulating the immune system. Its active components, including polysaccharides, saponins, and flavonoids, contribute to its immune-boosting, anti-inflammatory, and antioxidant effects. These compounds enhance the production of white blood cells, particularly T-cells, and help in protecting the body against stress.
How to use	Tea: Astragalus root can be boiled in water to make tea. This can be consumed daily, especially during cold and flu season. Capsules/Tablets: These are available for those who prefer a more convenient form. They contain powdered Astragalus root or extract. Tincture: A liquid extract of Astragalus can be taken directly or added to water or tea.
Dosage	Tea: 3-6 grams of Astragalus root boiled in 12 ounces (about 350 ml) of water, consumed once or twice daily. Capsules/Tablets: 500-1000 mg of Astragalus extract, taken once or twice daily. Tincture: Follow the manufacturer's recommended dosage, usually 1-2 ml, three times a day.
How long to use	Astragalus is considered safe for long-term use as a general tonic to support immune health. However, for specific conditions or more acute use, it's often recommended for periods ranging from a few weeks to several months. It's important to take breaks or reassess its use periodically to ensure it continues to meet your health needs.

Barberry

Barberry (Berberis vulgaris) is a shrub that bears sour-tasting berries, known for its rich content of berberine, a compound with significant medicinal properties. It's been used traditionally to treat a variety of ailments, particularly those related to the digestive system and infections.

Properties	Antimicrobial: Berberine in barberry has been shown to possess broad-spectrum antimicrobial activity against bacteria, viruses, fungi, and parasites. Anti-inflammatory: Barberry can help reduce inflammation, beneficial for inflammatory conditions and supporting overall immune health. Digestive Aid: Stimulates bile secretion, which improves digestion and helps in the management of gallbladder and liver issues. Blood Sugar Regulation: Berberine has been found to help regulate blood sugar levels, making it beneficial for individuals with diabetes or metabolic syndrome.
What disease it fights	Gastrointestinal Infections: Including diarrhea caused by bacteria like E. coli and other gastrointestinal pathogens. Urinary Tract Infections (UTIs): Its antimicrobial properties make it useful in preventing and treating UTIs. Metabolic Syndrome: Can aid in managing components of metabolic syndrome, such as high blood sugar and lipid levels. Liver and Gallbladder Issues: Improves bile flow, supporting liver health and preventing gallstones.
How it works	The primary mechanism behind barberry's medicinal properties is attributed to berberine. This compound interferes with the ability of bacteria to adhere to human cells, reducing infection risk. Berberine also stimulates bile secretion and has a beneficial effect on glucose and lipid metabolism, aiding in blood sugar regulation and supporting digestive health.
How to use	Capsules/Supplements: Barberry is commonly taken in capsule form, providing a concentrated dose of berberine. Tea: The dried root, bark, or berries can be used to make tea. Tincture: A liquid extract of barberry can be used for its therapeutic benefits, especially for digestive health.
Dosage	Capsules/Supplements: Typical dosages of barberry (specifically for its berberine content) range from 500-2000 mg per day, divided into two or three doses. Tea: Boil 1-2 teaspoons of dried barberry in a cup of water for about 15 minutes. Drink up to 2 cups daily. Tincture: Follow the manufacturer's instructions, generally 2-4 ml three times a day.
How long to use	Barberry should be used with caution and typically for short durations—no longer than a few weeks for acute conditions—due to the potent effects of berberine. For chronic conditions or ongoing health support, consultation with a healthcare provider is recommended to ensure safety and monitor for any potential side effects, especially concerning its impact on blood sugar and liver function.

Bay Laurel

Bay laurel (Laurus nobilis), also known as sweet bay, is a fragrant evergreen tree or shrub from the Lauraceae family, native to the Mediterranean region. Its leaves are commonly used in cooking for their aromatic properties but also have a long history in traditional medicine for various health benefits.

Properties	Antimicrobial: Bay laurel possesses antimicrobial properties that can fight certain bacteria and fungi. Anti-inflammatory: Contains compounds that help reduce inflammation, useful in treating conditions such as arthritis. Antioxidant: Rich in antioxidants that combat oxidative stress and support overall health. Digestive Aid: Traditionally used to improve digestion and alleviate digestive disorders.
What disease it fights	Respiratory Infections: The antimicrobial properties can help treat infections in the respiratory system. Joint Pain and Inflammation: Its anti-inflammatory effects are beneficial for conditions like arthritis and rheumatism. Digestive Issues: Can stimulate digestion and relieve symptoms of indigestion, flatulence, and bloating. Skin Health: Applied topically, bay laurel oil can help treat skin infections and wounds due to its antimicrobial and anti-inflammatory properties.
How it works	The active compounds in bay laurel, including eucalyptol and cineole, contribute to its antimicrobial and anti-inflammatory effects. These compounds help inhibit the growth of pathogens and reduce inflammation, aiding in the relief of various health conditions.
How to use	Culinary Use: Dried or fresh bay leaves are used to flavor soups, stews, and other dishes. Tea: A tea made from bay leaves can be consumed for its digestive and respiratory benefits. Essential Oil: Bay laurel oil, diluted with a carrier oil, can be applied topically for joint pain, skin conditions, or used in aromatherapy.
Dosage	Tea: Steep 2-3 dried bay leaves in boiling water for about 5-10 minutes. Drink 1-2 cups daily. Essential Oil: For topical application, dilute a few drops of bay laurel oil in a carrier oil before applying to the skin. For aromatherapy, follow the diffuser's guidelines.
How long to use	Bay laurel can be used safely in culinary amounts on a daily basis. For therapeutic uses such as teas or essential oil applications, it may be used for short-term relief (a few weeks) of specific conditions. Long-term use should be approached with caution, and it's advisable to consult a healthcare professional for guidance, especially when using essential oils or supplements.

Basil

Basil (Ocimum basilicum), commonly known as Sweet Basil, is highly regarded in culinary and herbal medicine traditions for its aromatic leaves. Beyond its widespread use in cooking, basil has been recognized for its medicinal properties, including anti-inflammatory, antioxidant, and antimicrobial effects.

Properties	Antioxidant: Basil is rich in compounds like flavonoids and volatile oils, which have potent antioxidant properties that help protect the body from oxidative stress. Anti-inflammatory: Contains eugenol, a compound that mimics the action of anti-inflammatory medications. Antimicrobial: Effective against a wide range of bacteria, yeasts, molds, and viruses. Adaptogenic: Helps the body adapt to stress and to restore balance. Antidiabetic: Some studies suggest basil can help lower blood sugar levels.
What disease it fights	Respiratory Disorders: Thanks to its antimicrobial properties, basil can help fight infections that cause coughs, colds, and other respiratory issues. Inflammatory Conditions: Its anti-inflammatory effects make it beneficial for people suffering from arthritis or other inflammatory conditions. Oxidative Stress-Related Diseases: The antioxidant content can help prevent diseases caused by oxidative stress, including heart disease and certain cancers. Stress: As an adaptogen, basil can help the body manage stress more effectively. Digestive Issues: It can help alleviate stomach spasms, gas, and bloating.
How it works	The therapeutic properties of basil come from its rich array of essential oils, flavonoids, and other phytonutrients. These compounds work in various ways, such as neutralizing free radicals, blocking inflammatory enzymes, fighting microbes, and modulating blood sugar levels, thus offering a multi-faceted approach to health promotion and disease prevention.
How to use	Culinary Uses: Fresh or dried basil leaves can be incorporated into a variety of dishes, including soups, salads, and sauces. Tea: Basil leaves can be steeped in hot water to make a soothing tea, beneficial for respiratory health or digestion. Essential Oil: Basil essential oil can be used in aromatherapy or diluted and applied topically for its antimicrobial and anti-inflammatory effects.
Dosage	Tea: Use about 2-3 teaspoons of fresh basil leaves (or 1 teaspoon of dried leaves) per cup of boiling water. Steep for 5-8 minutes. Culinary: There's no specific dosage for culinary use; it can be used according to taste preferences. Essential Oil: Always dilute with a carrier oil (about 1 drop of basil oil in 1 tablespoon of carrier oil) before topical application. For aromatherapy, follow the diffuser's instruction manual.
How long to use	Basil can be consumed safely in culinary amounts daily. For medicinal uses, such as teas or essential oil applications, it's generally considered safe to use for short periods—typically up to a few weeks. As with any herbal remedy, it's wise to take breaks or vary the herbs used to promote overall health and avoid potential side effects.

Bay Leaf

Bay leaf, known scientifically as Laurus nobilis, is a fragrant leaf from the laurel tree, commonly used as a spice in cooking but also valued for its medicinal properties. Traditional uses include aiding digestion, relieving respiratory conditions, and reducing inflammation.

Properties	Antioxidant: Contains compounds like cineol and eugenol, which have potent antioxidant properties. Anti-inflammatory: The eugenol in bay leaves also acts as a natural anti-inflammatory agent. Antimicrobial: Effective against a range of bacteria, fungi, and yeast. Digestive Aid: Traditionally used to stimulate digestion and relieve digestive disorders. Analgesic: Can help relieve pain, including headaches and migraines. Diuretic: Helps promote urine production, aiding in detoxification and reducing bloating.
What disease it fights	Digestive Issues: Improves digestion, relieves gas, bloating, and stomach pain. Respiratory Conditions: Used in herbal steams or teas to alleviate respiratory issues and infections. Inflammatory Conditions: The anti-inflammatory properties can help with arthritis and other inflammatory conditions. High Blood Sugar: Some studies suggest bay leaves could help improve insulin function and lower blood sugar levels. Infections: Due to its antimicrobial properties, it can help prevent and fight infections.
How it works	Bay leaf's health benefits stem from its rich composition of antioxidants, essential oils, and organic compounds. These substances can help reduce inflammation, neutralize free radicals, and kill bacteria and fungi. The leaf's compounds can also stimulate digestive enzymes, improving digestion and nutrient absorption.
How to use	Cooking: Bay leaves are commonly used to flavor soups, stews, and other dishes. The leaves are usually removed before serving. Tea: A bay leaf tea can be made by steeping 2-3 dried leaves in hot water for about 5 minutes. Essential Oil: Bay leaf essential oil can be used in aromatherapy or diluted and applied topically for pain relief and to address respiratory conditions.
Dosage	Tea: Drinking 1-2 cups of bay leaf tea per day is generally considered safe for most adults. Cooking: There are no specific dosage recommendations for culinary use, as the leaves are removed after cooking and contribute only trace amounts of bioactive compounds to the dish. Essential Oil: Always dilute with a carrier oil (typically 1-2 drops of essential oil per tablespoon of carrier oil) for topical use. For aromatherapy, follow the diffuser's guidelines.
How long to use	Bay leaves can be used safely in cooking daily. For medicinal uses like tea or essential oil, it's typically recommended to use them for a few weeks, then take a break or assess effectiveness. Continuous long-term use (especially of the essential oil) should be approached with caution to monitor for any potential side effects or interactions.

Bilberry

Bilberry (Vaccinium myrtillus), closely related to blueberries and cranberries, is a small, dark berry known for its high antioxidant content, particularly anthocyanins. These compounds give bilberries their deep blue color and are credited with numerous health benefits, especially for eye health and circulation.

Properties	Antioxidant: High in anthocyanins, which protect cells from oxidative damage. Anti-inflammatory: Helps reduce inflammation throughout the body. Vision Support: Traditionally used to improve night vision and overall eye health. Circulatory Health: Aids in improving blood flow and vascular health. Blood Sugar Regulation: May help manage blood sugar levels.
What disease it fights	Eye Disorders: Including night vision improvement, retinopathy, and macular degeneration. Circulatory Issues: Such as varicose veins, hemorrhoids, and atherosclerosis, by strengthening blood vessels and improving circulation. Diabetes: By aiding in blood sugar regulation. Oxidative Stress-Related Conditions: Protects against diseases linked to oxidative stress, including heart disease and certain cancers.
How it works	The anthocyanins in bilberry are powerful antioxidants that protect against cellular damage from free radicals. They also improve blood vessel elasticity and reduce blood clotting, enhancing circulatory health. For eye health, anthocyanins help regenerate rhodopsin, a protein in the eyes that's crucial for night vision and overall eye function.
How to use	Fresh or Frozen Berries: Can be consumed directly or added to cereals, yogurts, and smoothies. Supplements: Available in capsules, tablets, or tinctures for those who prefer a more concentrated form or can't access fresh berries. Tea: Bilberry leaves can be brewed into tea, though it's less common than using the fruit.
Dosage	Fresh Berries: No specific dosage; can be enjoyed as part of a healthy diet. Supplements: Typically, for eye health and circulation, 80-160 mg of standardized bilberry extract (containing 25% anthocyanins) twice daily is recommended. Tea: 1-2 teaspoons of dried leaves per cup of boiling water, steeped for 10 minutes, consumed up to three times a day. However, long-term use of the leaves is not recommended due to potential toxicity.
How long to use	Bilberry fruit can be consumed regularly as part of a balanced diet without specific time restrictions. For supplements, following the recommended duration on the product label or consulting with a healthcare provider is wise. Generally, supplements are used for specific health concerns rather than indefinitely, with periodic evaluations to assess effectiveness and need.

Black Cohosh

Black Cohosh (Actaea racemosa), a plant native to North America, is widely used for its potential benefits, especially in relation to women's health issues such as menopause symptoms and menstrual discomforts.

Properties	Phytoestrogenic: Black Cohosh contains compounds that can mimic the effects of estrogen, which is particularly useful in managing menopausal symptoms. Anti-inflammatory: Helps reduce inflammation, contributing to its effectiveness in treating joint pain and arthritis-related symptoms. Nervine: May have a calming effect on the nervous system, which can help in reducing anxiety and improving sleep quality. Antispasmodic: Can relieve muscle spasms, including those associated with menstrual cramps.
What disease it fights	Menopause Symptoms: Including hot flashes, night sweats, mood swings, and vaginal dryness. Menstrual Discomfort: Helps in alleviating PMS and menstrual cramps. Mood Disorders: Its potential effects on the nervous system can help in managing anxiety and depression symptoms associated with menopause. Bone Health: Some research suggests Black Cohosh could have a beneficial effect on bone density.
How it works	The exact mechanism of how Black Cohosh works is not fully understood, but it's believed its phytoestrogens interact with estrogen receptors, helping to balance hormone levels without the risks associated with hormone replacement therapy. Its anti-inflammatory and antispasmodic properties also contribute to its effectiveness in relieving pain and discomfort.
How to use	Black Cohosh is available in various forms, including capsules, tinctures, and teas. The method of use often depends on personal preference and the specific health concern being addressed.
Dosage	Capsules/Tablets: The common dosage is between 20 to 40 mg twice daily of standardized extract, but it can vary based on the product. Tincture: Typically, 1-2 ml three times a day is recommended for the tincture form. Tea: While less common due to its bitter taste, tea can be made from the dried root.
How long to use	Black Cohosh should not be used for extended periods without breaks or oversight from a healthcare provider. A common practice is to use it for up to six months, then assess its effectiveness and safety before continuing. Some sources suggest taking a break after six months of use.

Black Seed (Nigella Sativa)

Black seed, also known as Nigella sativa, has been used for thousands of years for its therapeutic benefits. It's renowned for its potent anti-inflammatory, antioxidant, antimicrobial, and immune-boosting properties.

Properties	Anti-inflammatory: Helps reduce inflammation in the body, beneficial for conditions like arthritis and autoimmune diseases. Antioxidant: Contains thymoquinone, an antioxidant that protects cells from damage caused by free radicals. Antimicrobial: Exhibits antibacterial, antiviral, and antifungal properties, useful in fighting various infections. Immune Booster: Can enhance the immune response, helping the body fight off illnesses more effectively. Anti-diabetic: Helps regulate blood sugar levels, making it beneficial for people with diabetes.
What disease it fights	Asthma and Allergies: Its anti-inflammatory and immune-boosting effects can help manage asthma and allergic reactions. High Blood Pressure and Cholesterol: May aid in lowering blood pressure and cholesterol levels, contributing to cardiovascular health. Digestive Health: Supports digestion and can alleviate symptoms of bloating, gas, and stomach ulcers. Skin Conditions: The oil is used topically to improve various skin conditions, including eczema and acne.
How it works	The wide range of benefits from black seed is mainly attributed to its active compound, thymoquinone, which has been shown to have anti-inflammatory and antioxidant effects. It influences various pathways in the body to reduce inflammation, fight infection, and support the immune system.
How to use	Oil: Black seed oil can be taken orally or applied topically to the skin. It's also used in hair care products for its nourishing properties. Capsules: For those who prefer not to taste the oil, capsules containing black seed oil are available. Powdered Seeds: Can be added to food or beverages or taken in capsule form.
Dosage	Oil: 1-2 teaspoons daily, taken directly or mixed into beverages or food. Capsules: Follow the manufacturer's instructions, typically 500 mg of black seed oil per capsule, taken 1-2 times daily. Powdered Seeds: Use 1 teaspoon of the powder daily, mixed into foods or drinks.
How long to use	Black seed can be used as a daily supplement for general health benefits. For specific health conditions, it's often taken for several weeks to months. As with any supplement, it's wise to take breaks or consult a healthcare professional for long-term use, especially to monitor its effects on blood pressure, blood sugar, and overall health.

Black Walnut

Black Walnut (Juglans nigra) is valued not only for its nuts but also for its husk, shell, and leaves, all of which have been used in traditional medicine. It's particularly known for its antiparasitic, antifungal, and antibacterial properties.

Properties	Antiparasitic: Especially effective against intestinal parasites. Antifungal and Antibacterial: Useful in treating fungal and bacterial infections. Astringent: Due to its tannin content, it can help tighten and tone tissues, useful in conditions like diarrhea or excessive sweating. Detoxifying: Traditionally used to support detoxification processes in the body.
What disease it fights	Intestinal Parasites: Black Walnut hulls are widely used to expel worms and other parasites from the intestines. Fungal Infections: Including candida overgrowths and athlete's foot. Skin Conditions: Applied topically to treat eczema, psoriasis, and other skin infections. Digestive Issues: The astringent properties help in treating diarrhea and improving digestive health.
How it works	The juglone (a quinone compound) in Black Walnut has been identified as having strong antiparasitic and antifungal activities. Tannins present in the plant provide astringent properties that help in reducing inflammation and tightening tissues, while essential fatty acids contribute to its overall health benefits.
How to use	Hull Extract/Tincture: Often used for its antiparasitic and antifungal properties. It can be diluted in water or juice before consumption. Powder: Made from dried and ground hulls, it can be used in capsule form or added to liquids. Topical Applications: As a salve or lotion for skin conditions or fungal infections.
Dosage	Tincture: Typically, 1-2 ml of the tincture three times a day. Dilute in water or juice to reduce potential irritation to the stomach. Capsules/Powder: Dosages can vary depending on the product, but a general guideline for adults is around 500 mg twice daily. Always follow the manufacturer's instructions or the advice of a healthcare professional.
How long to use	Black Walnut should be used with caution and typically not for extended periods due to its potency. For acute conditions, such as expelling parasites or treating a fungal infection, a course of treatment might last from 2 to 6 weeks. It's essential to monitor for any adverse reactions, especially if used internally, as it can be irritating to the gastrointestinal tract in some individuals.

Bladderwrack

Bladderwrack (Fucus vesiculosus) is a type of seaweed found on the coasts of the North Sea, the western Baltic Sea, and the Atlantic and Pacific Oceans. It's been used traditionally for thyroid health, weight loss, and skin health due to its high iodine content.

Properties	Thyroid Support: The high iodine content in bladderwrack is essential for thyroid health, supporting the production of thyroid hormones. Metabolic Boost: May aid in weight loss by enhancing metabolism, attributed to its impact on thyroid function. Anti-inflammatory: Contains fucoidan, a compound known for its anti-inflammatory properties. Antioxidant: Offers antioxidant benefits, helping to protect cells from oxidative stress.
What disease it fights	Thyroid Disorders: Particularly useful for individuals with iodine deficiency hypothyroidism, supporting normal thyroid function. Obesity: By improving thyroid function and metabolism, it can contribute to weight management. Digestive Health: The polysaccharides in bladderwrack can have a prebiotic effect, supporting gut health. Joint Pain and Arthritis: Its anti-inflammatory properties may help reduce symptoms associated with joint pain and arthritis.
How it works	Bladderwrack's health benefits are primarily due to its iodine content, which is crucial for thyroid hormone synthesis. Proper thyroid function is essential for metabolism, growth, and development. Fucoidan, another significant compound in bladderwrack, contributes to its anti-inflammatory and antioxidant effects, supporting overall health and well-being.
How to use	Capsules: Bladderwrack is commonly taken in capsule form, providing a convenient way to consume this seaweed. Powder: Can be added to smoothies, teas, or foods. It's a versatile form for incorporating bladderwrack into the diet. Tincture: A liquid extract of bladderwrack can be used for its concentrated benefits.
Dosage	Capsules: Dosages can vary depending on the concentration, but a typical dose is 300-600 mg daily. Powder: Start with 1/4 teaspoon per day, gradually increasing to no more than 1 teaspoon daily to monitor tolerance. Tincture: Follow the manufacturer's instructions, typically 1-2 ml three times a day.
How long to use	Short to medium-term use of bladderwrack is recommended, ranging from a few weeks to a few months, especially when addressing specific health issues like thyroid support or weight management. Long-term use should be approached with caution due to potential iodine overload and should be monitored by a healthcare professional.

Blessed Thistle

Blessed Thistle (Cnicus benedictus) is a plant that has been traditionally used in herbal medicine for centuries, recognized for its digestive, antimicrobial, and anti-inflammatory properties.

Properties	Digestive Stimulant: Blessed Thistle is known to stimulate the appetite and aid digestion by increasing saliva and gastric juice production. Galactagogue: Traditionally used to increase milk supply in breastfeeding mothers. Antimicrobial: Exhibits some antimicrobial activity, which may help fight certain infections. Anti-inflammatory: Contains compounds that may reduce inflammation.
What disease it fights	Digestive Disorders: Including indigestion, constipation, and gas. Poor Appetite: Used to stimulate appetite in those with loss of appetite for various reasons. Menstrual Disorders: May help relieve menstrual cramps and promote menstrual flow. Infections: Its antimicrobial properties may help in combating bacterial and fungal infections.
How it works	The active components in Blessed Thistle, including cnicin and polyacetylenes, are believed to stimulate digestive secretions and possess antimicrobial and anti-inflammatory effects. By stimulating the production of digestive juices, it can help improve digestion and relieve gastrointestinal discomfort. Its galactagogue effect is thought to be due to its overall stimulating effect on the body's systems, although the exact mechanism is not fully understood.
How to use	Tea: A common method for consuming Blessed Thistle, made by steeping the dried herb in hot water. Capsules: For those who prefer not to taste the herb, capsules are a convenient option. Tincture: A liquid extract of Blessed Thistle can be taken in water or juice.
Dosage	Tea: 1–2 teaspoons of dried Blessed Thistle per cup of boiling water, steeped for 10–15 minutes, consumed 2-3 times daily. Capsules: Follow the manufacturer's instructions, typically 1-2 capsules taken 2-3 times daily. Tincture: 1-2 ml three times a day.
How long to use	Blessed Thistle is generally used on a short-term basis for digestive issues or to stimulate milk production, usually not exceeding 8 weeks. Long-term use is not well-documented and may not be recommended due to the lack of extensive safety data.

Blue Cohosh

Blue Cohosh (Caulophyllum thalictroides) is a plant traditionally used in Native American medicine and later adopted by other herbal medicine traditions. It's known for its strong properties affecting women's reproductive systems, but due to its potent nature, it must be used with caution.

Properties	Uterine Stimulant: Blue Cohosh is known for its ability to stimulate uterine contractions, which is why it has been used to induce labor. Antispasmodic: Helps relieve muscle spasms and cramping, which can be useful for menstrual cramps. Anti-inflammatory: Offers some degree of inflammation reduction, potentially benefiting conditions such as arthritis. Diuretic: Assists in the removal of excess fluid from the body, which can help with conditions like edema.
What disease it fights	Menstrual Disorders: It's used to relieve menstrual cramps and regulate menstrual flow. Labor Induction: Traditionally used to induce labor in pregnant women who are past their due date. Arthritis: The anti-inflammatory properties can help alleviate arthritis pain.
How it works	Blue Cohosh contains several active compounds, including saponins and alkaloids like caulophylline, which contribute to its effects. These compounds are believed to stimulate the uterus and affect other smooth muscles, either by inducing contractions or by relieving spasms, depending on the dosage and the body's current state.
How to use	Due to its potent nature and potential risks, the use of Blue Cohosh should be under the guidance of a healthcare provider or an experienced herbalist, especially when used for inducing labor or treating gynecological issues.
Dosage	Given the potent effects and possible risks associated with Blue Cohosh, including its potential impact on blood pressure and glucose levels, a standardized dosage recommendation is not provided here. The dosage can vary significantly based on the form (e.g., dried herb, tincture, capsule) and the individual's specific circumstances.
How long to use	The duration of use for Blue Cohosh should be as short as necessary and closely monitored by a healthcare professional, especially when used for labor induction or menstrual disorders. Long-term use is generally not recommended due to the lack of comprehensive safety data.

Blue Vervain

Blue Vervain (Verbena hastata) is a perennial plant known for its medicinal properties, historically used in various traditional medicine systems.

Properties	Nervine: Supports the nervous system, helps alleviate stress and anxiety. Antispasmodic: Relieves muscle spasms and cramps. Diaphoretic: Promotes sweating and helps reduce fevers. Sedative: Mild sedative properties can aid sleep and relaxation. Digestive Aid: Stimulates appetite and aids digestion. Anti-inflammatory: Helps reduce inflammation in the body.
What disease it fights	Anxiety and Stress: Its nervine properties make it beneficial for relieving stress and anxiety. Insomnia: The sedative effects can help improve sleep quality. Digestive Issues: Can stimulate digestion and relieve symptoms like bloating and indigestion. Muscle Spasms and Cramps: The antispasmodic properties can help alleviate muscle tension and menstrual cramps. Respiratory Conditions: Used traditionally to treat colds and flu by inducing sweating and reducing fever.
How it works	The beneficial effects of Blue Vervain are attributed to its various active compounds, including iridoid glycosides, which have been shown to have anti-inflammatory and nervine properties. These compounds can help soothe the nervous system and reduce inflammation, making Blue Vervain useful for a variety of conditions.
How to use	Tea: A common method of consumption, made by steeping the dried herb in hot water. Tincture: A concentrated liquid form that can be diluted in water or taken directly in small amounts. Capsules: For those who prefer not to taste the herb, capsules are an alternative.
Dosage	Tea: Typically, 1-2 teaspoons of dried Blue Vervain herb per cup of boiling water, steeped for 10-15 minutes, consumed 1-3 times daily. Tincture: 2-4 ml up to three times daily. Capsules: Follow the manufacturer's instructions, as potency can vary.
How long to use	Blue Vervain is generally considered safe for short-term use, typically a few weeks up to a couple of months. Long-term use should be approached with caution, and it's wise to consult with a healthcare professional, especially for continuous use beyond a few months.

Borage

Borage (Borago officinalis), also known as starflower, is a herb notable for its high gamma-linolenic acid (GLA) content, a type of Omega-6 fatty acid. It's been traditionally used for its anti-inflammatory properties, to improve skin health, and as a natural remedy for respiratory and mood disorders.

Properties	Anti-inflammatory: GLA in borage oil can help reduce inflammation in the body. Mood Enhancer: Traditionally used to lift spirits and ease depression. Respiratory Health: Used in folk medicine to treat coughs and bronchitis. Skin Health: Borage oil is often used topically to treat eczema, psoriasis, and improve overall skin health.
What disease it fights	Skin Disorders: Including eczema, psoriasis, and acne, due to its anti-inflammatory properties. Arthritis: The GLA in borage may reduce joint pain and symptoms of rheumatoid arthritis. Stress and Anxiety: Can have a calming effect, helping to alleviate stress and anxiety. Respiratory Conditions: Used to relieve coughs and respiratory infections.
How it works	Borage oil's high GLA content is converted by the body into dihomo-gamma-linolenic acid (DGLA), an anti-inflammatory substance. This process can help alleviate inflammation associated with skin disorders, arthritis, and other inflammatory conditions. Additionally, borage has been thought to have a diuretic effect, which can help in reducing symptoms of premenstrual syndrome (PMS).
How to use	Oil: Borage oil can be taken orally in capsule form or used topically on the skin. Herbal Tea: The leaves can be used to make tea, though they should be used with caution due to potential liver toxicity with excessive consumption. Leaves: Young, tender borage leaves can be eaten in salads or cooked as greens, in moderation.
Dosage	Oil (capsules): Typically, 1 to 2 grams of borage oil per day, which should provide about 240 to 480 mg of GLA. Follow the specific product's recommendation. Tea: 1 to 2 teaspoons of dried borage leaves steeped in hot water for about 10 minutes, once daily. Due to potential toxicity, borage tea should be consumed only occasionally, not as a daily supplement.
How long to use	Borage oil can be used for several weeks to months, depending on the condition being treated and the individual's response. However, due to concerns about liver toxicity and the potential effect of pyrrolizidine alkaloids (PAs) found in the plant, long-term use of borage leaves, especially in high doses, should be avoided.

Boswellia (Frankincense)

Boswellia, also known as Frankincense, is derived from the resin of the Boswellia tree species. It has been used for thousands of years in traditional medicines for its anti-inflammatory, analgesic, and antiseptic properties.

Properties	Anti-inflammatory: Boswellia acids can significantly reduce inflammation and are often used in conditions like arthritis. Analgesic: Offers pain relief, particularly in inflamed areas. Antiseptic: Can prevent the growth of bacteria and infections. Astringent: Helps tighten the tissues, which can be beneficial for skin health.
What disease it fights	Chronic Inflammatory Conditions: Such as rheumatoid arthritis and osteoarthritis, by reducing inflammation and pain. Inflammatory Bowel Diseases (IBD): Including Crohn's disease and ulcerative colitis, by helping to reduce intestinal inflammation. Asthma: Boswellia can help reduce the frequency and severity of asthma attacks. Skin Conditions: Used topically to heal wounds, scars, and improve overall skin condition.
How it works	Boswellia works primarily through its active components, boswellic acids. These compounds inhibit 5-lipoxygenase (5-LO), an enzyme that produces leukotriene, which is involved in the inflammatory process. By inhibiting this pathway, Boswellia effectively reduces inflammation and pain without the side effects commonly associated with conventional anti-inflammatory drugs.
How to use	Oral Supplements: Boswellia is available in capsules or tablets, which are taken orally. Topical Applications: Creams or ointments containing Boswellia can be applied to the skin for localized issues. Incense: While not used for direct healing, burning Boswellia resin as incense can have calming effects.
Dosage	Oral Supplements: The typical dosage ranges from 300 to 500 mg of standardized extract (containing 60% boswellic acids) taken two to three times daily. Topical Applications: Follow the instructions on the product label for creams or ointments.
How long to use	Boswellia can be used for several weeks to months, depending on the condition being treated and the individual's response. Some studies on osteoarthritis have used Boswellia supplements for up to 90 days. Continuous use beyond several months should be monitored by a healthcare professional to assess effectiveness and safety.

Burdock Root

Burdock root (Arctium lappa) is a plant that has been used in traditional medicine across various cultures for centuries, primarily for its detoxifying and blood-purifying properties.

Properties	Detoxifying: Burdock root is believed to help detoxify the blood and promote lymphatic drainage. Diuretic: It can help increase urine output, assisting in the removal of waste from the body. Antioxidant: Contains powerful antioxidants, such as quercetin and luteolin, that help protect cells from oxidative stress. Anti-inflammatory: Offers anti-inflammatory benefits, which can help reduce swelling and pain. Blood Sugar Regulation: Some studies suggest it can help in managing blood sugar levels.
What disease it fights	Skin Conditions: Including acne, eczema, and psoriasis, by helping to remove toxins from the blood that may contribute to these issues. Digestive Issues: Used to improve digestion and treat issues like bloating and constipation. Arthritis: The anti-inflammatory properties can help reduce symptoms of arthritis. Diabetes: Its potential to regulate blood sugar levels may be beneficial for those managing diabetes.
How it works	The beneficial effects of burdock root are attributed to its high content of inulin, a type of soluble fiber, which can help improve digestion and lower blood sugar levels. Its diuretic properties assist in flushing toxins from the body, while its antioxidants and anti-inflammatory compounds support overall health by protecting against oxidative stress and reducing inflammation.
How to use	Tea: Made by steeping dried burdock root in boiling water, typically consumed 2-3 times daily. Capsules: Dried, powdered burdock root is available in capsule form, offering a more convenient option for some. Tincture: A liquid extract of burdock root, which can be diluted in water or taken directly in small amounts.
Dosage	Tea: 1-2 teaspoons of dried root per cup of boiling water, steeped for about 10 minutes. Drink up to 3 cups daily. Capsules: Follow the manufacturer's recommendations, typically around 1-2 grams per day in divided doses. Tincture: 2-4 ml three times daily, diluted in water.
How long to use	Burdock root can be used over a period of several weeks to a few months, depending on the condition being treated and the individual's response. For chronic conditions or ongoing wellness support, it may be used in cycles (e.g., 4 weeks on, 1 week off) to prevent potential side effects from long-term use.

Calendula

Calendula, scientifically known as Calendula officinalis, is a medicinal herb with vibrant yellow-orange flowers, widely recognized for its healing properties.

Properties	Anti-inflammatory: Calendula contains flavonoids and saponins that help reduce inflammation, making it effective for wounds, ulcers, and swollen tissues. Antimicrobial: It has the ability to fight bacteria, viruses, and fungi, protecting wounds from infection. Healing: Promotes tissue regeneration, speeding up the healing process of cuts, burns, and bruises. Astringent: Can tighten and tone the skin, useful in treating acne and minimizing pores. Antispasmodic: Relieves muscle spasms and menstrual cramps.
What disease it fights	Skin Disorders: Including cuts, wounds, burns, eczema, and acne, due to its healing and anti-inflammatory properties. Oral Health Issues: Such as gingivitis and mouth ulcers, thanks to its antimicrobial action. Inflammatory Conditions: Calendula's anti-inflammatory effects make it beneficial for treating conditions like diaper rash and hemorrhoids. Menstrual Cramps: Its antispasmodic properties can help ease menstrual discomfort.
How it works	Calendula works by promoting the production of collagen at wound sites, which enhances healing. Its anti-inflammatory compounds reduce inflammation, while its antimicrobial properties prevent wound infections. Additionally, its astringent actions help in tightening the skin and tissues, providing relief in various skin conditions.
How to use	Topical Application: Calendula can be applied directly to the skin in the form of creams, ointments, or gels. Tea: For internal health benefits or as a soothing wash for wounds or skin conditions. Tincture: Can be diluted with water and used as a mouth rinse or applied to the skin for healing purposes.
Dosage	Creams/Ointments: Apply to the affected area 2-3 times daily, or as needed. Tea: 1-2 teaspoons of dried calendula flowers steeped in hot water for 10 minutes. Drink or use as a wash 2-3 times daily. Tincture: For external use, dilute 1 part tincture with 3 parts water and apply to the skin or use as a mouth rinse 2-3 times daily.
How long to use	For acute conditions like wounds, burns, or skin irritations, Calendula can be used until symptoms improve, typically within a few days to a week. For chronic conditions or for ongoing support, such as menstrual cramps or eczema, it may be used for longer periods, with periodic evaluation to monitor effectiveness and any potential skin sensitivities.

California Poppy

California Poppy (Eschscholzia californica) is an herb native to the United States and Mexico, known for its bright orange flowers. It has been used traditionally to support sleep, relieve pain, and ease anxiety due to its mild sedative and analgesic properties.

Properties	Sedative: Helps to promote relaxation and improve sleep quality. Anxiolytic: Can reduce anxiety and stress levels. Analgesic: Offers pain relief, particularly for acute and neuropathic pain. Antispasmodic: Relieves muscle spasms or cramps.
What disease it fights	Insomnia: Aids in improving the quality of sleep without the grogginess often associated with pharmaceutical sleep aids. Anxiety and Stress: Helps to calm the mind and reduce symptoms of anxiety. Pain Management: Can be used to alleviate various types of pain, including headaches and nerve pain. ADHD: Some use it as a natural remedy to manage ADHD symptoms, particularly in children, due to its calming effects.
How it works	The sedative and anxiolytic effects of California Poppy are believed to be due to a combination of its alkaloid content, which includes californidine, eschscholtzine, and other bioactive compounds. These compounds interact with the central nervous system to promote relaxation and reduce pain signaling without the addictive properties of stronger sedatives.
How to use	Tea: Dried leaves and flowers can be steeped in hot water to make a relaxing tea. Tincture: A liquid extract can be used for more precise dosing, especially when addressing anxiety or sleep issues. Capsules: Available for those who prefer not to taste the herb but wish to benefit from its properties.
Dosage	Tea: 1-2 teaspoons of dried herb per cup of boiling water, steeped for 10-15 minutes. Drink 30 minutes before bedtime or when needed to relieve anxiety. Tincture: Typically, 30-40 drops in a little water, taken 1-3 times daily, or before bed for sleep support. Capsules: Follow the manufacturer's instructions, as potency can vary significantly.
How long to use	California Poppy can be used as needed for acute issues like trouble sleeping or temporary anxiety. For chronic conditions, it's typically used for a few weeks to a few months, followed by an evaluation period to assess its effectiveness. Continuous long-term use is not commonly recommended without consulting a healthcare provider, especially for children or if used in conjunction with other medications.

Cardamom

Cardamom (Elettaria cardamomum) is a spice native to India, known for its aromatic seeds and used both in cooking and traditional medicine. Its health benefits stem from its antioxidant, anti-inflammatory, and digestive properties.

Properties	Antioxidant: Cardamom contains compounds that can protect cells from damage and reduce inflammation. Digestive Aid: It can help manage digestive problems like bloating, gas, and indigestion. Diuretic: Promotes urination to remove water, toxins, and prevent urinary tract infections. Antimicrobial: Fights infections, especially in the mouth; used traditionally for oral health. Anti-inflammatory: Reduces inflammation in the body, potentially benefiting conditions like arthritis.
What disease it fights	Digestive Disorders: Including indigestion, gas, and bloating. Respiratory Conditions: Its expectorant properties can help relieve symptoms of colds and coughs. High Blood Pressure: Some studies suggest cardamom may help lower blood pressure levels. Oral Health Issues: Can combat bad breath and prevent oral infections due to its antimicrobial properties.
How it works	The therapeutic effects of cardamom are attributed to its rich blend of essential oils, antioxidants, and phytonutrients. These compounds can improve digestive enzyme activity, neutralize harmful free radicals, reduce inflammation, and exhibit antimicrobial activity against various pathogens.
How to use	Culinary Uses: Cardamom can be added to dishes, both sweet and savory, or used in teas and baked goods for flavor and health benefits. Tea: Cardamom pods can be steeped in hot water to make a soothing tea that aids digestion and respiratory health. Chewing Pods: Fresh cardamom pods can be chewed as a natural breath freshener and to promote oral health.
Dosage	Culinary and Tea: There is no specific dosage for culinary uses or tea; it can be used according to taste and preference. For tea, 2-3 pods per cup is a common ratio. Supplements: If taking cardamom as a supplement, follow the manufacturer's dosage recommendations, typically ranging from 250–500 mg per day.
How long to use	As a culinary spice or in tea, cardamom can be consumed regularly without specified duration limits. For specific health conditions or when taking supplements, it might be used for a few weeks to a few months, depending on individual needs and responses. Continuous long-term use of high doses in supplement form should be monitored by a healthcare professional.

Cat's Claw

Cat's Claw (Uncaria tomentosa) is a vine commonly found in the Amazon rainforest and other tropical areas of South and Central America. It's recognized for its immune-boosting, anti-inflammatory, and antioxidant properties.

Properties	Immune Booster: Enhances immune system response. Anti-inflammatory: Helps reduce inflammation, beneficial for arthritis and autoimmune diseases. Antioxidant: Protects against oxidative stress and cellular damage. Antiviral: Exhibits potential antiviral properties against some viruses.
What disease it fights	Arthritis and Joint Pain: Reduces symptoms of osteoarthritis and rheumatoid arthritis. Autoimmune Disorders: Modulates the immune system, potentially benefiting conditions like lupus and multiple sclerosis. Digestive Issues: Used for inflammatory bowel diseases (IBD) such as Crohn's disease and ulcerative colitis.
How it works	Cat's claw works by modulating the immune system to enhance its response to threats while also exerting anti-inflammatory effects that can help manage arthritis and autoimmune conditions. Its antioxidants protect cells from damage.
How to use	Capsules/Supplements: The most common form, providing a controlled dosage. Tea: Made from the bark or root, can be consumed for general health benefits.
Dosage	Capsules/Supplements: Typically, 250-350 mg taken twice daily. Tea: 1 gram of powdered bark per cup of boiling water, steeped for 10-15 minutes, drunk 2-3 times daily.
How long to use	Cat's claw is generally used for several weeks to months, depending on the condition being treated. Long-term use should be monitored by a healthcare professional to ensure safety and effectiveness.

Catnip

Catnip (Nepeta cataria) is a perennial herb belonging to the mint family and is known for its sedative and relaxing properties in humans, despite its stimulating effects on cats.

Properties	Sedative: Helps in reducing anxiety and promoting relaxation, making it beneficial for sleep disorders. Antispasmodic: Offers relief from muscle spasms and cramps. Digestive Aid: Can soothe the stomach and relieve symptoms of indigestion, gas, and bloating. Diaphoretic: Promotes sweating, which can help in reducing fevers. Mild Analgesic: Provides pain relief for minor aches and pains.
What disease it fights	Insomnia and Sleep Disorders: Its sedative properties help improve sleep quality. Anxiety and Stress: Catnip has a calming effect on the nervous system, reducing anxiety and stress. Digestive Issues: Helps in relieving indigestion, gas, and bloating. Cold and Flu: The diaphoretic action helps in managing fevers associated with colds and flu.
How it works	The active compounds in Catnip, including nepetalactone, are believed to have a mild sedative effect on humans, which contributes to its ability to promote relaxation and sleep. These compounds can also relax muscles, ease digestive discomfort, and support the body in managing fevers.
How to use	Tea: Catnip leaves can be steeped in hot water to make a soothing tea. This is particularly effective for relaxation and aiding digestion. Tincture: A concentrated liquid form that can be used for more precise dosing. Fresh or Dried Leaves: Can be used to prepare herbal remedies or added to food.
Dosage	Tea: 1–2 teaspoons of dried catnip per cup of boiling water, steeped for 10 minutes. Drink up to 3 cups daily, especially before bedtime for sleep disorders. Tincture: 1–2 ml, up to three times daily. Always start with the lower dose to assess tolerance.
How long to use	Catnip can be used as needed for immediate relief from anxiety, indigestion, or sleeplessness. For chronic conditions, it might be used for several weeks, followed by a period of assessment to determine its effectiveness. Continuous long-term use should be approached with caution, and it's beneficial to consult with a healthcare provider, especially if symptoms persist.

Cayenne

Cayenne pepper (Capsicum annuum) is a type of chili pepper celebrated not only for its culinary uses but also for its therapeutic properties. It contains capsaicin, a compound that gives it its heat and is responsible for many of its health benefits.

Properties	Pain Relief: Capsaicin in cayenne is known for its pain-relieving properties, used topically and internally. Circulatory Stimulant: Helps improve blood flow and reduce blood clots. Digestive Aid: Stimulates digestion by increasing gastric juices and enzyme production. Anti-inflammatory: Reduces inflammation in the body. Metabolic Booster: Can increase metabolic rate, aiding in weight loss.
What disease it fights	Pain: Effective against joint pain, migraines, and nerve pain. Poor Circulation: Helps in conditions like Raynaud's disease and reduces the risk of heart disease by improving blood flow. Digestive Issues: Alleviates indigestion, gas, and cramps. Weight Management: Its thermogenic properties help in weight loss efforts. Infections: The antimicrobial properties can fight certain pathogens.
How it works	Cayenne works primarily through its active ingredient, capsaicin. Capsaicin binds to a receptor on nerve cells that normally responds to heat. This binding action initiates various responses, including pain relief, increased blood flow, and reduced inflammation. It also stimulates digestion by encouraging the secretion of gastric juices and enzymes.
How to use	Dietary: Cayenne can be added to foods for flavor and its metabolic benefits. Start with a small amount and adjust according to tolerance. Capsules: For those who want the health benefits without the heat, cayenne is available in capsule form. Topical Creams and Ointments: For pain relief, especially for arthritis and neuropathic pain.
Dosage	Dietary: There is no specific dosage; use according to personal tolerance and culinary preference. Capsules: Typically, 30–120 mg three times daily, but dosages can vary based on the product's capsaicin content. Topical Applications: Apply as directed on the product label, usually 2-4 times daily.
How long to use	Dietary: Cayenne can be used indefinitely in culinary amounts. Capsules and Topical Forms: For chronic conditions, cayenne supplements can be used continuously, with periodic evaluation for effectiveness and side effects. For acute pain relief, use as needed.

Celery Seed

Celery seed (Apium graveolens) is derived from the celery plant and has been used for centuries in traditional medicine for various health issues, particularly those related to inflammation and the urinary tract. It's known for its antioxidant, anti-inflammatory, diuretic, and antihypertensive properties.

Properties	Anti-inflammatory: Can help reduce inflammation, making it beneficial for conditions such as arthritis and gout. Antioxidant: Contains compounds that protect the body from oxidative stress and support overall cellular health. Diuretic: Promotes the elimination of excess water from the body, supporting urinary tract health and blood pressure regulation. Antihypertensive: Some compounds in celery seed may help lower blood pressure.
What disease it fights	Arthritis and Gout: The anti-inflammatory and diuretic effects can help manage symptoms and reduce uric acid levels. Urinary Tract Infections (UTIs): Its diuretic action helps flush the urinary tract, potentially preventing infections. High Blood Pressure: The antihypertensive properties may contribute to lowering blood pressure. Inflammatory Conditions: May provide relief for various inflammatory conditions beyond arthritis, such as asthma or inflammatory bowel disease (IBD).
How it works	The beneficial effects of celery seed are attributed to its various phytochemicals, including flavonoids, coumarins, and linoleic acid. These compounds work synergistically to reduce inflammation, combat oxidative stress, promote urine production, and possibly lower blood pressure by relaxing the blood vessels.
How to use	Capsules/Supplements: Celery seed is available in capsule form, providing a convenient and concentrated dosage. Tea: Celery seed can be brewed into a tea, often used for its diuretic and anti-inflammatory benefits. Spice: While less concentrated than supplements, using celery seed as a spice in cooking can still offer health benefits.
Dosage	Capsules/Supplements: The dosage can vary depending on the concentration; a common recommendation is 500-1000 mg taken once or twice daily. Tea: Boil 1 teaspoon of celery seeds in a cup of water for 10-15 minutes. Drink up to 2 cups daily
How long to use	Celery seed can be used for short-term relief of specific conditions like a UTI or an acute gout flare-up, typically for a few weeks. For chronic conditions such as arthritis or hypertension, it may be used longer but should be monitored by a healthcare professional to assess effectiveness and adjust the approach as needed.

Chamomile

Chamomile (Matricaria recutita for German chamomile or Chamaemelum nobile for Roman chamomile) is one of the most ancient medicinal herbs known to mankind, distinguished by its apple-like scent and flavor. It's widely recognized for its calming, anti-inflammatory, and antispasmodic properties.

Properties	Sedative: Chamomile is well-regarded for its mild sedative effects, helping to promote relaxation and improve sleep quality. Anti-inflammatory: Contains several compounds that reduce inflammation. Antispasmodic: Eases muscle spasms, including those associated with menstrual cramps and gastrointestinal discomfort. Gastrointestinal Relief: Offers relief from digestive issues, such as indigestion, gas, and mild gastrointestinal infections. Wound Healing: Applied topically, it can speed the healing of cuts, scrapes, and burns.
What disease it fights	Sleep Disorders: Chamomile tea is commonly used to improve sleep quality and manage insomnia. Anxiety and Stress: Its calming effects can help reduce anxiety and promote relaxation. Digestive Issues: Helps in treating various digestive ailments, including indigestion, gas, and diarrhea. Menstrual Pain: Can alleviate menstrual cramps due to its antispasmodic properties. Skin Conditions: Used topically to soothe skin irritations, eczema, and wounds.
How it works	Chamomile contains several active compounds, such as bisabolol, flavonoids, and apigenin, which contribute to its medicinal properties. Apigenin, in particular, binds to benzodiazepine receptors in the brain, exerting a mild sedative effect. Its anti-inflammatory and antispasmodic effects are beneficial for soothing the digestive system and reducing pain.
How to use	Tea: The most common method of consumption. Steep 2-3 grams of dried chamomile flowers in hot water for 5-10 minutes. Tincture: A concentrated liquid form that can be taken orally or added to water. Topical Applications: Chamomile creams or ointments can be applied to the skin to soothe irritations and accelerate healing.
Dosage	Tea: 1-2 cups before bedtime for sleep or throughout the day for digestive or menstrual discomfort. Tincture: Generally, 1-4 ml three times daily, but follow specific product instructions. Topical: Apply as needed, according to the product's directions.
How long to use	Chamomile can be used safely for extended periods; many people consume chamomile tea daily as part of their evening routine to promote relaxation and sleep. For acute conditions like menstrual pain or gastrointestinal upset, use as needed. If symptoms persist, consult a healthcare provider.

Chaparral

Chaparral (Larrea tridentata) is a plant native to the southwestern United States and parts of Mexico, known for its potent antioxidant properties primarily attributed to the compound nordihydroguaiaretic acid (NDGA). It has been traditionally used for a variety of purposes, including as an antimicrobial, anti-inflammatory, and detoxifying agent. However, it is crucial to approach chaparral with caution due to concerns about its potential hepatotoxicity (liver toxicity).

Properties	Antioxidant: Chaparral contains powerful antioxidants that can help neutralize free radicals. Antimicrobial: Exhibits antimicrobial activities against a range of bacteria, fungi, and viruses. Anti-inflammatory: Can reduce inflammation, offering potential benefits for conditions associated with inflammation. Detoxifying: Traditionally used to support the body's detoxification pathways.
What disease it fights	Skin Conditions: Applied topically to treat issues such as eczema, psoriasis, and fungal infections. Respiratory Conditions: Used for its expectorant properties to aid in the relief of respiratory ailments like colds and bronchitis. Inflammatory Conditions: May help manage arthritis and other inflammatory health issues. Antioxidant Support: Offers general antioxidant support, which can contribute to overall health.
How it works	Chaparral's primary active component, NDGA, is thought to inhibit the activity of certain enzymes and reduce the production of reactive oxygen species, thereby exerting its antioxidant, anti-inflammatory, and antimicrobial effects. These actions can help in managing various health conditions, especially those related to oxidative stress and inflammation.
How to use	Given the potential risks associated with chaparral, particularly to liver health, its use should be approached with caution: Topical Application: Chaparral can be applied externally in the form of creams or ointments for skin conditions. This method minimizes systemic absorption and associated risks. Tea or Tincture: Although traditional uses include making tea or tinctures from the leaves, internal use is generally not recommended without strict supervision from a healthcare professional due to safety concerns.
Dosage	Due to the potential for liver toxicity, there is no recommended dosage for the internal use of chaparral. For topical applications, follow product-specific guidelines to ensure safe use.
How long to use	For topical applications, chaparral can be used until symptoms improve, typically not exceeding a few weeks without evaluating its effects and side effects. Internal use should be avoided or closely monitored by a healthcare provider, considering the significant concerns about safety.

Chaste Tree (Vitex)

Chaste Tree, also known as Vitex (Vitex agnus-castus), is an herb that has been used for centuries, particularly for women's health issues. It's best known for its ability to regulate hormonal imbalances, especially those related to the menstrual cycle and menopause.

Properties	Hormonal Balance: Vitex is widely recognized for its ability to normalize hormone levels, particularly progesterone and estrogen. PMS Relief: Helps alleviate symptoms of premenstrual syndrome (PMS), such as mood swings, breast tenderness, and cramps. Fertility Support: May improve female fertility by regulating menstrual cycles. Menopause Symptom Relief: Helps in reducing symptoms of menopause like hot flashes and sleep disturbances. Acne Treatment: For some women, balancing hormones can lead to an improvement in hormonal acne.
What disease it fights	Menstrual Disorders: Including PMS, menstrual irregularities, and fertility issues. Menopause Symptoms: Helps ease the transition and alleviate common symptoms. Hormonal Acne: By regulating hormones, it can improve skin condition.
How it works	Vitex operates primarily by influencing the hypothalamus and pituitary gland, leading to an increased production of luteinizing hormone (LH) and a slight reduction in follicle-stimulating hormone (FSH). This action promotes a balance between estrogen and progesterone levels. It also affects dopamine levels, which can help alleviate PMS symptoms and support overall hormonal balance.
How to use	Capsules/Tablets: The most common and convenient form for taking Vitex, ensuring a consistent dosage. Tincture: Liquid extract forms are available and can be mixed with water or juice.
Dosage	Capsules/Tablets: Typically, 150-500 mg once daily in the morning. Dosages can vary depending on the concentration of the active ingredients. Tincture: 1-2 ml three times daily. It's important to note that Vitex requires some time to show effects. It might take up to three months to notice significant changes, with continued use recommended for the best results.
How long to use	Vitex is best used for a minimum of three to six months to achieve noticeable hormonal balance. Some may find continued use beneficial for maintaining hormonal equilibrium and managing symptoms. However, usage beyond 18 months should be evaluated for necessity and effectiveness.

Chickweed

Chickweed (Stellaria media) is a common herb often regarded as a weed in many gardens, yet it holds a variety of medicinal and nutritional properties. It's rich in vitamins and minerals and has been traditionally used for its soothing, anti-inflammatory, and mildly diuretic effects. Chickweed is notable for its ability to help with skin conditions, support digestive health, and offer relief from respiratory issues.

Properties	Anti-inflammatory: Helps reduce inflammation, making it beneficial for skin conditions and joint pain. Emollient: Soothes irritated skin, providing relief from eczema, psoriasis, and other skin irritations. Expectorant: Aids in the relief of coughs and colds by helping to loosen phlegm. Diuretic: Promotes the production of urine, helping in the detoxification process and relieving urinary tract issues. Nutritive: High in vitamins A and C, minerals, and flavonoids, supporting overall health and wellness.
What disease it fights	Skin Conditions: Effective in treating rashes, eczema, psoriasis, and insect bites due to its soothing and anti-inflammatory properties. Digestive Issues: Can relieve indigestion and constipation; its mild laxative effect helps maintain digestive regularity. Respiratory Problems: Acts as an expectorant, making it useful in treating colds, coughs, and bronchitis. Weight Management: Its diuretic effect aids in reducing water retention, supporting weight loss efforts.
How it works	Chickweed contains saponins, which have been shown to possess anti-inflammatory and expectorant properties. These compounds help in soothing the skin, reducing inflammation, and aiding in the removal of mucus from the respiratory tract. Its nutritional content supports the body's overall health, while its emollient properties moisturize and soothe irritated skin.
How to use	Salad Green: Fresh chickweed can be washed and added to salads for its nutritional benefits. Tea: Dried chickweed can be steeped in boiling water to make tea. This can be consumed or used as a wash for skin irritations. Poultice: Fresh, crushed leaves can be applied directly to the skin to soothe irritations and inflammations. Tincture: A concentrated liquid form can be taken orally for internal health benefits.
Dosage	Tea: Steep 1-2 teaspoons of dried herb in boiling water for about 10 minutes. Drink 2-3 cups daily. Tincture: Typically, 1-2 ml three times a day, but follow specific product instructions. Fresh: As a salad green, chickweed can be consumed liberally as part of a regular diet.
How long to use	For acute conditions like skin irritations or mild respiratory issues, chickweed can be used until symptoms improve, typically for a few days to weeks. For ongoing support, such as digestive health or as a nutritive supplement, chickweed can be included as part of a regular diet over an extended period.

Cilantro

Cilantro (Coriandrum sativum), also known as coriander (its seeds) in some parts of the world, is a herb commonly used in culinary dishes for its distinctive flavor. Beyond its culinary uses, cilantro has various medicinal properties, including anti-inflammatory, digestive, and detoxifying effects.

Properties	Detoxifying: Cilantro has been cited for its ability to chelate heavy metals from the body, supporting detoxification processes. Antioxidant: Contains antioxidants that protect against oxidative stress. Antimicrobial: Exhibits antimicrobial properties against harmful bacteria. Digestive Aid: Can aid in relieving indigestion and settling the stomach. Anti-inflammatory: Helps reduce inflammation in the body.
What disease it fights	Heavy Metal Toxicity: Its chelating properties are utilized to help remove heavy metals from the body. Digestive Disorders: Aids in relieving symptoms of indigestion, gas, and bloating. Inflammatory Conditions: May help in reducing inflammation related to arthritis and other inflammatory conditions. Infections: The antimicrobial properties can help fight bacterial infections, particularly foodborne pathogens.
How it works	Cilantro contains compounds like linalool and geranyl acetate, which contribute to its digestive, anti-inflammatory, and antimicrobial effects. Its potential to chelate heavy metals, such as lead, mercury, and aluminum, makes it valuable in detoxifying the body, although the exact mechanisms and effectiveness are subjects of ongoing research.
How to use	Fresh Leaves: Can be incorporated into salads, salsas, and various dishes for both flavor and health benefits. Juice or Smoothies: Fresh cilantro can be juiced or blended into smoothies as a detoxifying agent. Tea: Leaves can be steeped in hot water to make a soothing tea.
Dosage	Fresh Leaves: There is no specific dosage for cilantro when used in cooking; it can be consumed according to personal taste preferences. Juice/Smoothies: A small handful of fresh cilantro can be added to juices or smoothies. Tea: Steep 1-2 teaspoons of fresh or dried cilantro leaves in boiling water for 5-10 minutes. Drink 1-2 cups daily.
How long to use	For general health purposes and as part of a balanced diet, cilantro can be consumed regularly without specific time restrictions. When using cilantro specifically for detoxification purposes, such as heavy metal chelation, it might be consumed daily for a few weeks to months, but it's important to monitor for any adverse reactions and consult with a healthcare professional to ensure safety and effectiveness.

Cinnamon

Cinnamon is a highly cherished spice, derived from the inner bark of trees from the genus Cinnamomum, known for its distinctive aroma and flavor, as well as its impressive array of health benefits.

Properties	Antioxidant: High in antioxidants which protect the body from oxidative damage caused by free radicals. Anti-inflammatory: Contains compounds that help reduce inflammation. Antidiabetic: Can improve insulin sensitivity and lower blood sugar levels. Antimicrobial: Effective against bacteria and fungi, it can help prevent infection. Cardioprotective: Promotes heart health by reducing high blood pressure and improving cholesterol levels.
What disease it fights	Diabetes: Helps in managing blood sugar levels and improving insulin sensitivity. Heart Disease: Aids in reducing risk factors for heart disease, such as high cholesterol and high blood pressure. Infections: Its antimicrobial properties can help fight against bacterial and fungal infections. Inflammation: Can alleviate chronic inflammation, which is linked to various health conditions.
How it works	The health benefits of cinnamon stem primarily from two compounds: cinnamaldehyde, which is responsible for its flavor and smell, and has potent antioxidant and anti-inflammatory properties, and polyphenols, which enhance insulin sensitivity. Together, these compounds contribute to cinnamon's protective effects against diabetes, heart disease, and more.
How to use	Dietary Incorporation: Cinnamon can be added to beverages, baked goods, and savory dishes. It's versatile and enhances flavor while providing health benefits. Cinnamon Water or Tea: Steeping cinnamon sticks in hot water makes a healthy drink that can be consumed daily. Supplements: Cinnamon capsules are available for those seeking a concentrated form.
Dosage	Culinary Use: There are no strict dosage guidelines; it can be used according to taste preferences. Tea: One cinnamon stick or 1-2 teaspoons of ground cinnamon per cup of boiling water; can be consumed 1-2 times daily. Supplements: Typically, 500 mg twice daily, but it's essential to follow the product's specific recommendations.
How long to use	Cinnamon can be safely incorporated into the diet daily when consumed in food quantities. For specific health goals like managing blood sugar levels or reducing inflammation, several weeks to months of consistent use may be necessary to observe benefits. For high-dose supplements, it's important to limit use to a few weeks to avoid potential adverse effects, unless monitored by a healthcare provider.

Cleavers

Cleavers (Galium aparine) is a herb recognized for its sticky or 'clingy' nature, which has been traditionally used for its lymphatic, diuretic, and detoxifying properties. It supports the lymphatic system, urinary tract health, and skin conditions, among other benefits.

Properties	Lymphatic Support: Cleavers is particularly valued for its ability to stimulate the lymphatic system, promoting the drainage of lymph and the detoxification of the body. Diuretic: Helps promote urine production and the elimination of waste, supporting kidney and urinary tract health. Anti-inflammatory: Offers relief from inflammation and can soothe skin conditions like eczema and psoriasis. Detoxifying: Assists in the removal of toxins from the body, supporting overall detoxification processes.
What disease it fights	Lymphatic Congestion: Helps in conditions related to lymphatic congestion and edema. Urinary Tract Infections (UTIs): Its diuretic effect can help flush out bacteria from the urinary tract. Skin Conditions: Used topically to soothe and treat various skin issues, including cuts, wounds, and burns. Detoxification: Supports the body's natural detoxification processes through its effects on the lymphatic and urinary systems.
How it works	Cleavers works by stimulating the lymphatic system, helping to facilitate the removal of waste and toxins from the body. Its diuretic properties aid in increasing urine output, which helps in the elimination of waste and supports urinary tract health. Additionally, the anti-inflammatory compounds present in cleavers can help soothe skin irritation and inflammation.
How to use	Tea: Cleavers can be brewed into a tea by steeping the fresh or dried aerial parts in boiling water. Tincture: A concentrated liquid form of cleavers can be taken orally for internal detoxification and lymphatic support. Topical Application: Fresh, crushed cleavers can be applied directly to the skin to soothe irritation or used as a wash.
Dosage	Tea: Steep 2-3 teaspoons of dried cleavers in a cup of boiling water for 10-15 minutes. Drink 1-3 cups daily. Tincture: Typically, 1-4 ml of tincture three times a day. Topical Application: Use as needed on the affected area. For a wash, use the tea preparation.
How long to use	Cleavers is generally safe for short-term use, ranging from a few days to several weeks, depending on the condition being treated. For ongoing support of the lymphatic system or for chronic conditions, it's best to consult a healthcare professional for guidance on appropriate duration and monitoring.

Clove

Clove (Syzygium aromaticum) is a potent spice and medicinal herb known for its powerful antioxidant, antimicrobial, and analgesic properties. It's been used historically in various traditional medicines around the world to treat a range of conditions.

Properties	Antioxidant: Clove is high in antioxidants, which help protect the body against oxidative stress and free radical damage. Antimicrobial: Effective against a wide range of bacteria, fungi, and viruses, especially in oral health. Analgesic and Anti-inflammatory: Provides relief from pain and inflammation, particularly in dental applications. Digestive Aid: Can stimulate digestion and relieve digestive issues such as gas and bloating.
What disease it fights	Dental Issues: Including toothaches, gum disease, and oral infections, due to its pain-relieving and antimicrobial effects. Infections: Its antimicrobial properties make it useful in fighting various microbial infections. Inflammation: Can help reduce inflammation in the body, beneficial for conditions like arthritis. Digestive Problems: Aids in relieving indigestion, bloating, and stomach discomfort.
How it works	Clove's medicinal properties are primarily attributed to the compound eugenol, which has been extensively studied for its analgesic, anti-inflammatory, and antimicrobial effects. Eugenol can block pain receptors and reduce inflammation, making it effective for pain relief, especially in dental care. Its antimicrobial action helps in treating and preventing infections.
How to use	Topical Application for Dental Pain: A small amount of clove oil can be applied directly to the affected tooth or gum area using a cotton swab. Ingestion for Digestive Health: Clove can be used as a spice in cooking or made into a tea to help with digestion. Aromatherapy for General Well-being: The essential oil can be used in a diffuser to benefit from its antimicrobial and soothing properties.
Dosage	Clove Oil (Topical for Dental Use): Apply 2-3 drops on a cotton swab to the affected area up to 3 times a day. Clove Tea: Steep 1-2 cloves in a cup of boiling water for 10 minutes. Drink 1-2 times daily for digestive health. Essential Oil for Aromatherapy: Use according to the diffuser's instructions.
How long to use	For Acute Dental Pain: Use clove oil for short-term relief (a few days) until dental treatment can be obtained. For Digestive Support and General Use: Clove can be used in culinary amounts daily. For therapeutic uses like teas or essential oil diffusion, use for periods of a few weeks to a month, then assess for effectiveness and any adverse reactions.

Comfrey

Comfrey (Symphytum officinale) is a perennial herb known for its healing properties, particularly in relation to skin, bone, and tissue repair. It's been used historically in traditional medicine for its ability to speed up the healing of bruises, sprains, fractures, and wounds due to its high content of allantoin, a substance that helps with cell regeneration and inflammation reduction. However, it's important to note that while comfrey has potent medicinal properties, it also contains pyrrolizidine alkaloids (PAs) that can be harmful to the liver if ingested or applied to open wounds.

Properties	Cell Regeneration: Comfrey's allantoin stimulates the growth of new cells, aiding in wound healing and the repair of damaged tissue. Anti-inflammatory: Reduces inflammation and swelling, providing relief from sprains, strains, and other injuries. Pain Relief: Offers analgesic properties that can alleviate pain associated with injuries and joint problems. Astringent: Helps tighten and tone the skin, which can be beneficial in healing minor wounds.
What disease it fights	Skin Conditions: Used topically for bruises, cuts, dermatitis, and other skin irritations. Musculoskeletal Injuries: Effective in treating sprains, strains, fractures, and back pain due to its anti-inflammatory and cell-regenerating properties. Arthritis and Joint Pain: Its anti-inflammatory and pain-relieving effects can help manage arthritis symptoms.
How it works	Comfrey works primarily through its allantoin content, which promotes cell growth and repair. This accelerates the healing process for skin and tissue injuries. Its rosmarinic acid content contributes to its anti-inflammatory properties, helping reduce swelling and pain.
How to use	Given the concerns regarding the toxicity of PAs found in comfrey, it is recommended to use comfrey only externally and never on open wounds. The safest forms include: Comfrey Creams and Ointments: For topical application on unbroken skin, to support the healing of bruises and sprains. Compresses or Poultices: Made from the leaves, applied to the affected area to reduce swelling and pain.
Dosage	Creams/Ointments: Follow the manufacturer's instructions, generally applied 2-3 times daily to the affected area. Compresses/Poultices: A fresh poultice can be applied 1-2 times daily. Ensure the skin is intact to prevent PA absorption.
How long to use	Comfrey should be used with caution and for short durations—typically no longer than 4-6 weeks for any given injury or condition. Continuous monitoring during this period is important to ensure that there are no adverse reactions.

Coriander

Coriander (Coriandrum sativum), also known as cilantro, particularly in the Americas, is a versatile herb widely used in culinary traditions around the world, both for its leaves and seeds. Beyond its culinary uses, coriander offers a variety of health benefits, including digestive, anti-inflammatory, and antimicrobial properties.

Properties	Digestive Aid: Coriander is known to aid in digestion and relieve digestive issues such as bloating, gas, and discomfort. Antioxidant: Contains antioxidants that help protect cells from damage by free radicals. Antimicrobial: Exhibits antimicrobial properties against a range of bacteria and fungi. Anti-inflammatory: Helps reduce inflammation in the body, which can alleviate symptoms of arthritis and other inflammatory conditions. Blood Sugar Regulation: Some studies suggest that coriander can help manage blood sugar levels.
What disease it fights	Digestive Disorders: Including indigestion, gas, and irritable bowel syndrome (IBS). Urinary Tract Infections (UTIs): The antimicrobial properties can help prevent and treat UTIs. Skin Conditions: Applied topically, it can help relieve eczema, rashes, and fungal infections. Cardiovascular Health: May help lower bad cholesterol (LDL) and raise good cholesterol (HDL).
How it works	The health benefits of coriander stem from its rich content of essential oils and bioactive compounds, including linalool, which aids digestion, and cineole, among others with anti-inflammatory and antiseptic effects. These components work synergistically to improve health by enhancing digestion, fighting infection, and reducing inflammation.
How to use	Culinary Use: Both the leaves and seeds can be used in cooking to add flavor and health benefits to dishes. Tea: A tea made from coriander seeds can help with digestive issues and lower blood sugar levels. Topical Application: Coriander seed oil can be used topically for its antifungal and anti-inflammatory properties.
Dosage	Culinary Use: As desired, according to personal taste preferences. Tea: Steep 1-2 teaspoons of crushed coriander seeds in boiling water for 5-10 minutes. Drink up to 2 cups daily. Topical Use: Dilute coriander seed oil with a carrier oil (e.g., coconut or almond oil) before application to the skin. Follow product-specific recommendations for dilution ratios.
How long to use	For Digestive Benefits and General Health: Coriander can be consumed regularly as part of a balanced diet without specific time restrictions. For Specific Health Issues: Use for a few weeks to a few months, monitoring for any improvements or side effects. For long-term use, especially in higher medicinal dosages or for topical applications, it's best to consult a healthcare professional.

Corn Silk

Corn silk (Zea mays) refers to the long, silky fibers that grow atop a corncob, inside its husk. Traditionally, it's been used in herbal medicine for its diuretic, anti-inflammatory, and blood sugar-regulating properties.

Properties	Diuretic: Enhances urine production, helping to flush toxins from the body and support urinary tract health. Anti-inflammatory: Can reduce inflammation, potentially benefiting conditions such as arthritis or urinary tract inflammations. Blood Sugar Regulation: Some studies suggest that corn silk may help manage blood sugar levels, making it beneficial for individuals with diabetes. Antioxidant: Contains compounds that fight oxidative stress, supporting overall health.
What disease it fights	Urinary Tract Infections (UTIs) and Bladder Issues: Its diuretic and soothing properties can help prevent and treat UTIs and promote bladder health. High Blood Pressure: The diuretic effect can contribute to lowering blood pressure by reducing fluid volume in the body. Diabetes: May help in regulating blood glucose levels. Inflammation: Its anti-inflammatory properties can provide relief for conditions like gout, arthritis, and prostate issues.
How it works	Corn silk contains several compounds, including flavonoids, polyphenols, and polysaccharides, which contribute to its health benefits. The diuretic action helps eliminate excess fluid and toxins, reducing the burden on the kidneys and urinary tract. Anti-inflammatory effects can help soothe irritated tissues, and the potential regulation of blood sugar levels is attributed to its antioxidant content and other bioactive compounds that may influence insulin sensitivity.
How to use	Tea: Corn silk can be brewed into a tea by steeping the fresh or dried silks in hot water. Tincture: A more concentrated form that can be taken orally. Capsules: Dried corn silk is also available in capsule form for those who prefer not to drink the tea.
Dosage	Tea: Use 1-2 teaspoons of dried corn silk per cup of boiling water. Steep for 10-15 minutes and drink 2-3 cups daily. Tincture: Typically, 1-2 ml three times a day, but follow the specific product instructions. Capsules: Follow the manufacturer's recommendations, usually around 400-500 mg taken 2-3 times daily.
How long to use	Corn silk can be used safely for short-term relief of symptoms, such as during a UTI, for periods up to 2 weeks. For chronic conditions like diabetes or hypertension, it's best used under the guidance of a healthcare provider, who can offer advice on long-term use and monitor for any potential interactions or side effects.

Cranberry

Cranberries are widely known for their nutrient-rich content and antioxidant properties, making them a valuable addition to the diet for promoting health and preventing diseases.

Properties	Antioxidant: High in vitamins C and E, as well as other antioxidants, cranberries can help protect the body from oxidative stress and reduce inflammation. Anti-adhesive: Contains proanthocyanidins (PACs) that prevent bacteria from adhering to the urinary tract walls, effectively reducing the risk of urinary tract infections (UTIs). Antimicrobial: Can inhibit the growth of various bacteria, including those that cause UTIs and stomach ulcers. Cardiovascular Health: May improve cardiovascular health by reducing blood pressure, improving cholesterol levels, and increasing blood flow.
What disease it fights	Urinary Tract Infections (UTIs): Cranberries are best known for their role in preventing UTIs. Digestive Health: May help prevent H. pylori infections, which can cause ulcers and gastritis. Cardiovascular Disease: The antioxidants in cranberries can help lower the risk of cardiovascular disease.
How it works	The primary mechanism by which cranberries exert their beneficial effects is through the presence of PACs, which prevent harmful bacteria from adhering to the urinary tract walls, thus preventing infections. Additionally, the antioxidants in cranberries help neutralize harmful free radicals, reducing oxidative stress and inflammation in the body.
How to use	Juice: Unsweetened cranberry juice is a popular way to consume cranberries for health benefits, especially for UTI prevention. Whole Berries: Fresh or frozen cranberries can be incorporated into the diet in various recipes, including salads, sauces, and baked goods. Supplements: Cranberry supplements are available in the form of capsules, tablets, or extracts.
Dosage	Juice: For UTI prevention, drinking 8-16 ounces (about 240-480 ml) of pure, unsweetened cranberry juice daily is often recommended. Whole Berries: There is no specific dosage; consumption as part of a healthy diet is encouraged. Supplements: Follow manufacturer's recommendations, typically around 400-500 mg of cranberry extract taken twice daily for UTI prevention.
How long to use	For UTI prevention, cranberry products can be used on an ongoing basis, especially for those with recurrent infections. However, for acute treatment of UTIs, it's crucial to consult with a healthcare provider, as cranberries are preventive, not curative, and antibiotics may be necessary.

Curly dock

Curly dock (Rumex crispus) is a perennial weed commonly found in many parts of the world, valued in traditional herbal medicine for its nutritional and medicinal properties. Known for its high vitamin C and iron content, it's been used to treat various conditions, including skin diseases, digestive issues, and as a general detoxifier.

Properties	Detoxifying: Traditionally used to cleanse the blood and liver, supporting the body's natural detoxification processes. Digestive Aid: Helps in relieving digestive issues such as constipation, indigestion, and bloating due to its mild laxative effect. Anti-inflammatory: Contains antioxidants and compounds that may reduce inflammation, beneficial for skin conditions and internal inflammation. Nutritional: High in vitamins (especially vitamin C) and minerals like iron, making it supportive of overall health.
What disease it fights	Skin Conditions: Applied topically or used internally to help treat skin issues like eczema, psoriasis, and acne. Digestive Disorders: Its laxative and digestive properties can aid in improving digestive health and relieving symptoms of constipation and indigestion. Anemia: The high iron content can help in managing and preventing iron-deficiency anemia. Liver and Blood Detoxification: Supports liver health and helps in the detoxification of the blood.
How it works	Curly dock works through several mechanisms, depending on the condition being treated. Its digestive aid and mild laxative effects come from anthraquinones, which stimulate bowel movements. The plant's high content of antioxidants and nutrients supports overall health by reducing oxidative stress and improving nutritional status.
How to use	Leaves: Young leaves can be eaten raw in salads or cooked like spinach. However, older leaves become more bitter and may require cooking to reduce their oxalic acid content. Tea: Dried leaves or roots can be steeped in boiling water to make a tea, consumed for internal health benefits. Topical Application: A poultice made from curly dock can be applied to the skin to treat various skin conditions.
Dosage	Tea: Use 1-2 teaspoons of dried leaves or root per cup of boiling water, steep for 10-15 minutes. Drink 2-3 cups daily. Topical Application: Apply the poultice to affected skin areas as needed. Fresh leaves can be crushed and applied directly, or dried leaves can be rehydrated for use.
How long to use	Curly dock can be used as needed for acute conditions, typically for a few days to a week. For chronic issues or general health maintenance, it may be incorporated into the diet or used periodically, under the guidance of a healthcare professional, to monitor for any potential side effects or interactions with other treatments.

Dandelion

Dandelion (Taraxacum officinale) is a versatile herb celebrated for its nutritional and medicinal properties. Every part of the dandelion, from its yellow flowers to its roots, can be used for health benefits. It's known for its detoxifying properties, support of liver function, diuretic effects, and nutritional content, including vitamins A, C, K, and minerals such as potassium.

Properties	Diuretic: Promotes the production of urine, aiding in detoxification and reducing water retention. Liver Support: Enhances liver function by helping to detoxify the liver and increase bile production. Anti-inflammatory: Contains compounds that reduce inflammation in the body. Nutritional: High in vitamins and minerals, it can supplement the diet to improve overall health. Digestive Aid: Stimulates appetite and aids digestion.
What disease it fights	Liver Disorders: Supports liver health and helps in conditions like jaundice and liver congestion. Digestive Issues: Improves appetite and digestion and helps in treating constipation and indigestion. Water Retention: Acts as a natural diuretic, aiding in conditions related to water retention and urinary tract infections. Inflammation: Can be used to alleviate inflammatory conditions and joint pain.
How it works	Dandelion works through a variety of active compounds including taraxacin, taraxacerin, and high levels of potassium and other vitamins and minerals. Its diuretic effect helps to eliminate toxins from the body through increased urine production, while its bitter compounds stimulate digestive functions and liver activity.
How to use	Tea: Both the leaves and roots can be dried and steeped in boiling water to make tea. Fresh Leaves: Can be used in salads or as a cooked green for their nutritional benefits. Root Decoction: The roots can be boiled and consumed as a drink. Supplements: Available in capsule or tincture form for those who prefer not to consume it directly.
Dosage	Tea: 1–2 teaspoons of dried herb per cup of boiling water, steeped for 10 minutes. Drink 2–3 cups daily. Fresh Leaves: As desired in salads. Aim for a small handful (1–2 ounces) daily for health benefits. Root Decoction: Simmer 1–2 teaspoons of dried root in a cup of water for 10 minutes. Drink 2–3 times daily. Supplements: Follow manufacturer's recommendations, typically 500–1,500 mg of dandelion root extract per day.
How long to use	Dandelion can be used safely over the long term for ongoing support of liver and kidney function. For specific health issues like edema or a detoxification program, it might be used for a shorter duration, such as several weeks. Continuous use should be monitored for any potential side effects or interactions with medications.

Devil's Claw

Devil's Claw (Harpagophytum procumbens) is a plant native to southern Africa, renowned for its anti-inflammatory and analgesic properties. It's primarily used to treat conditions related to inflammation and pain, such as arthritis, back pain, and other musculoskeletal complaints. The active ingredients in Devil's Claw, including harpagoside, contribute to its therapeutic effects.

Properties	Anti-inflammatory: Significantly reduces inflammation, making it beneficial for arthritis and other inflammatory conditions. Analgesic: Offers pain relief, particularly for joint pain and discomfort. Digestive Aid: Although less commonly used for this purpose, it can stimulate appetite and aid digestion.
What disease it fights	Arthritis: Both osteoarthritis and rheumatoid arthritis sufferers may find relief from the pain and inflammation with regular use. Back Pain: Effective in reducing low back pain and improving mobility. Other Inflammatory Conditions: May help with conditions like gout, fibromyalgia, and tendinitis.
How it works	The primary mechanism is believed to be through the inhibition of inflammatory pathways in the body, notably by reducing the activity of genes that produce inflammatory cytokines. Harpagoside, one of the key active compounds, is primarily credited with these effects.
How to use	Devil's Claw is available in several forms, including capsules, tablets, tinctures, and teas. The form you choose may depend on personal preference, the specific condition being treated, and ease of use.
Dosage	Capsules/Tablets: Dosages can vary, but a typical dose is between 600 to 1200 mg of Devil's Claw extract divided into two or three daily doses. Products should contain around 50 to 100 mg of harpagoside to ensure effectiveness. Tincture: Follow manufacturer's guidelines, but generally, 1-2 ml three times a day is recommended. Tea: Made by steeping 1-2 teaspoons of the root in a cup of boiling water for 8-10 minutes. Drink up to three cups a day.
How long to use	Devil's Claw can be used over the medium to long term for chronic conditions. Many studies have assessed its use over periods of 8-12 weeks, showing significant benefits without serious side effects. However, as with any herbal remedy, it's important to periodically evaluate its effectiveness and any side effects.

Dill

Dill (Anethum graveolens) is a culinary herb known for its aromatic seeds and feathery leaves. Beyond its kitchen uses, dill has a variety of health benefits rooted in its rich content of vitamins, minerals, and antioxidants.

Properties	Digestive Aid: Dill has been traditionally used to ease digestion, prevent gas, and soothe stomach discomfort. Antimicrobial: Contains compounds that can help fight off bacterial and fungal infections. Antioxidant: Offers protection against cell damage caused by free radicals, thanks to its high antioxidant content. Sedative: Some components of dill may have mild sedative effects, aiding in sleep and reducing anxiety. Bone Health: The calcium content in dill can contribute to the maintenance of bone strength and health.
What disease it fights	Digestive Issues: Helps in relieving indigestion, flatulence, and colic, especially in infants. Insomnia and Anxiety: Its sedative properties can help improve sleep quality and reduce feelings of anxiety. Infections: The antimicrobial effects may prevent and fight infections, particularly in the digestive tract. Bone Degradation: By supplying calcium, dill can play a role in preventing osteoporosis and supporting overall bone health.
How it works	Dill works through several mechanisms: The essential oils in dill, including carvone and limonene, contribute to its digestive and antimicrobial benefits by soothing the digestive system and inhibiting the growth of harmful microbes. Antioxidants in dill protect against oxidative stress, reducing inflammation and supporting cellular health. The calming effects might be due to the modulation of neurotransmitter activity in the brain.
How to use	Culinary Use: Fresh or dried dill can be added to salads, soups, fish dishes, and sauces to enhance flavor and nutritional value. Tea: Dill tea, made from seeds or leaves, can be consumed for digestive relief or to promote relaxation. Essential Oil: Dill oil can be used in aromatherapy or diluted and applied topically for its calming effects.
Dosage	Culinary Use: There's no specific dosage; use according to taste preferences in cooking. Tea: Steep 1-2 teaspoons of dill seeds or a small handful of leaves in boiling water for 5-10 minutes. Drink 1-2 cups daily. Essential Oil: For topical use, dilute a few drops in a carrier oil and apply as needed. For aromatherapy, follow the diffuser's instructions.
How long to use	Dill can be consumed regularly as part of a healthy diet. For specific issues like digestive discomfort or insomnia, it might be used for shorter periods, such as a few days to weeks, until symptoms improve. Continuous use, especially of essential oil or concentrated extracts, should be monitored for any potential side effects.

Dong Quai

Dong Quai (Angelica sinensis) is a traditional Chinese medicinal herb often referred to as "female ginseng" due to its widespread use for female reproductive health issues. It's recognized for its ability to regulate menstrual cycles, alleviate menstrual pain, and manage menopausal symptoms. Dong Quai contains compounds that may act on the circulatory, immune, and nervous systems, offering a broad range of health benefits.

Properties	Hormonal Regulation: Helps balance estrogen levels, beneficial for menstrual and menopausal issues. Blood Tonic: Traditionally used to nourish and invigorate the blood, improving circulation. Anti-inflammatory: Contains compounds that reduce inflammation. Antispasmodic: Alleviates muscle spasms, useful for menstrual cramps.
What disease it fights	Menstrual Disorders: Such as irregular cycles, dysmenorrhea (painful menstruation), and premenstrual syndrome (PMS). Menopausal Symptoms: Helps manage hot flashes, night sweats, and mood swings. Anemia: Its blood tonic properties can be beneficial in treating anemia, especially when related to menstrual issues.
How it works	Dong Quai's mechanisms are attributed to its complex composition, including phytoestrogens, which are plant-based compounds that can mimic estrogen in the body, helping to stabilize hormonal fluctuations. Its blood-nourishing properties are linked to compounds that may improve blood quality and circulation, enhancing overall vitality and energy.
How to use	Tea: Dong Quai can be brewed as a tea, often combined with other herbs to enhance its effects. Capsules/Supplements: Available in capsule form for more consistent dosing. Tincture: A liquid extract that can be taken directly or diluted in water.
Dosage	Tea: Steep 1 teaspoon of dried Dong Quai root in a cup of boiling water for 10-15 minutes. Drink once daily. Capsules/Supplements: Dosages can vary widely; a common recommendation is 500-1000 mg per day, taken in divided doses. Tincture: 1-2 ml three times daily but follow specific product instructions.
How long to use	Dong Quai is typically used over several months to fully realize its benefits, especially for menstrual and menopausal issues. It's often recommended to take a break after 6 months of continuous use to evaluate its effects and your body's response.

Echinacea

Echinacea is a group of herbaceous plants that have been used traditionally to enhance the immune system and reduce symptoms of colds, flu, and other infections.

Properties	Immunostimulant: Echinacea is known for its ability to boost the immune system, making it more effective in fighting infections. Anti-inflammatory: Helps reduce inflammation, which can be beneficial in treating symptoms of colds and flu. Antiviral and Antibacterial: Exhibits antiviral and antibacterial properties, aiding in the prevention and treatment of infections. Antioxidant: Contains compounds that fight oxidative stress, supporting overall health.
What disease it fights	Common Colds and Flu: Echinacea is widely used to prevent and reduce the duration and severity of cold and flu symptoms. Respiratory Infections: Can help alleviate symptoms associated with respiratory tract infections. Urinary Tract Infections (UTIs): Its antimicrobial properties may help in treating UTIs. Skin Conditions: Topically, echinacea can be used to heal wounds, burns, and other skin inflammations.
How it works	Echinacea enhances the immune system partly by increasing the production of white blood cells, which are essential for fighting off infections. It also stimulates the activity of other immune cells like T-cells and macrophages. The anti-inflammatory effects are beneficial in reducing the symptoms and discomfort associated with colds, flu, and other inflammatory conditions.
How to use	Tea: Made from the dried herb (leaves, flowers, and roots) to support immune health, especially during cold and flu season. Capsules/Tablets: Contain powdered echinacea, convenient for daily supplementation. Tincture: A liquid extract that can be taken directly under the tongue or diluted in water. Topical Creams/Ointments: For treating skin conditions and wounds.
Dosage	Tea: 1-2 teaspoons of dried echinacea per cup of boiling water, steeped for 10-15 minutes. Drink 2-3 cups daily when feeling ill. Capsules/Tablets: 300-500 mg of echinacea extract three times daily at the first sign of symptoms. Tincture: 2-4 ml of echinacea tincture three times daily. Topical: Apply as directed on the product label, several times daily as needed.
How long to use	Echinacea is typically used at the onset of cold or flu symptoms and continued for 7-10 days. For immune system support during peak cold and flu seasons, it might be used for a few weeks. Continuous long-term use is generally not recommended without breaks, as it may lead to diminishing effectiveness and overstimulation of the immune system.

Elderberry

Elderberry (Sambucus nigra) is a fruit known for its immune-boosting and antiviral properties, making it highly effective in the prevention and treatment of colds and flu.

Properties	Immune Boosting: Rich in vitamins and antioxidants that can enhance the immune system. Antiviral: Has been shown to inhibit the replication of viruses, including those that cause the flu. Anti-inflammatory: Helps reduce inflammation throughout the body. Antioxidant: Contains anthocyanins, which have strong antioxidant effects.
What disease it fights	Colds and Flu: Elderberry is most commonly used for its effectiveness against the common cold and flu. Respiratory Health: Helps alleviate symptoms associated with respiratory ailments, such as bronchitis and sinus infections. Immune Support: Regular consumption can support overall immune function, potentially reducing the incidence of viral infections.
How it works	Elderberry works primarily by boosting the body's immune response. Its antiviral compounds prevent the virus from entering and replicating in human cells. The high antioxidant content also helps to reduce oxidative stress and inflammation, supporting overall health and well-being.
How to use	Syrup: Elderberry syrup is a popular preparation for both adults and children and can be taken directly or mixed into a beverage. Tea: Made by steeping dried elderberries (and often the flowers) in boiling water. Capsules and Lozenges: Available for those who prefer a more convenient form of supplementation. Homemade Preparations: Elderberries can be cooked down into a syrup or jelly at home, often combined with honey for additional benefits.
Dosage	Syrup: 1 tablespoon (15 ml) of syrup taken 4 times daily during active cold or flu symptoms. For prevention during peak cold and flu seasons, 1 tablespoon daily. Tea: 1–2 teaspoons of dried elderberries per cup of boiling water, steeped for 15 minutes. Drink 2-3 cups daily when fighting off an illness. Capsules/Lozenges: Follow the manufacturer's instructions, typically 1-2 capsules twice daily.
How long to use	Elderberry is generally used for short-term relief and prevention of colds and flu. It's typically taken for the duration of the illness or for up to 5 days at the first sign of symptoms. For preventive use during cold and flu season, elderberry can be used for several weeks to a few months, with periodic breaks.

Elecampane

Elecampane (Inula helenium) is a perennial herb known for its tall stature, large leaves, and yellow daisy-like flowers. It has been used in traditional medicine for centuries, primarily for its expectorant, antiseptic, and anti-inflammatory properties, making it particularly effective for respiratory ailments.

Properties	Expectorant: Helps clear mucus from the respiratory tract, making it beneficial for conditions like bronchitis, asthma, and whooping cough. Antiseptic and Antibacterial: Can combat microbial and bacterial infections in the respiratory system. Anti-inflammatory: Reduces inflammation, which is helpful for irritated respiratory passages and conditions like asthma. Digestive Aid: Stimulates digestion and can help relieve gastrointestinal discomfort, such as indigestion and bloating.
What disease it fights	Respiratory Conditions: Its expectorant and antiseptic properties make it valuable for treating coughs, bronchitis, asthma, and other respiratory infections. Digestive Issues: Can be used to improve digestive health and relieve symptoms of indigestion and bloating. Skin Conditions: When applied topically, it may help treat fungal infections and skin irritations.
How it works	The root of elecampane contains several active compounds, including inulin, sesquiterpene lactones (such as alantolactone), and sterols, which contribute to its medicinal properties. Inulin supports respiratory health by soothing irritated tissues and promoting mucus clearance, while sesquiterpene lactones offer antimicrobial and anti-inflammatory benefits.
How to use	Tea: A tea can be made from the dried root to aid with respiratory conditions. Tincture: A more concentrated form that can be taken orally for respiratory and digestive support. Decoction: Boiled root preparation, stronger than tea, often used for more severe respiratory issues.
Dosage	Tea: 1-2 teaspoons of dried elecampane root per cup of boiling water, steeped for 10 minutes. Drink up to 3 cups daily. Tincture: 1-2 ml three times a day. Decoction: Half to one teaspoon of the root simmered in a cup of water for about 10-15 minutes, taken 1-3 times daily.
How long to use	Elecampane is typically used for the duration of respiratory symptoms, which may be a few days to a few weeks. For chronic conditions or as a digestive aid, it might be used for longer periods, but it's wise to consult with a healthcare provider for guidance on long-term use.

Eucalyptus

Eucalyptus (Eucalyptus globulus) is a fast-growing evergreen tree native to Australia, widely recognized for its medicinal properties. The leaves of the eucalyptus tree are used to produce an essential oil that has been utilized in traditional medicine to treat a variety of conditions, particularly those involving the respiratory system.

Properties	Antimicrobial: Eucalyptus oil is known for its ability to kill bacteria, viruses, and fungi, making it effective in treating infections. Anti-inflammatory: Reduces inflammation, particularly beneficial for respiratory conditions. Decongestant: Helps clear nasal congestion and relieve sinus pressure. Analgesic: Offers pain relief, useful in treating headaches and muscle pain. Expectorant: Aids in loosening and expelling mucus from the lungs.
What disease it fights	Respiratory Conditions: Including asthma, bronchitis, COPD, and sinusitis. Eucalyptus is effective in clearing congestion and reducing inflammation in the airways. Cold and Flu: The oil can alleviate symptoms of the common cold and flu, such as cough and sore throat. Joint and Muscle Pain: Its analgesic properties are beneficial in soothing pain from conditions like arthritis and rheumatism. Skin Infections: When applied topically, it can treat wounds, burns, and skin infections due to its antimicrobial action.
How it works	The primary active component in eucalyptus oil, 1,8-cineole (also known as eucalyptol), is responsible for most of its therapeutic effects. This compound has been shown to reduce inflammation, act as an expectorant, and possess antimicrobial properties that help fight respiratory infections and alleviate symptoms associated with colds and flu.
How to use	Inhalation: Add a few drops of eucalyptus oil to hot water and inhale the steam, or use in a diffuser to help clear nasal passages and relieve respiratory symptoms. Topical Application: Dilute eucalyptus oil with a carrier oil (like coconut or olive oil) and apply to the skin to treat pain or skin infections. Do not apply undiluted eucalyptus oil directly to the skin. Sprays and Rubs: Eucalyptus oil can be found in over-the-counter chest rubs and sprays, which can be used according to product instructions.
Dosage	Inhalation: For steam inhalation, add 2-3 drops of eucalyptus oil to a bowl of hot water. For a diffuser, follow the manufacturer's instructions. Topical Application: Use a 2-5% dilution of eucalyptus oil in a carrier oil for muscle pain or skin conditions (about 12-30 drops of eucalyptus oil per ounce of carrier oil).
How long to use	Eucalyptus oil can be used as needed to alleviate symptoms of respiratory conditions, colds, and flu, typically not exceeding 7-10 days for acute symptoms. For chronic pain relief or ongoing respiratory support, use should be intermittent, with breaks to prevent potential irritation or sensitization.

Evening Primrose

Evening Primrose (Oenothera biennis) is valued for its oil, extracted from the plant's seeds, which is rich in gamma-linolenic acid (GLA), a type of omega-6 fatty acid. This plant is widely recognized for its potential health benefits, particularly for women's health issues such as premenstrual syndrome (PMS), menopause symptoms, and breast pain. Evening Primrose Oil (EPO) also has anti-inflammatory properties that can benefit skin conditions and arthritis.

Properties	Hormonal Balance: EPO can influence hormonal activity, which may alleviate PMS and menopause symptoms. Anti-inflammatory: Beneficial for inflammatory conditions, including eczema, psoriasis, and rheumatoid arthritis. Skin Health: Promotes healthy skin, potentially improving conditions like acne and improving overall skin texture and elasticity. Nerve Function: GLA in EPO is thought to support healthy nerve function and may help with conditions like diabetic neuropathy.
What disease it fights	PMS and Menopause Symptoms: Eases symptoms such as mood swings, hot flashes, and breast tenderness. Skin Disorders: Can help manage eczema, acne, and improve skin health. Rheumatoid Arthritis: Its anti-inflammatory action can reduce joint pain and stiffness. Diabetic Neuropathy: May improve symptoms in some individuals.
How it works	The GLA in Evening Primrose Oil gets converted in the body to dihomo-gamma-linolenic acid (DGLA), a substance that can reduce inflammation. For hormonal balance, EPO may influence prostaglandin synthesis, which plays a role in regulating menstrual cycles and menopausal symptoms.
How to use	Supplementation: Evening Primrose Oil is most commonly taken in capsule form to ensure a precise dosage of GLA. Topical Application: EPO can be applied directly to the skin for eczema, acne, and to improve overall skin health.
Dosage	Capsules: The typical dosage for adults ranges from 500 mg to 1300 mg taken 1-3 times daily. The exact dosage can depend on the condition being treated. Topical Application: There is no specific dosage; apply a few drops to the affected area of the skin as needed.
How long to use	Evening Primrose Oil can be used over several months to fully realize its benefits, especially for chronic conditions. For menstrual or menopausal symptoms, some women use EPO regularly, while others may use it cyclically or as symptoms arise.

Eyebright

Eyebright (Euphrasia officinalis) is a small herb native to Europe, traditionally used for eye-related conditions thanks to its name suggesting its primary use. It has been utilized in herbal medicine to treat eye inflammation, eye irritation, and to relieve symptoms of conjunctivitis, blepharitis, and allergies affecting the eyes.

Properties	Anti-inflammatory: Helps reduce inflammation, beneficial for treating eye conditions and irritations. Astringent: The astringent properties of eyebright can help tighten and tone tissues, reducing discharge in conditions like conjunctivitis. Antiseptic: Can help in preventing and fighting infections due to its antimicrobial activity. Antihistamine: May provide relief from allergy symptoms affecting the eyes.
What disease it fights	Conjunctivitis and Blepharitis: Due to its anti-inflammatory and antiseptic properties, it's traditionally used for these conditions. Eye Irritations: Helps relieve irritation from environmental factors, such as dust and smoke. Eye Strain and Fatigue: Can provide relief for eyes tired from extended periods of screen use.
How it works	Eyebright's efficacy for eye health is attributed to its complex mixture of tannins, flavonoids, and iridoid glycosides, which contribute to its anti-inflammatory, astringent, and antiseptic properties. These compounds work together to reduce inflammation, tighten mucous membranes, and combat microbial infections.
How to use	Tea Wash: A cooled tea made from eyebright can be used as a wash to soothe and cleanse the eyes. Compress: Soaked cotton pads in eyebright tea can be applied as a compress for relief of irritation and inflammation. Tincture: Diluted in water, it can be used as an eye drop or wash.
Dosage	Tea: 1-2 teaspoons of dried eyebright herb steeped in boiling water for 10 minutes, cooled, and strained meticulously before use. Can be used several times a day as an eye wash or compress. Tincture: Must be diluted before use; typically, 1 part eyebright tincture to 10 parts boiled and cooled water. Use a few drops in each eye or as a wash 1-2 times daily.
How long to use	Eyebright is generally used for short-term relief of eye conditions and symptoms. It might be used for a few days to several weeks, depending on the severity and improvement of symptoms. Continuous use should be approached with caution, and consultation with a healthcare provider is recommended, especially for persistent or severe eye conditions.

Fennel

Fennel (Foeniculum vulgare) is a flavorful culinary herb and medicinal plant with a long history of use in traditional medicine, particularly for digestive health. Rich in potent phytonutrients and essential oils, fennel offers a range of health benefits, from anti-inflammatory and antioxidant effects to estrogenic activities.

Properties	Digestive Aid: Fennel is well-known for its ability to relieve gas, bloating, and indigestion, thanks to its antispasmodic properties. Antioxidant: Contains antioxidants that protect cells from oxidative stress. Anti-inflammatory: Offers anti-inflammatory effects that can benefit overall health. Estrogenic: Contains phytoestrogens, which can influence estrogen balance and may help manage menstrual symptoms.
What disease it fights	Digestive Disorders: Such as irritable bowel syndrome (IBS), gas, bloating, and indigestion. Menstrual Discomfort: May help alleviate menstrual cramps and regulate the menstrual cycle. Respiratory Conditions: The seeds have been used traditionally to help loosen and expel phlegm. Eye Health: Ancient remedies use fennel for its potential to improve vision and treat eye conditions.
How it works	Fennel's benefits are largely attributed to its essential oil components, including anethole, which is known for its antispasmodic and anti-inflammatory effects. These properties make fennel effective in soothing the digestive tract, relieving gas and bloating, and reducing inflammation.
How to use	Tea: Fennel tea, made from crushed seeds, is a common method for digestive relief and can be enjoyed after meals. Raw or Cooked: Fennel bulb can be consumed raw in salads or cooked in various dishes for both its flavor and health benefits. Supplements: Fennel is available in capsules or tinctures for more concentrated dosages.
Dosage	Tea: Steep 1-2 teaspoons of fennel seeds in boiling water for 10-15 minutes. Drink 2-3 cups daily for digestive health or menstrual discomfort. Capsules/Tinctures: Follow manufacturer's instructions, as potency can vary widely.
How long to use	Fennel can be used safely as a culinary herb daily. For medicinal purposes, such as teas or supplements for digestive health or menstrual discomfort, fennel is often used for short-term relief but can also be incorporated over longer periods if well tolerated. Always listen to your body, and if symptoms persist or adverse effects occur, consult a healthcare provider.

Fenugreek

Fenugreek (Trigonella foenum-graecum) is a versatile herb that has been used in traditional medicine for centuries, notably for its digestive, anti-inflammatory, and lactation-enhancing properties. Its seeds are rich in fiber, vitamins, and minerals, making it beneficial for various health conditions.

Properties	Galactagogue: Enhances milk production in breastfeeding mothers. Digestive Aid: Improves digestion and relieves gastrointestinal issues like constipation and inflammation. Anti-diabetic: Helps in managing blood sugar levels by improving insulin sensitivity. Antimicrobial: Exhibits antibacterial and antifungal activities. Anti-inflammatory: Contains compounds that reduce inflammation.
What disease it fights	Lactation Issues: Used by nursing mothers to increase milk supply. Diabetes: Helps in the management of blood glucose levels. Digestive Disorders: Aids in relieving digestive problems including indigestion, constipation, and gastritis. High Cholesterol: Can help lower cholesterol levels, thereby supporting cardiovascular health.
How it works	Fenugreek contains a variety of active compounds, including soluble fiber, saponins, and phytoestrogens. These contribute to its health benefits by stimulating milk production, slowing down the absorption of sugars in the stomach, and promoting insulin. Its fiber content aids in digestion, and its anti-inflammatory properties help alleviate various conditions.
How to use	Tea: Steeping fenugreek seeds in hot water to make tea is a common method for digestive health and lactation support. Capsules: Fenugreek supplements are available for those seeking to manage diabetes, cholesterol levels, or enhance lactation. Sprouts: Fenugreek seeds can be sprouted and added to salads for nutritional benefits. Powder: The seeds can be ground into a powder and used in cooking or as a supplement.
Dosage	Tea: Use 1 teaspoon of fenugreek seeds per cup of boiling water, steeped for 5-10 minutes. Drink 1-3 cups daily. Capsules: Typically, 500-1000 mg of fenugreek capsules taken three times daily with meals. However, dosages can vary based on the condition being treated. Powder: 1/2 to 1 teaspoon daily, mixed into food or beverages.
How long to use	Fenugreek can be used both for short-term relief of issues like digestive discomfort and for longer durations (several weeks to months) for conditions like diabetes management or lactation support. For long-term use, especially at higher dosages, monitoring and consultation with a healthcare provider are recommended to assess efficacy and safety.

Feverfew

Feverfew (Tanacetum parthenium) is a medicinal herb traditionally used for preventing migraine headaches, reducing fever, and treating arthritis and digestive problems. Its active compounds, including parthenolide, have anti-inflammatory and anti-migraine properties.

Properties	Anti-migraine: Feverfew is best known for its ability to prevent and reduce the severity of migraine headaches. Anti-inflammatory: Offers anti-inflammatory benefits that can alleviate arthritis and joint pain. Antipyretic: Historically used to reduce fever, though this is not its primary use in modern herbal medicine.
What disease it fights	Migraines: Regular use can decrease the frequency and intensity of migraine headaches. Arthritis: Its anti-inflammatory properties can help relieve arthritis-related discomfort. Menstrual Cramps: May alleviate menstrual pain due to its anti-inflammatory action.
How it works	Feverfew's efficacy, particularly against migraines, is attributed to its ability to inhibit the release of serotonin and prostaglandins, which are involved in the inflammation process. This inhibition can reduce the severity of migraines and other inflammation-related symptoms.
How to use	Fresh Leaves: Some people chew fresh feverfew leaves daily for migraine prevention. Capsules/Tablets: A more common and palatable option, capsules or tablets ensure a consistent dosage of the active ingredients. Tea: Feverfew leaves can be brewed into a tea, though the bitter taste might not be suitable for all.
Dosage	Fresh Leaves: Chewing 2-3 leaves daily is traditional but not commonly recommended due to potential mouth sores and bitterness. Capsules/Tablets: Typically, 50-100 mg daily, containing at least 0.2% parthenolide, the active compound. Follow the product's specific dosage recommendations. Tea: Steep 1 teaspoon of dried leaves in boiling water for 5-10 minutes. Due to its bitterness, tea is less commonly used for migraine prevention.
How long to use	Feverfew is often used for extended periods, as its benefits, particularly for migraine prevention, accumulate over time. Many users take feverfew for several months to years, but it's important to evaluate its effectiveness periodically. If using feverfew continuously for more than four months, consulting a healthcare provider for guidance and monitoring is advisable.

Field scabious

Field scabious (Knautia arvensis) is a perennial plant known for its attractive flowers and medicinal properties. It has been traditionally used in herbal medicine to treat skin conditions, coughs, and as a diuretic.

Properties	Anti-inflammatory: Helps reduce inflammation, beneficial for skin conditions and internal inflammation. Antitussive: Can soothe coughs and is useful in treating respiratory conditions. Diuretic: Promotes the production of urine, aiding in the removal of toxins from the body. Vulnerary: Supports the healing of wounds and skin irritations.
What disease it fights	Skin Conditions: Traditionally used to treat eczema, scabies, and other skin irritations due to its anti-inflammatory and vulnerary properties. Respiratory Conditions: Its antitussive properties can help soothe coughs and potentially assist with other respiratory issues. Urinary Tract Health: As a diuretic, it can support kidney function and urinary health.
How it works	The mechanisms behind field scabious's benefits are thought to be linked to its content of tannins, saponins, and flavonoids, which contribute to its anti-inflammatory, diuretic, and healing properties. These compounds can help soothe irritated skin, reduce inflammation, promote wound healing, and support the elimination of bodily toxins.
How to use	Infusion/Tea: Leaves and flowers can be used to make an infusion or tea, beneficial for internal use, especially for coughs or urinary tract support. Topical Application: A poultice made from the leaves and flowers can be applied to the skin to treat wounds, cuts, and skin irritations. Tincture: A more concentrated form, useful for targeted therapeutic applications.
Dosage	Tea: Steep 1-2 teaspoons of dried flowers or leaves in boiling water for 10 minutes. Drink 2-3 times daily. Topical Application: Apply the poultice directly to the affected area as needed. Tincture: Typically, 1-2 ml three times daily, but follow specific product recommendations or consult a healthcare provider.
How long to use	Field scabious can be used for the duration of acute conditions, such as a cough or skin irritation, usually for a few days to a week. For chronic issues, it may be part of a longer-term herbal strategy, under the guidance of a healthcare professional, to ensure effectiveness and monitor for potential interactions or side effects.

Flaxseed

Flaxseed, known scientifically as Linum usitatissimum, is a rich source of dietary fiber, omega-3 fatty acids, and lignans. These components contribute to its numerous health benefits, including improving digestive health, reducing the risk of heart disease, and potentially aiding in the management of certain hormone-related conditions.

Properties	Omega-3 Fatty Acids: Flaxseed is a rich plant source of alpha-linolenic acid (ALA), a type of omega-3 fatty acid, beneficial for heart health. Dietary Fiber: Contains both soluble and insoluble fiber, supporting digestive health and regularity. Lignans: Offers antioxidant and estrogenic properties, potentially reducing the risk of certain types of cancer. Anti-inflammatory: The omega-3s and lignans in flaxseed have anti-inflammatory effects.
What disease it fights	Cardiovascular Diseases: Omega-3 fatty acids help reduce blood pressure, cholesterol, and the risk of heart disease. Constipation and Digestive Disorders: High fiber content supports bowel regularity and digestive health. Breast and Prostate Cancer: Lignans may have protective effects against cancer cell growth. Menopausal Symptoms: Flaxseed may help manage hot flashes and hormonal imbalances.
How it works	Flaxseed's health benefits are primarily due to its rich composition of ALA omega-3 fatty acids, which can reduce inflammation and improve heart health, dietary fiber that aids in digestion and prevents constipation, and lignans that offer antioxidant protection and may modulate hormone levels favorably.
How to use	Whole or Ground: Ground flaxseed is more easily digested, allowing for better absorption of its nutrients compared to whole flaxseed. It can be added to smoothies, yogurts, cereals, and baked goods. Flaxseed Oil: Contains a high concentration of ALA but lacks the fiber and lignans found in whole or ground seeds. Can be used as a dietary supplement or salad dressing. Soaked Flaxseed: Soaking in water can make flaxseed gelatinous, which is beneficial for digestive health.
Dosage	Ground Flaxseed: 1-2 tablespoons per day, mixed into foods or beverages. Flaxseed Oil: 1 tablespoon per day as a supplement or incorporated into foods.
How long to use	Flaxseed can be incorporated into the daily diet on a long-term basis as part of a healthy eating plan. For specific health conditions, it's wise to monitor your health and adjust as necessary under the guidance of a healthcare provider.

Fumitory

Fumitory (Fumaria officinalis) is a plant with a long history in herbal medicine, traditionally used to treat a variety of ailments, including skin conditions, digestive problems, and liver disorders. Its effectiveness is attributed to its content of alkaloids, flavonoids, and other phytochemicals that contribute to its medicinal properties.

Properties	Detoxifying: Traditionally used to support liver function and promote detoxification. Diuretic: Helps increase urine production, aiding in the removal of toxins from the body. Antispasmodic: Can relieve spasms in the digestive tract, reducing discomfort from conditions like irritable bowel syndrome (IBS). Anti-inflammatory: May help reduce inflammation in the body, contributing to overall health and well-being.
What disease it fights	Digestive Disorders: Its antispasmodic and detoxifying effects are beneficial for improving digestion and treating conditions such as IBS and constipation. Skin Conditions: By supporting liver and digestive health, fumitory can indirectly benefit skin health, potentially improving conditions like eczema and acne. Liver Disorders: Supports liver health and function, which is crucial for overall body detoxification.
How it works	The alkaloids and other phytochemicals in fumitory exert a detoxifying effect on the liver, promoting bile flow and enhancing the liver's ability to process and eliminate toxins. Its diuretic properties further aid in the elimination of these toxins through urine. Additionally, its antispasmodic effects can soothe the digestive tract, reducing symptoms of digestive discomfort.
How to use	Tea: Dried fumitory herb can be steeped in hot water to make tea, commonly used for its digestive and liver-supporting benefits. Tincture: A concentrated form of fumitory, useful for more targeted therapeutic effects. Capsules: Dried fumitory herb is also available in capsule form, providing an alternative for those who prefer not to drink tea.
Dosage	Tea: Steep 1-2 teaspoons of dried herb in a cup of boiling water for 10-15 minutes. Drink 2-3 times daily. Tincture: Typically, 1-2 ml three times daily, but follow specific product recommendations. Capsules: Follow the manufacturer's instructions, usually taken once or twice daily.
How long to use	Fumitory is generally used for short to medium-term support, especially for acute digestive issues or to support a detoxification program, typically not exceeding a few weeks. For long-term use or chronic conditions, consultation with a healthcare professional is advised to monitor effectiveness and adjust the approach as needed.

Garlic

Garlic (Allium sativum) has been used for centuries for its medicinal properties, celebrated for its cardiovascular, antimicrobial, and antioxidant benefits.

Properties	Antimicrobial: Garlic has been shown to fight a wide array of bacteria, viruses, fungi, and parasites. Cardiovascular Health: It can lower blood pressure and cholesterol levels, reducing the risk of heart disease. Antioxidant: Contains antioxidants that protect against cell damage and aging. It may reduce the risk of Alzheimer's disease and dementia. Anti-inflammatory: Offers anti-inflammatory effects that may help manage conditions like arthritis. Immune Support: Boosts the immune system, potentially reducing the severity and frequency of colds and other infections.
What disease it fights	Cardiovascular Diseases: Including hypertension and high cholesterol. Common Colds and Infections: Its immune-boosting properties can help reduce the occurrence of colds and other infections. Digestive Health Issues: May help prevent certain types of cancer, especially those in the digestive system. Type 2 Diabetes: Can help regulate blood sugar levels.
How it works	The health benefits of garlic are primarily attributed to its sulfur compounds, which are released when a garlic clove is chopped, crushed, or chewed. These compounds, including allicin (which is quite transient), have various effects on the body, from fighting harmful microorganisms to improving heart health and enhancing immune function.
How to use	Raw: Eating raw garlic, finely chopped or crushed, maximizes its health benefits. It can be added to salads, dips, or spreads. Cooked: While cooking can reduce some beneficial compounds, garlic still contributes flavor and health properties to cooked dishes. Supplements: Garlic supplements are available for those who prefer not to eat raw garlic. These might be in the form of capsules, tablets, or extracts.
Dosage	Raw Garlic: 1-2 cloves per day, eaten raw or added to food after cooking to retain medicinal properties. Supplements: The dosage can vary widely depending on the form; standardized extracts should be taken as directed on the package. Typically, doses up to 1200 mg per day of garlic extract have been used for heart health.
How long to use	Garlic can be consumed daily as part of a regular diet for ongoing health benefits. When used for specific health conditions, such as to lower blood pressure or cholesterol, it may take several weeks to observe benefits. For acute conditions like colds, garlic is often used for shorter periods, such as several days to a week.

Ginger

Ginger (Zingiber officinale) is a widely used spice and medicinal herb known for its potent anti-inflammatory, antioxidant, and digestive properties. It has been used throughout history in various forms of traditional medicine, including Ayurveda and Chinese Medicine, to treat a range of conditions.

Properties	Anti-inflammatory: Ginger contains gingerols and shogaols, compounds known to reduce inflammation, making it effective for pain relief. Antioxidant: Offers protection against oxidative stress and free radical damage. Digestive Aid: Promotes digestion, helps relieve nausea, and can soothe stomach discomfort. Antiemetic: Effective in preventing or alleviating nausea and vomiting, including morning sickness and motion sickness. Antimicrobial: Exhibits antibacterial and antiviral properties.
What disease it fights	Digestive Issues: Alleviates indigestion, bloating, and gas. Nausea and Vomiting: Used to treat motion sickness, pregnancy-related nausea, and chemotherapy-induced nausea. Pain and Inflammation: Helps reduce pain and inflammation in conditions like arthritis, menstrual pain, and exercise-induced muscle soreness. Colds and Flu: Its antimicrobial properties can help fight infections.
How it works	Ginger works primarily through its bioactive compounds, gingerols, and shogaols, which have anti-inflammatory and antioxidative effects. These compounds can inhibit the synthesis of pro-inflammatory molecules, thereby reducing inflammation and pain. Ginger also stimulates digestion and enhances gastric motility, aiding in the relief of digestive discomfort.
How to use	Fresh Ginger: Can be consumed raw, cooked, or as an addition to teas and smoothies. Ginger Tea: Made by steeping sliced or grated fresh ginger in boiling water. Supplements: Available in capsules, extracts, and powders for those who prefer a more concentrated form without the strong taste. Topical Application: Ginger oil can be diluted and applied to the skin to relieve pain and inflammation.
Dosage	Fresh Ginger: 2-4 grams per day of fresh ginger root for most conditions. Ginger Tea: Use about 1 inch of fresh ginger root per cup of tea, up to 3 times daily. Supplements: Follow the manufacturer's recommendations, typically around 500 mg to 1 gram per day.
How long to use	Ginger can be used daily as part of a regular diet for its general health benefits. For specific health conditions, such as nausea or pain relief, ginger is often used on an as-needed basis. Long-term supplementation should be discussed with a healthcare provider to ensure safety, especially for those on medications or with medical conditions.

Ginkgo Biloba

Ginkgo biloba, one of the oldest living tree species, has been used in traditional Chinese medicine for thousands of years and is widely recognized for its potential cognitive and circulatory benefits.

Properties	Cognitive Enhancement: Ginkgo is best known for its potential to improve memory, cognitive speed, and overall brain function. Circulatory Support: It can enhance blood circulation, which is beneficial for both brain health and cardiovascular function. Antioxidant: Contains potent antioxidants that protect cells from oxidative damage. Anti-inflammatory: Offers anti-inflammatory effects that may help reduce the risk of certain chronic diseases.
What disease it fights	Cognitive Decline: Used to slow down age-related memory loss and improve cognitive functions. Dementia and Alzheimer's Disease: May offer benefits in early stages or as a preventive measure. Peripheral Artery Disease (PAD): Improves symptoms related to poor circulation. Anxiety and Depression: Some studies suggest Ginkgo can help alleviate symptoms of anxiety and depression.
How it works	Ginkgo biloba works primarily by improving blood flow to various parts of the body, including the brain, which can enhance cognitive function and memory. Its antioxidants help combat oxidative stress, a factor in cognitive decline and aging. Ginkgo also affects neurotransmitter systems, potentially improving mental health conditions like anxiety and depression.
How to use	Supplements: Ginkgo biloba is most commonly taken in capsule or tablet form for cognitive and circulatory support. Tea: Leaves can be steeped to make tea, although supplements are preferred for therapeutic doses. Extract: A concentrated form can be taken as a liquid by dropper.
Dosage	Supplements: The typical dosage for cognitive enhancement and circulatory health ranges from 120 mg to 240 mg per day, usually divided into two or three doses. Supplements should be standardized to contain 24% flavone glycosides and 6% terpene lactones. Tea/Extract: Due to variability in concentration, follow product-specific recommendations or consult a healthcare provider for guidance.
How long to use	Ginkgo biloba can be used long-term, but it may take several weeks to notice benefits. Continuous use for up to six months has been studied, but effectiveness and safety beyond six months should be evaluated with a healthcare professional.

Ginseng

Ginseng, known for its two primary varieties, Asian (Panax ginseng) and American (Panax quinquefolius), has been a cornerstone in traditional medicine for centuries, particularly in Asia and North America. It's celebrated for its antioxidant, anti-inflammatory, and energy-boosting properties.

Properties	Energy Enhancement: Ginseng is reputed to boost energy levels and physical stamina. Cognitive Function: Can improve mental clarity, focus, and cognitive performance. Immune Support: Enhances the immune system, possibly reducing the frequency of colds and other infections. Blood Sugar Regulation: Some types of ginseng have been shown to help manage blood sugar levels, beneficial for people with diabetes. Stress Reduction: Acts as an adaptogen, helping the body cope with physical and emotional stress.
What disease it fights	Fatigue: Helps combat general fatigue and chronic fatigue syndrome. Cognitive Decline: May slow the progression of cognitive impairment in conditions like Alzheimer's disease. Diabetes: Assists in glucose regulation for type 2 diabetes. Common Cold and Flu: Regular intake can reduce the incidence and severity of respiratory infections.
How it works	Ginseng contains active compounds known as ginsenosides, which are thought to be responsible for its health benefits. These compounds affect various bodily systems, enhancing energy production, modulating the immune response, and improving cellular health. Ginsenosides also have a beneficial impact on the brain's neurotransmitter systems, potentially improving mood and cognitive function.
How to use	Tea: Dried ginseng root can be steeped in hot water to make tea. Capsules/Supplements: Ginseng extract is available in capsules or tablets, offering a convenient way to consume it. Slices: Fresh or dried ginseng can be sliced and added to soups, stews, or brewed as a tea.
Dosage	Tea: 1-2 grams of dried ginseng root in hot water, steeped for 5-10 minutes. Drink 1-2 cups daily. Capsules/Supplements: The dosage can vary depending on the extract's concentration, but a general recommendation is 200-400 mg of standardized extract daily.
How long to use	Ginseng is best used in cycles to prevent adaptation and maximize its benefits. A common cycle is 2-3 weeks on, followed by a 2-week break. For chronic conditions or general wellness, it might be used for several months, monitoring for any side effects.

Goldenrod

Goldenrod (Solidago spp.) is a flowering plant recognized for its bright yellow flowers and medicinal properties. It's traditionally used for urinary tract health, inflammation, and as a diuretic to help flush out the kidneys and bladder.

Properties	Diuretic: Promotes the production of urine, aiding in the flushing of the urinary tract. Anti-inflammatory: Helps reduce inflammation, beneficial for conditions like arthritis and allergies. Antimicrobial: Exhibits actions against certain bacteria and fungi, supporting urinary tract health. Antispasmodic: Can relieve muscle spasms, including those in the urinary tract.
What disease it fights	Urinary Tract Infections (UTIs): Its diuretic and antimicrobial properties support urinary tract health and can help prevent UTIs. Kidney Stones: Helps prevent the formation of kidney stones by promoting fluid flow. Arthritis and Rheumatism: The anti-inflammatory properties may provide relief from inflammation and pain. Allergies: Can relieve allergy symptoms due to its anti-inflammatory action.
How it works	Goldenrod's health benefits are attributed to its bioactive compounds, including saponins, flavonoids, and phenolic acids, which provide its diuretic, anti-inflammatory, and antimicrobial effects. By promoting urine production, it helps flush out bacteria and reduce inflammation in the urinary tract, while its antimicrobial components can help prevent infections.
How to use	Tea: Goldenrod can be brewed as a tea from dried leaves and flowers, consumed to support urinary tract health and reduce inflammation. Tincture: A concentrated liquid form that can be taken orally, providing a more potent dose. Capsules: Available for those who prefer a convenient, standardized dosage.
Dosage	Tea: Steep 1-2 teaspoons of dried goldenrod in a cup of boiling water for about 10 minutes. Drink 2-3 cups daily. Tincture: Typically, 1-2 ml three times daily, but follow the specific product instructions. Capsules: Follow the manufacturer's recommendations, usually 1-2 capsules two or three times daily.
How long to use	Goldenrod is generally used for short-term relief of conditions, such as during a UTI or allergy season, often for a few weeks. For ongoing issues like chronic UTIs or kidney stones, it may be used under supervision for longer periods, with periodic evaluations to assess effectiveness and tolerance.

Goldenseal

Goldenseal (Hydrastis canadensis) is a perennial plant native to North America, valued in traditional medicine for its antimicrobial, anti-inflammatory, and astringent properties. It has been used to treat a variety of conditions, particularly those involving infections and inflammation.

Properties	Antimicrobial: Goldenseal is widely recognized for its broad-spectrum antimicrobial properties, effective against bacteria, fungi, and protozoa. Anti-inflammatory: Helps reduce inflammation, which can be beneficial in treating conditions like gastritis and other inflammatory diseases. Astringent: The astringent qualities of Goldenseal make it useful for skin conditions, promoting healing and reducing secretion in wounds. Mucous Membrane Support: Particularly effective in treating respiratory tract infections and aiding in the health of mucous membranes.
What disease it fights	Digestive Issues: Including diarrhea, gastritis, and peptic ulcers due to its antimicrobial and anti-inflammatory effects. Respiratory Infections: Used to treat colds, flu, and sinus infections. Skin Conditions: Effective in treating skin infections and promoting wound healing. Urinary Tract Infections (UTIs): Its antimicrobial action makes it useful for treating UTIs.
How it works	The primary active components in Goldenseal, including berberine, hydrastine, and canadine, contribute to its therapeutic effects. Berberine, in particular, has been extensively studied for its antimicrobial activity, which inhibits the growth of bacteria and other pathogens. The compounds in Goldenseal also work to reduce inflammation and support the health of mucous membranes throughout the body.
How to use	Capsules/Tablets: This is the most common form for internal use, providing a controlled dosage of Goldenseal's active compounds. Tincture: A liquid form that can be taken orally or added to water. Topical Applications: Creams and ointments containing Goldenseal can be applied to skin infections and wounds.
Dosage	Capsules/Tablets: Typically, 400-500 mg taken two to three times daily. Tincture: 0.5-1 ml three times daily, diluted in water or juice. Topical Applications: Apply as directed on the product label, usually 2-3 times daily.
How long to use	Goldenseal is usually used for short-term treatments, not exceeding two to three weeks, due to concerns about its long-term safety and potential impact on beneficial gut flora. For ongoing conditions or repeated use, it's important to consult a healthcare provider.

Gotu Kola

Gotu Kola (Centella asiatica) is a herb revered in Ayurvedic and traditional Chinese medicine for its wide-ranging health benefits, including enhancing cognitive function, promoting wound healing, and supporting skin health. It is known for its anti-inflammatory, neuroprotective, and adaptogenic properties.

Properties	Cognitive Enhancement: Supports memory and cognitive function, making it popular for improving mental clarity and focus. Wound Healing: Promotes the healing of wounds and burns by increasing blood supply to the affected areas and boosting the production of collagen. Anti-inflammatory: Offers relief for inflammatory conditions, potentially beneficial for arthritis and skin inflammation. Skin Health: Enhances the synthesis of collagen, contributing to healthier skin and aiding in the treatment of various skin conditions, including psoriasis and eczema. Adaptogenic: Helps the body adapt to stress and restore balance.
What disease it fights	Cognitive Disorders: May help in preventing or managing cognitive decline and improving overall brain health. Skin Conditions: Effective in treating wounds, ulcers, eczema, and psoriasis through enhanced collagen production. Varicose Veins and Hemorrhoids: Strengthens vascular tissues and improves circulation, aiding in the treatment of varicose veins and hemorrhoids. Anxiety and Stress: Its adaptogenic properties can help reduce stress and anxiety levels.
How it works	Gotu Kola contains several active compounds, including triterpenoid saponins (such as asiaticoside, madecassoside) that are thought to contribute to its healing, anti-inflammatory, and cognitive-enhancing effects. These compounds improve collagen synthesis, promote new tissue growth, and increase antioxidant defense, thereby supporting wound healing and enhancing cognitive functions.
How to use	Tea: Dried leaves can be steeped in hot water to make a calming tea. Capsules/Supplements: Available for those who prefer a more convenient and controlled dosage. Topical Applications: Creams and ointments containing Gotu Kola extract can be applied to the skin to aid in healing and improve skin health.
Dosage	Tea: Steep 1-2 teaspoons of dried Gotu Kola leaves in boiling water for 10-15 minutes. Drink 1-2 cups daily. Capsules/Supplements: Dosages can vary widely; however, 500-1000 mg per day is common. It's essential to follow the manufacturer's recommendations or consult a healthcare provider. Topical Applications: Apply as directed on the product label, typically 2-3 times daily to the affected area.
How long to use	Gotu Kola can be used over extended periods for chronic conditions, with some traditional practices recommending its use for several weeks to months. However, it's important to monitor for any adverse effects over time, especially when consumed internally.

Grape Seed Extract

Grape Seed Extract (GSE) is derived from the ground-up seeds of red wine grapes and is celebrated for its potent antioxidant properties. It's rich in oligomeric proanthocyanidin complexes (OPCs), which are known to provide extensive health benefits, including cardiovascular protection, anti-inflammatory effects, and support for skin health.

Properties	Antioxidant: GSE is highly regarded for its strong antioxidant properties, which help neutralize free radicals and reduce oxidative stress. Anti-inflammatory: Can help reduce inflammation in the body, potentially benefiting conditions associated with chronic inflammation. Cardiovascular Health: Supports heart health by improving circulation, strengthening blood vessels, and reducing high blood pressure. Anti-cancer: Some studies suggest that the antioxidants in GSE may have anti-cancer properties. Skin Health: Promotes skin elasticity and can protect against sun damage due to its antioxidant content.
What disease it fights	Cardiovascular Diseases: By improving circulation and protecting the blood vessels, GSE can reduce the risk of heart disease. Chronic Inflammation: Its anti-inflammatory effects can be beneficial in managing conditions like arthritis. Skin Damage: Helps in protecting the skin from UV radiation and improving skin health. Cancer: The antioxidant properties may contribute to cancer prevention, though more research is needed in this area.
How it works	The OPCs in grape seed extract are thought to be responsible for most of its health benefits. These compounds can improve blood flow and have a strengthening effect on collagen, supporting skin and vascular health. Their antioxidant capacity helps in reducing oxidative damage to cells, which is linked to various chronic diseases.
How to use	Supplements: GSE is most commonly taken in capsule or tablet form for internal health benefits. Topical Applications: Available in some skin care products for its antioxidant and protective properties.
Dosage	Supplements: The typical dosage of grape seed extract is between 100 to 300 mg per day, taken in divided doses. However, dosages can vary based on the concentration of the extract and the specific health concern being addressed.
How long to use	GSE can be used as a long-term supplement for general health and cardiovascular support. For specific conditions, such as improving skin health or reducing inflammation, it might be used for several months to evaluate its effectiveness. Continuous monitoring and consultation with a healthcare provider are recommended, especially when using supplements for chronic conditions.

Green Tea

Green Tea Extract, derived from the Camellia sinensis plant, is rich in antioxidants, particularly catechins like epigallocatechin gallate (EGCG), which are believed to be responsible for most of its health benefits.

Properties	Antioxidant: Offers powerful antioxidant properties, protecting cells from oxidative stress and damage. Metabolic Enhancement: Can boost metabolism and aid in weight loss efforts. Cardiovascular Health: Improves cardiovascular health by lowering bad cholesterol levels and increasing antioxidant capacity in the blood. Anti-cancer: The high levels of catechins have been linked to a reduced risk of certain types of cancer. Brain Health: Contains compounds that can cross the blood-brain barrier, potentially improving brain health and lowering the risk of neurodegenerative diseases.
What disease it fights	Obesity and Metabolic Syndrome: Aids in weight management and can improve markers of metabolic health. Cardiovascular Diseases: Helps reduce factors contributing to heart disease, such as high cholesterol and hypertension. Cancer: May offer protective effects against certain cancers through its antioxidant mechanisms. Type 2 Diabetes: Improves insulin sensitivity and reduces blood sugar levels. Cognitive Decline: The antioxidants in green tea can protect against brain aging and diseases like Alzheimer's.
How it works	Green Tea Extract works primarily through its high content of polyphenols, especially EGCG, which exert significant antioxidant effects. These compounds help neutralize harmful free radicals, reducing oxidative damage and inflammation. EGCG has also been shown to enhance metabolic rate and fat oxidation, supporting weight loss.
How to use	Supplements: Available in capsule or liquid extract form, providing a concentrated dose of the tea's active ingredients. Beverage: While not as concentrated as the extract, drinking green tea can also provide health benefits.
Dosage	Supplements: The recommended dosage can vary, but generally, 250–500 mg per day is used for health benefits. It's important to choose a supplement standardized for EGCG content to ensure potency. Beverage: Drinking 3–5 cups of green tea daily can offer health benefits, though this provides a lower dose of catechins compared to supplements.
How long to use	Green Tea Extract can be used over the long term for ongoing health benefits, such as cardiovascular health support and antioxidant protection. However, due to concerns about liver toxicity with high doses or prolonged use of concentrated extracts, it's important to follow recommended dosages and consult with a healthcare provider for personalized advice.

Ground-ivy

Ground-ivy (Glechoma hederacea), also known as creeping Charlie, is a perennial herb that has been used in traditional herbal medicine for centuries. It's recognized for its expectorant, anti-inflammatory, and astringent properties.

Properties	Expectorant: Helps clear mucus from the respiratory tract, making it beneficial for conditions such as bronchitis, coughs, and colds. Anti-inflammatory: Can reduce inflammation, helpful for soothing sore throats and arthritis. Astringent: Its astringent properties make it useful for treating wounds and skin conditions. Diuretic: Promotes the elimination of fluids from the body, aiding in detoxification and urinary tract health.
What disease it fights	Respiratory Conditions: Its expectorant properties are valuable in treating coughs, colds, and bronchitis by helping to clear mucus. Arthritis and Inflammatory Conditions: Can help alleviate inflammation associated with arthritis and similar conditions. Skin Disorders: The astringent qualities may benefit certain skin conditions by tightening tissues and reducing irritation. Urinary Tract Issues: As a diuretic, it can support urinary tract health by promoting fluid elimination.
How it works	Ground-ivy's medicinal effects are attributed to its various active compounds, including flavonoids, terpenoids, and saponins. These components work together to exert expectorant, anti-inflammatory, and astringent actions, helping to clear mucus, reduce inflammation, and tighten and tone tissues, respectively.
How to use	Tea: A common method for internal use, benefiting respiratory and urinary tract health. Tincture: Can be taken orally for a more concentrated form, useful for its expectorant and anti-inflammatory effects. Topical Application: Infused oils or poultices from the plant can be applied to the skin for wounds and skin irritations.
Dosage	Tea: Steep 1-2 teaspoons of dried ground-ivy in a cup of boiling water for 10-15 minutes. Drink 2-3 times daily. Tincture: Generally, 1-2 ml three times a day, but follow specific product instructions or consult a healthcare provider. Topical Application: Use as needed, applying directly to the affected area.
How long to use	Ground-ivy is typically used for the duration of acute symptoms, such as during a respiratory infection or for urinary issues, usually not exceeding a few weeks. For chronic conditions or for ongoing support, such as in arthritis, it may be used longer under the guidance of a healthcare professional to monitor effectiveness and ensure safety.

Gum Arabic

Gum arabic, also known as acacia gum (derived from the Acacia tree species), is a natural gum consisting of the hardened sap of various species of the acacia tree. It's been used for centuries in traditional medicine and food preparation for its health benefits.

Properties	High in Soluble Fiber: Gum arabic is rich in soluble fiber, which can aid digestion, improve gut health, and regulate blood sugar levels. Prebiotic: Acts as a food source for beneficial gut bacteria, supporting a healthy microbiome. Anti-inflammatory: Contains compounds that may help reduce inflammation in the body. Wound Healing: Traditionally used for its wound-healing properties when applied topically.
What disease it fights	Digestive Disorders: Its prebiotic and fiber content supports digestive health, potentially relieving symptoms of IBS (Irritable Bowel Syndrome) and constipation. Diabetes Management: By slowing glucose absorption, it can help regulate blood sugar levels, beneficial for people with diabetes. Obesity and Weight Management: The fiber in gum arabic can promote feelings of fullness, helping with weight control.
How it works	The health benefits of gum arabic stem from its high soluble fiber content, which can absorb water in the gut to form a gel-like substance, easing bowel movements and supporting overall digestive health. Its prebiotic nature fosters a healthy gut microbiota, essential for digestion, immune function, and possibly mood regulation. Additionally, its anti-inflammatory properties may contribute to reduced inflammation in various parts of the body.
How to use	Dietary Supplement: Gum arabic is available in powder form, which can be dissolved in water or added to smoothies and other foods as a fiber supplement. Prebiotic: Taken orally to support gut health and digestion. Topical Application: Applied to the skin to aid in the healing of minor wounds and skin irritations.
Dosage	Dietary Supplement: The typical dosage for gum arabic as a supplement is about 5-30 grams per day, dissolved in water or another liquid. It's best to start with a lower dose to assess tolerance. Topical Application: There is no specific dosage; it can be applied as needed, directly to the skin or as part of a cream or gel formulation.
How long to use	As a dietary supplement for digestive health or weight management, gum arabic can be used daily for several weeks to months, observing how your body responds. For topical applications, use until the desired healing effect is achieved.

Hawthorn

Hawthorn (Crataegus species) is a plant whose leaves, berries, and flowers are used to make medicines, especially for heart and cardiovascular diseases. It's recognized for its ability to strengthen heart function, improve circulation, and manage blood pressure.

Properties	Cardiovascular Support: Hawthorn is well-regarded for its cardiovascular benefits, including strengthening the heart muscle, improving cardiac output, and enhancing circulation. Antioxidant: Contains powerful antioxidants that help neutralize free radicals and reduce oxidative stress. Blood Pressure Regulation: Can help lower high blood pressure by relaxing blood vessels. Cholesterol Management: Some evidence suggests hawthorn can improve cholesterol levels by reducing the formation of blood fats.
What disease it fights	Heart Failure: Used to manage symptoms of heart failure, such as shortness of breath and fatigue. Angina: May reduce symptoms of angina (chest pain) by improving blood flow to the heart. Hypertension: Helps in managing high blood pressure. Atherosclerosis: The antioxidant properties may help prevent the formation of plaques in the arteries.
How it works	The beneficial effects of hawthorn are attributed to its unique blend of bioactive compounds, including flavonoids, oligomeric proanthocyanidins, and phenolic acids. These compounds work together to improve heart muscle tone, enhance blood flow, expand blood vessels, and provide antioxidant protection.
How to use	Extracts and Supplements: Hawthorn is commonly taken in the form of capsules, tablets, or liquid extracts for cardiovascular support. Tea: Made from hawthorn berries, leaves, or flowers, it can be consumed as a mild tonic for heart health. Tincture: A concentrated liquid form that can be taken directly or diluted in water.
Dosage	Supplements: Typical dosages of hawthorn extract range from 250 to 500 mg three times daily, standardized to contain about 2% flavonoids or 18-20% oligomeric procyanidins. Tea: 1-2 teaspoons of dried hawthorn plant per cup of boiling water, steeped for 10-15 minutes. Drink up to 3 cups daily. Tincture: Generally, 0.5-1 ml three times daily, but follow specific product instructions.
How long to use	Hawthorn is often used for long-term support of cardiovascular health. It may take several weeks or even months to notice significant benefits. Continuous use is generally considered safe, but it's important to monitor your condition and consult with a healthcare provider, especially if you are using hawthorn in conjunction with other heart medications.

Henna

Henna (Lawsonia inermis) is a plant with a long history of use in traditional medicine, beauty, and body art across many cultures. Known primarily for its natural dye properties, henna also possesses medicinal qualities.

Properties	Antimicrobial: Henna has been shown to have antibacterial and antifungal properties, making it useful in treating skin infections and conditions. Anti-inflammatory: Can help reduce inflammation, beneficial for soothing skin irritations and conditions like eczema. Cooling Effect: When applied topically, henna has a cooling effect, which can soothe burns, sunburns, and reduce fever. Astringent: Its astringent qualities can be beneficial in skin care, particularly for oily or acne-prone skin.
What disease it fights	Skin Conditions: Used topically to treat fungal infections, eczema, and acne due to its antimicrobial and anti-inflammatory properties. Fever: The cooling effect of henna can help lower body temperature in cases of fever. Headaches: Applied to the skin, it can help relieve headaches due to its cooling effect.
How it works	The medicinal effects of henna are attributed to its active compounds, including lawsone (hennotannic acid), which has antimicrobial and anti-inflammatory properties. These compounds can inhibit the growth of certain bacteria and fungi, reduce inflammation, and provide a cooling sensation on the skin, which can be soothing in various conditions.
How to use	Topical Application: Henna paste is applied to the skin for its medicinal and cooling effects. For skin conditions, a paste made from henna powder and water can be applied directly to the affected area. Hair Treatment: Henna is widely used as a natural dye for hair and to strengthen and condition the hair. Body Art: Henna paste is used for temporary body art, known as Mehndi, especially in cultural ceremonies.
Dosage	Topical Application: There is no specific "dosage" for henna when used topically. Apply as needed, allowing the paste to dry on the skin before removal. For cooling effects or to treat fever, henna can be applied to the palms and soles. Hair Treatment: The amount of henna needed depends on hair length and thickness. Generally, 100-200 grams of henna powder may be needed for one application on hair.
How long to use	For medicinal purposes, henna should be used as needed or until symptoms improve. For ongoing conditions like eczema or fungal infections, monitoring the skin's response and adjusting frequency of application accordingly is advisable. Continuous use for hair or skin health can be part of a regular beauty regimen.

Hibiscus

Hibiscus extract, derived from the flowers of the Hibiscus sabdariffa plant, is celebrated for its vibrant color, tart flavor, and a wide array of health benefits. Rich in powerful antioxidants such as vitamin C and anthocyanins, hibiscus has been traditionally used to support heart health, manage blood pressure, and enhance liver health.

Properties	Antihypertensive: Hibiscus has been shown to lower blood pressure in several studies, making it beneficial for heart health. Antioxidant: Offers strong antioxidant properties, helping to combat oxidative stress and reduce inflammation. Diuretic: Promotes the excretion of salt from the body, which can help in lowering blood pressure. Hepatoprotective: Supports liver health and can aid in liver enzyme regulation.
What disease it fights	Hypertension (High Blood Pressure): Hibiscus tea has been widely studied for its effectiveness in reducing high blood pressure. High Cholesterol: May help in lowering bad LDL cholesterol and raising good HDL cholesterol. Liver Disorders: Supports liver health by improving liver enzyme levels and protecting against liver damage. Metabolic Syndrome: Its antioxidant properties can benefit those dealing with metabolic syndrome by improving cholesterol levels, blood pressure, and obesity.
How it works	The health benefits of hibiscus are primarily attributed to its high content of anthocyanins, polyphenols, and vitamin C, which provide antioxidant and anti-inflammatory effects. These compounds can help reduce blood pressure by relaxing the blood vessels and acting as a natural diuretic, reducing blood volume and salt content.
How to use	Tea: Hibiscus tea, made from dried hibiscus flowers, is the most common and easy way to enjoy its benefits. It can be consumed hot or cold. Supplements: Hibiscus is available in capsules or liquid extracts for those seeking a more concentrated form. Tincture: A liquid form that can be diluted in water.
Dosage	Tea: 1-2 teaspoons (5-10 grams) of dried hibiscus flowers steeped in 1 cup (240 ml) of boiling water for 5-10 minutes. Drink 1-3 cups daily. Supplements: Follow the manufacturer's recommendations, but dosages typically range from 500 mg to 1000 mg daily. Tincture: Follow product-specific guidelines for proper dosage.
How long to use	Hibiscus tea and supplements can be used daily as part of a routine health regimen. For managing specific conditions like hypertension, it may be necessary to consume hibiscus regularly for several weeks to observe significant benefits. Long-term use should be monitored for effectiveness and any potential side effects.

Holy Basil (Tulsi)

Holy Basil, also known as Tulsi (Ocimum sanctum), is a revered plant in Ayurvedic medicine, known for its adaptogenic properties that help the body adapt to stress and promote mental balance. It's also celebrated for its anti-inflammatory, antioxidant, antimicrobial, and blood sugar-regulating benefits.

Properties	Adaptogenic: Helps the body cope with stress, reducing the physical and psychological impact. Antioxidant: Offers protection against oxidative stress and cellular damage. Anti-inflammatory: Can reduce inflammation throughout the body, aiding in the relief of inflammatory conditions. Antimicrobial: Exhibits antibacterial, antiviral, and antifungal properties. Blood Sugar Regulation: May help in managing blood glucose levels, beneficial for those with diabetes or at risk.
What disease it fights	Stress and Anxiety: By reducing cortisol levels and modulating the body's stress response. Infections: Its antimicrobial action can help prevent and fight infections. Inflammatory Conditions: Useful in managing arthritis, cardiovascular diseases, and other inflammatory conditions. Diabetes: Assists in regulating blood sugar levels, contributing to diabetes management.
How it works	Holy Basil contains a wide range of bioactive compounds, including eugenol, ursolic acid, and oleanolic acid, which contribute to its health benefits. These compounds work together to enhance the body's natural response to physical and emotional stress, reduce inflammation, combat harmful microbes, and regulate blood sugar levels.
How to use	Tea: Fresh or dried leaves can be used to brew a soothing cup of tea. Supplements: Capsules or liquid extracts provide a more concentrated form of Holy Basil for therapeutic use. Fresh Leaves: Can be chewed or added to foods for a health boost.
Dosage	Tea: Use 1-2 teaspoons of dried Holy Basil leaves per cup of boiling water, steeped for 5-10 minutes. Drink 2-3 cups daily. Supplements: Dosages can vary; typically, 300-600 mg of extract per day, divided into two or three doses, is recommended for stress reduction and general health. Fresh Leaves: 2-3 leaves chewed daily can provide health benefits.
How long to use	Holy Basil can be used daily as part of a health maintenance routine, with some people incorporating it continuously for its stress-reducing and health-promoting benefits. For specific health conditions, such as managing stress or blood sugar levels, it might be used for several weeks to months, observing for effectiveness and any changes in symptoms.

Hollyhock

Hollyhock (Alcea rosea) is a flowering plant that belongs to the mallow family and is closely related to hibiscus and marshmallow plants. It has been used traditionally in herbal medicine for its soothing, anti-inflammatory, and emollient properties, particularly for skin and respiratory conditions.

Properties	Soothing and Demulcent: The mucilage content provides a soothing effect on irritated mucous membranes, helpful for coughs and sore throats. Anti-inflammatory: Can help reduce inflammation, making it beneficial for treating skin irritations and inflammatory conditions. Emollient: Softens and moisturizes the skin, useful for dry or irritated skin conditions. Diuretic: Some traditional uses include acting as a mild diuretic, promoting the elimination of fluids from the body.
What disease it fights	Respiratory Conditions: Its demulcent properties can relieve symptoms of coughs, sore throats, and bronchitis by soothing irritated mucous membranes. Skin Conditions: Effective in treating and soothing skin irritations, eczema, and other inflammatory skin disorders. Digestive Issues: The soothing mucilage can also benefit the digestive tract, alleviating irritation and inflammation.
How it works	Hollyhock's healing effects are primarily due to its high mucilage content, which forms a protective layer over irritated tissues, soothing inflammation and irritation. This action is beneficial for both internal and external use, providing relief for the skin, throat, and digestive system.
How to use	Tea: Made from the flowers or leaves, hollyhock tea can be drunk to soothe respiratory or digestive ailments. Topical Application: A poultice or infusion of the flowers or leaves can be applied directly to the skin to soothe irritation and inflammation. Bath Additive: Flowers and leaves can be added to bathwater for a soothing and emollient effect on the skin.
Dosage	Tea: Steep 1-2 teaspoons of dried flowers or leaves in boiling water for 10-15 minutes. Drink 2-3 cups daily for internal relief. Topical Application: Apply as needed to the affected area, using fresh or rehydrated dried flowers and leaves. Bath Additive: Add a handful of flowers or leaves to a warm bath and soak to relieve skin irritation.
How long to use	For acute conditions like sore throats or skin irritation, hollyhock can be used until symptoms improve, typically for a few days to a week. For chronic conditions or for ongoing support, such as in skincare routines, it may be used longer, under the guidance of a healthcare professional to monitor effectiveness and prevent any potential reactions.

Hops

Hops (Humulus lupulus) are best known for their role in beer brewing, but they also possess various medicinal properties, making them beneficial for health beyond their flavoring contributions. They have been traditionally used for their sedative, anti-inflammatory, and estrogenic effects.

Properties	Sedative and Sleep Aid: Hops are widely recognized for their sedative properties, helping to improve sleep quality and ease insomnia. Estrogenic Effects: Contains phytoestrogens, which may help alleviate menopausal symptoms and menstrual discomfort. Anti-inflammatory: Beneficial for reducing inflammation, potentially aiding in the treatment of conditions like arthritis. Antibacterial: Exhibits antibacterial activity, particularly against gram-positive bacteria.
What disease it fights	Sleep Disorders: Especially effective in treating insomnia and improving overall sleep quality. Menopausal and Menstrual Symptoms: May alleviate symptoms like hot flashes and mood swings. Anxiety and Stress: The sedative effects can help reduce anxiety and promote relaxation. Digestive Issues: Used in traditional medicine to treat indigestion and other gastrointestinal problems.
How it works	The sedative effects of hops are primarily attributed to the compound methylbutenol, which is known to exert a calming effect on the brain, enhancing sleep quality. Additionally, the presence of phytoestrogens contributes to its beneficial effects on menopausal and menstrual symptoms. Its anti-inflammatory and antibacterial properties further support its use in managing inflammation and preventing infection.
How to use	Tea: Hops can be brewed into a tea, often combined with other herbs like valerian for enhanced sleep aid effects. Tinctures and Extracts: Concentrated forms of hops are available for those seeking stronger or more consistent dosages. Pillows: Dried hops are sometimes filled in small pillows or sachets to aid sleep through inhalation of their sedative aromas.
Dosage	Tea: 1-2 teaspoons of dried hops per cup of boiling water, steeped for 5-10 minutes. Drink 30 minutes before bedtime. Tinctures and Extracts: Follow the manufacturer's instructions, typically a few drops to a milliliter taken before bedtime or as needed for relaxation. Pillows: No dosage applies, but using a hops pillow nightly may help improve sleep quality.
How long to use	Hops can be used as needed for improving sleep or managing anxiety and stress. For chronic conditions or ongoing use, it's wise to periodically evaluate the effects and consult with a healthcare provider, especially when using for more than a few months.

Horse chestnut

Horse chestnut (Aesculus hippocastanum) is a plant whose seeds, leaves, bark, and flowers have been used in traditional medicine. It's best known for its ability to improve venous health, particularly in treating varicose veins, hemorrhoids, and chronic venous insufficiency (CVI).

Properties	Venotonic: Improves the tone of veins, enhancing blood flow and reducing venous insufficiency. Anti-inflammatory: Reduces inflammation in the veins, helping to alleviate symptoms associated with varicose veins and hemorrhoids. Antiedematous: Reduces swelling and fluid retention in the legs. Antioxidant: Contains antioxidants that protect the veins from damage caused by free radicals.
What disease it fights	Chronic Venous Insufficiency (CVI): Effective in reducing symptoms like swelling, pain, fatigue, and itching in the legs. Varicose Veins: Helps alleviate the discomfort and appearance of varicose veins. Hemorrhoids: Reduces inflammation and discomfort caused by hemorrhoids.
How it works	The active compound in horse chestnut is aescin (or escin), which strengthens the walls of veins and capillaries, reducing permeability and improving blood flow. This action helps to decrease swelling, pain, and the sensation of heaviness in the legs associated with poor venous circulation.
How to use	Extracts and Supplements: Horse chestnut is commonly taken as an oral supplement, either in capsule or liquid form, standardized to contain a specific amount of aescin. Topical Creams: For external symptoms like varicose veins and hemorrhoids, horse chestnut can also be applied topically as a cream or gel.
Dosage	Oral Supplements: The typical dosage for horse chestnut seed extract (standardized to contain 16-20% aescin) is 300 mg twice daily. Topical Creams: Apply as directed on the product label, usually 2-3 times daily to the affected area.
How long to use	Horse chestnut is generally used for several weeks to months depending on the severity of the condition and response to treatment. For chronic conditions like CVI, use may be ongoing under the supervision of a healthcare provider to manage symptoms effectively.

Horsetail

Horsetail (Equisetum arvense) is a perennial fern that has been used in traditional medicine for centuries, notably for its diuretic, anti-inflammatory, and bone health-promoting properties. This herb is rich in minerals, especially silica, which is essential for bone and tissue health.

Properties	Diuretic: Promotes the excretion of urine, aiding in detoxification and the management of fluid retention. Bone Health: High silica content supports the formation and maintenance of healthy bones, cartilage, and connective tissue. Antioxidant and Anti-inflammatory: Contains antioxidants that combat oxidative stress and anti-inflammatory compounds that can reduce inflammation. Hair, Skin, and Nail Health: Silica also supports the health and strength of hair, skin, and nails.
What disease it fights	Urinary Tract and Kidney Issues: Its diuretic effect is useful in treating urinary tract infections and kidney stones. Osteoporosis and Bone Fractures: Silica helps in the formation of collagen and bone remineralization. Edema: Can help reduce swelling and fluid retention. Brittle Nails and Hair Loss: The mineral content can improve the condition and strength of hair and nails.
How it works	Horsetail's beneficial effects are primarily attributed to its high silica content, which is crucial for the synthesis of collagen, an essential protein found in bones, cartilage, and connective tissue. Its diuretic properties help in flushing out toxins from the body, while its anti-inflammatory compounds reduce inflammation.
How to use	Tea: Dried horsetail can be steeped in hot water to make a tea for internal use. Capsules/Supplements: For those who prefer not to drink the tea, horsetail is available in capsule form. Topical Applications: Horsetail extract can be used in lotions or shampoos for hair and skin health.
Dosage	Tea: Steep 1-2 teaspoons of dried horsetail in a cup of boiling water for 5-10 minutes. Drink 1-3 cups daily. Capsules/Supplements: Follow the manufacturer's recommendations, typically 300-500 mg daily in divided doses.
How long to use	Horsetail can be used for specific periods depending on the health issue being addressed. For conditions like edema or urinary tract infections, short-term use (a few weeks) is common. For supporting bone health or hair and nail strength, longer-term use may be necessary. Always monitor your body's response and consult with a healthcare provider, especially for long-term use.

Hyssop

Hyssop (Hyssopus officinalis) is an herb known for its aromatic leaves and flowers, historically used in both medicinal and culinary applications. It possesses a variety of therapeutic properties including expectorant, antiviral, antibacterial, and digestive benefits.

Properties	Expectorant: Helps clear mucus from the respiratory tract, aiding in the treatment of coughs and colds. Antiviral and Antibacterial: Exhibits activity against certain viruses and bacteria, supporting its use in infectious conditions. Digestive Aid: Can soothe the digestive system and relieve issues like gas and bloating. Anti-inflammatory: Reduces inflammation, which can be beneficial for conditions like asthma and arthritis.
What disease it fights	Respiratory Conditions: Useful in treating coughs, colds, and bronchitis by helping to expel mucus. Digestive Disorders: Aids in relieving symptoms of indigestion, gas, and bloating. Skin Conditions: Applied topically, it can help treat skin irritations and infections due to its antiseptic properties. Mild Hypertension: There are indications that hyssop can help regulate blood pressure, though more research is needed.
How it works	Hyssop's therapeutic benefits are attributed to its diverse range of compounds, including volatile oils, flavonoids, and tannins. These compounds work together to provide expectorant, antiviral, and anti-inflammatory effects, among others, helping to relieve symptoms of various conditions.
How to use	Tea: Hyssop leaves and flowers can be steeped in boiling water to make a tea, which can be drunk to relieve respiratory and digestive issues. Tincture: A concentrated liquid form that can be taken orally or added to water. Essential Oil: Used in aromatherapy for respiratory benefits or diluted and applied topically for skin conditions (Note: essential oils should be used with caution and never ingested without professional guidance). Dried Herb: Can be used in cooking or to make homemade remedies.
Dosage	Tea: 1-2 teaspoons of dried hyssop per cup of boiling water, steeped for 10 minutes. Drink 2-3 cups daily. Tincture: Typically, 1-2 ml taken three times daily. Essential Oil: For topical use, essential oil should be diluted with a carrier oil (usually 1-2 drops of essential oil per tablespoon of carrier oil).
How long to use	Hyssop is generally considered safe for short-term use (up to two weeks) at the recommended dosages. For ongoing conditions or extended use, it's wise to consult with a healthcare provider to monitor for any potential side effects and ensure continued safety.

Jasmine

Jasmine, known botanically as Jasminum spp., is celebrated not only for its fragrant flowers but also for its therapeutic properties in herbal medicine and aromatherapy.

Properties	Antidepressant and Anxiolytic: Jasmine's fragrance is known to have a calming effect, potentially reducing anxiety and depression symptoms. Antiseptic and Antibacterial: Certain compounds in jasmine, such as benzoic acid and benzyl benzoate, have been shown to possess antibacterial properties. Antispasmodic: Can provide relief from spasms in the body, such as coughs or muscle cramps. Aphrodisiac: Traditionally used to enhance libido and improve mood.
What disease it fights	Stress and Anxiety: The soothing aroma of jasmine can help alleviate stress and anxiety. Mild Depression: Aromatherapy with jasmine oil might have uplifting effects. Respiratory Infections: Its antiseptic properties can help in treating and preventing infections. Skin Conditions: Applied topically, jasmine can help improve skin health due to its antibacterial and antiseptic qualities.
How it works	The calming and uplifting effects of jasmine are largely attributed to its aromatic compounds, which can influence the central nervous system through inhalation. These compounds interact with brain chemicals and receptors that affect mood and stress levels. Its antibacterial properties help in treating and preventing infections when applied topically.
How to use	Aromatherapy: Jasmine oil can be used in diffusers or inhaled directly to benefit from its calming and uplifting properties. Topical Application: Jasmine-infused oils and creams can be applied to the skin to utilize its antiseptic and soothing effects. Tea: Jasmine flowers are often infused with green or black tea, providing a calming beverage with potential health benefits.
Dosage	Aromatherapy: There is no strict dosage for inhalation. Use a few drops in a diffuser as needed for relaxation and mood enhancement. Topical Application: When using jasmine oil topically, it should be diluted with a carrier oil (typically 1-2 drops of jasmine oil per tablespoon of carrier oil) to prevent irritation. Tea: Jasmine tea can be consumed 1-3 cups daily. The tea is generally safe and can be enjoyed as part of a daily routine.
How long to use	Jasmine can be used safely as part of a daily wellness routine, especially for aromatherapy and tea consumption. For topical applications, it's important to monitor for any skin reactions, especially with prolonged use. As with any herbal remedy, if symptoms persist or worsen, consulting a healthcare provider is recommended.

Juniper Berries

Juniper berries, derived from various species of the juniper bush, have been used for centuries in traditional medicine across many cultures, mainly for their diuretic, antiseptic, and digestive stimulant properties.

Properties	Diuretic: Juniper berries are well-known for their diuretic effect, helping to flush toxins from the body through increased urine production. Antiseptic: Possess antimicrobial properties, making them beneficial in treating urinary tract infections and cleansing the urinary tract. Digestive Stimulant: Can stimulate the digestive system, improving digestion and relieving gas and bloating. Anti-inflammatory: Contains compounds that help reduce inflammation in the body.
What disease it fights	Urinary Tract Infections (UTIs): The antiseptic properties help in preventing and treating UTIs. Digestive Disorders: Aid in relieving indigestion, gas, and bloating by stimulating the digestive system. Joint Pain and Inflammation: The anti-inflammatory effects can be beneficial for those with arthritis or other inflammatory joint conditions. Skin Conditions: When used topically, juniper berry oil can help treat skin irritations and infections due to its antiseptic properties.
How it works	The primary active components in juniper berries include volatile oils, terpenes, and flavonoids, which contribute to their diuretic, antiseptic, and anti-inflammatory effects. These compounds promote the elimination of waste products by increasing urine volume and possess antimicrobial activity that helps cleanse the urinary tract and improve overall urinary health.
How to use	Tea: Crushed juniper berries can be steeped in hot water to make a tea. This is a common method for consuming juniper for UTI prevention or digestive health. Tincture: A concentrated liquid form that can be taken orally, typically diluted in water. Essential Oil: Juniper berry essential oil can be used in aromatherapy or diluted and applied topically for skin conditions. It should never be ingested.
Dosage	Tea: Use 1 teaspoon of crushed juniper berries per cup of boiling water, steeped for 20 minutes. Drink 1-2 cups daily for up to four weeks. Tincture: Typically, 1-2 ml three times daily. Follow specific product instructions for best results. Essential Oil: For topical use, dilute with a carrier oil according to the product's guidelines.
How long to use	Juniper berries are generally used for short-term health interventions, such as during a UTI or for acute digestive issues, and should not be used for extended periods without a break. Long-term use can lead to kidney irritation and other side effects. A typical course of treatment would be no longer than four weeks.

Kanna

Kanna (Sceletium tortuosum) is a succulent plant native to South Africa, known for its mood-enhancing and sedative properties. Historically, it has been used by indigenous peoples for its psychoactive effects, including relaxation, mood elevation, and to combat stress and anxiety.

Properties	Mood Enhancement: Kanna is known for its ability to improve mood and reduce stress and anxiety, thanks to its serotonergic activity. Sedative: Can have a calming effect, aiding in relaxation and sleep. Cognitive Enhancer: Some users report improved focus and cognitive function at lower doses. Appetite Suppressant: Traditionally used to suppress appetite, although this effect may vary among individuals.
What disease it fights	Anxiety and Stress: The mood-enhancing and sedative properties make it beneficial for those experiencing anxiety and stress. Depression: While not a substitute for professional medical treatment, kanna has been used to alleviate mild to moderate depression symptoms. Insomnia: Its sedative effects may help improve sleep quality in some individuals.
How it works	Kanna's active compounds, including mesembrine and mesembrenone, function as serotonin reuptake inhibitors (SSRIs), similar to some antidepressants. This action increases serotonin levels in the brain, which can enhance mood and reduce anxiety. The exact mechanisms and all active compounds are not fully understood, and effects can vary widely among individuals.
How to use	Oral Ingestion: Kanna can be consumed orally in the form of capsules, tablets, or teas made from dried plant material. Sublingual: Powdered kanna placed under the tongue allows for quick absorption into the bloodstream. Smoking or Vaping: Some users smoke or vape kanna for its psychoactive effects, although this method is less studied and not recommended for health-focused use.
Dosage	Due to the variability in individual reactions and the lack of extensive clinical research, dosages can vary: Oral Ingestion: Start with a low dose, such as 50-100 mg of dried plant material, and adjust based on tolerance and effect. Some products may offer different concentrations, so follow label instructions. Sublingual: 50-150 mg of powdered plant can be used, adjusting for personal tolerance and response.
How long to use	Kanna should be used cautiously, especially considering its psychoactive properties. For stress, anxiety, or mood improvement, it may be used on an as-needed basis. Long-term use should be approached with caution, monitoring for potential side effects or interactions with other medications, especially those affecting serotonin levels.

Kava Kava

Kava Kava (Piper methysticum) is a plant native to the Pacific Islands, where it has been used for centuries in ceremonial drinks for its sedative, anxiolytic, and euphoriant properties. It is primarily used in herbal medicine to relieve anxiety, stress, and insomnia.

Properties	Anxiolytic: Kava Kava is well-known for its ability to reduce anxiety without impairing cognitive function. Sedative: Can promote relaxation and aid in the treatment of insomnia, helping to improve sleep quality. Muscle Relaxant: Offers muscle relaxant effects without the side effects associated with pharmaceutical relaxants. Neuroprotective: Some studies suggest Kava Kava may have neuroprotective benefits due to its interaction with the central nervous system.
What disease it fights	Anxiety Disorders: Effective in reducing symptoms of generalized anxiety disorder (GAD) and social anxiety. Insomnia: Helps improve sleep quality and duration for those struggling with sleep disorders. Stress: Can alleviate physical and mental symptoms of stress. Muscle Tension: Useful in relieving muscle tension and associated pain.
How it works	Kava Kava's active components, known as kavalactones, interact with several neurotransmitter systems in the brain, including GABA, dopamine, and serotonin pathways, which are involved in regulating mood and relaxation. The anxiolytic and sedative effects are thought to be primarily due to the modulation of GABA receptors, similar to how certain anti-anxiety medications work, but without the risk of dependency.
How to use	Beverage: Traditional preparation involves making a beverage from the ground root mixed with water. Capsules/Extracts: For those who prefer not to consume it as a drink, Kava Kava is available in capsules or liquid extracts, which provide a more controlled dosage. Tincture: A liquid form that can be used for easier dose adjustment according to individual needs.
Dosage	Capsules/Extracts: Typical dosages range from 100 to 300 mg of kavalactones per day. It's crucial to start with the lower end of the dosage range and adjust based on the response. Beverage/Tincture: Due to variations in preparation and concentration, follow specific instructions provided with the product or by a healthcare provider.
How long to use	Kava Kava is generally used on an as-needed basis for anxiety and stress, and for periods of a few weeks to a few months for chronic insomnia or anxiety disorders. Continuous long-term use is not recommended without the supervision of a healthcare provider, due to concerns about potential liver toxicity.

Konjac

Konjac (Amorphophallus konjac) is a plant native to Asia, known for its glucomannan content, a highly soluble dietary fiber. It's utilized in traditional Chinese medicine and has gained popularity in the West for weight loss, cholesterol management, and improving digestive health.

Properties	Weight Management: Glucomannan absorbs water and expands in the stomach, which can help to reduce appetite and support weight loss efforts. Digestive Health: Acts as a prebiotic, supporting the growth of beneficial gut bacteria and promoting healthy digestion. Cholesterol Reduction: May help lower cholesterol levels by binding with cholesterol and bile acids in the gut. Blood Sugar Regulation: Slows the absorption of sugar, helping to control blood sugar levels.
What disease it fights	Obesity: By promoting feelings of fullness, it aids in weight management. Constipation: The high fiber content improves bowel movements and prevents constipation. High Cholesterol: Helps reduce LDL (bad) cholesterol levels. Diabetes: Assists in regulating blood glucose levels, beneficial for people with type 2 diabetes.
How it works	Konjac's glucomannan content is key to its health benefits. When consumed, glucomannan absorbs water and expands, forming a bulky fiber in the stomach and intestines. This process can delay gastric emptying, induce satiety (fullness), and slow down glucose absorption, contributing to its effects on weight loss, cholesterol reduction, and blood sugar control.
How to use	Supplements: Konjac is available in capsule or tablet form, which should be taken with water before meals. Food Products: Konjac flour is used to make shirataki noodles, a low-calorie, high-fiber alternative to traditional pasta. Powder: Can be added to smoothies or used as a thickening agent in cooking.
Dosage	For weight loss and cholesterol management: The typical dosage is 1 gram of glucomannan taken with at least 8 ounces of water, 30 minutes to 1 hour before meals, three times a day. For constipation: Dosages may vary; it's important to adjust intake based on individual response and ensure adequate hydration.
How long to use	Konjac can be used as part of a weight management or cholesterol-lowering plan for several weeks to months, under the guidance of a healthcare provider. For chronic conditions like constipation or diabetes, long-term use may be beneficial but should be monitored for safety and effectiveness.

Lavender

Lavender (Lavandula angustifolia) is celebrated for its fragrance and myriad therapeutic properties, including its calming, sedative, anti-inflammatory, and antimicrobial effects. It's widely used in aromatherapy, herbal medicine, and skincare.

Properties	Anxiolytic and Sedative: Lavender oil is renowned for its ability to reduce anxiety and promote relaxation, making it beneficial for stress relief and sleep support. Anti-inflammatory and Analgesic: It can soothe inflammatory conditions and alleviate pain. Antimicrobial: Lavender has been shown to possess antimicrobial properties against a range of pathogens. Antioxidant: Offers protection against oxidative stress and free radical damage.
What disease it fights	Anxiety and Stress: Effective in reducing anxiety levels and managing stress. Insomnia and Sleep Disorders: Helps improve sleep quality and duration. Skin Conditions: Used to treat acne, eczema, and wound healing due to its antimicrobial and anti-inflammatory properties. Minor Burns and Insect Bites: Soothes skin and reduces inflammation.
How it works	Lavender's calming effects on the nervous system are primarily attributed to its volatile oils and compounds like linalool and linalyl acetate, which are absorbed through olfaction and skin application. These compounds interact with the limbic system to induce relaxation and reduce anxiety. Its anti-inflammatory and antimicrobial effects are beneficial for skin health and healing.
How to use	Aromatherapy: Lavender essential oil can be used in diffusers, inhaled directly, or applied to a pillow to promote relaxation and sleep. Topical Application: Diluted lavender oil can be applied to the skin to treat conditions like acne, eczema, or burns. Always dilute with a carrier oil to prevent irritation. Tea: Dried lavender flowers can be steeped in hot water to make a calming tea. Baths: Adding a few drops of lavender oil or dried flowers to bathwater can provide a relaxing and therapeutic experience.
Dosage	Essential Oil for Aromatherapy: A few drops in a diffuser or inhaled directly as needed for relaxation. Topical Application: Mix 1-2 drops of lavender essential oil with a tablespoon of carrier oil before application to the skin. Tea: 1-2 teaspoons of dried lavender flowers per cup of boiling water, steeped for 5-10 minutes. Drink 1-2 cups daily for relaxation.
How long to use	Lavender can be used as needed for immediate relaxation effects or as part of a regular routine for ongoing stress management and sleep support. For skin conditions, use should be evaluated over a few weeks to monitor effectiveness and skin tolerance.

Lemon Balm

Lemon balm (Melissa officinalis) is a perennial herb in the mint family, appreciated for its lemon-scented leaves and its gentle yet powerful health benefits. It's widely used for its calming effects on the nervous system, ability to improve digestion, and its antiviral properties.

Properties	Anxiolytic and Sedative: Lemon balm is well-regarded for its ability to reduce anxiety and promote sleep, making it a valuable herb for those with insomnia or stress-related issues. Digestive Aid: Can relieve symptoms of indigestion, bloating, and gas. Antiviral: Particularly effective against the herpes simplex virus, it can reduce the frequency and severity of outbreaks. Cognitive Enhancer: Some studies suggest lemon balm can improve cognitive function and memory.
What disease it fights	Anxiety and Stress: Helps to alleviate symptoms of anxiety and stress, promoting a sense of calm. Sleep Disorders: Its sedative properties can aid in improving sleep quality and duration. Herpes Virus Infections: Applied topically to treat cold sores or genital herpes lesions. Digestive Problems: Used to relieve various digestive complaints, including indigestion and gas.
How it works	The calming effects of lemon balm are attributed to its impact on the central nervous system, particularly its ability to modulate neurotransmitter activity, thereby reducing anxiety and promoting relaxation. The antiviral properties are mainly due to compounds such as rosmarinic acid, which have been shown to be effective against the herpes simplex virus. Lemon balm also contains terpenes, which contribute to its digestive and cognitive-enhancing benefits.
How to use	Tea: Dried lemon balm leaves can be steeped in hot water to make a soothing tea. This is an excellent way to enjoy its anxiolytic and digestive benefits. Topical Applications: For antiviral properties, particularly against herpes simplex, lemon balm can be applied in cream or ointment form directly to the affected area. Tincture: A concentrated liquid form can be used for stress and anxiety relief. Capsules: Available for those who prefer a more convenient form for anxiety and sleep support.
Dosage	Tea: 1-2 teaspoons of dried lemon balm leaves per cup of boiling water, steeped for 10 minutes. Drink up to 3 cups daily. Topical Cream/Ointment: Apply as directed on the product label, typically 2-4 times daily at the first sign of an outbreak. Tincture: 1-2 ml three times daily, but it's essential to follow specific product instructions. Capsules: Dosages can vary, but typically range from 300-500 mg taken 1-3 times daily for stress and anxiety relief.
How long to use	Lemon balm can be used as needed for relief from anxiety, stress, and indigestion. For sleep disorders, it may be used in the short term or as part of a nightly routine. When used for herpes outbreaks, it should be applied at the first sign of symptoms and continued until the outbreak resolves. As with any herbal remedy, it's wise to periodically assess the benefits and any potential side effects, especially with long-term use.

Lemongrass

Lemongrass (Cymbopogon citratus) is a tropical plant known for its strong lemon scent and flavor, widely used in cooking and herbal medicine. It boasts a range of medicinal properties, including anti-inflammatory, antimicrobial, and analgesic effects. Lemongrass is also appreciated for its ability to relieve anxiety, improve digestion, and boost oral health.

Properties	Antimicrobial: Lemongrass has strong antimicrobial properties, making it effective against various bacteria, fungi, and yeast. Anti-inflammatory: Can reduce inflammation, offering benefits for conditions like arthritis and other inflammatory disorders. Digestive Health: Aids digestion and helps relieve symptoms of bloating and discomfort. Anxiolytic: Exhibits mild sedative properties that can help reduce anxiety and promote relaxation. Antioxidant: Contains antioxidants that protect against oxidative stress and may support overall health.
What disease it fights	Digestive Disorders: Helps in managing digestive issues, including indigestion and gastritis. Anxiety and Stress: The calming effects can alleviate stress and anxiety symptoms. Infections: Its antimicrobial action can be useful in treating infections, including urinary tract infections and oral health issues. Inflammatory Conditions: May provide relief for inflammatory conditions, such as arthritis.
How it works	Lemongrass contains several compounds, including citral, which is responsible for its lemon scent and many of its health benefits. Citral and other components have antimicrobial and anti-inflammatory properties, helping to fight infections and reduce inflammation. The herb's essential oils can also affect the central nervous system, providing anxiolytic effects and aiding in relaxation and sleep.
How to use	Tea: Lemongrass leaves can be boiled or steeped in hot water to make a herbal tea, often consumed for digestive or calming effects. Essential Oil: Lemongrass oil can be used in aromatherapy or diluted and applied topically for pain relief, but it should not be ingested. Cooking: Fresh or dried lemongrass is widely used in culinary preparations for its flavor.
Dosage	Tea: Use 1-2 teaspoons of fresh or dried lemongrass per cup of boiling water, steeped for 5-10 minutes. Drink 2-3 cups daily. Essential Oil: For topical use, dilute 2-3 drops of lemongrass essential oil in a tablespoon of carrier oil. For aromatherapy, follow the diffuser's instructions.
How long to use	Lemongrass tea can be consumed daily as part of a healthy diet for its general health benefits. For specific health issues like digestive disorders or anxiety, it may be used for several weeks to monitor its effectiveness. Essential oils and topical applications should be used with caution, and long-term use should be discussed with a healthcare provider.

Licorice Root

Licorice root (Glycyrrhiza glabra) is an herb that has been used for thousands of years in various cultures for its medicinal properties. It's known for its ability to soothe gastrointestinal problems, relieve respiratory issues, reduce stress, and support adrenal function.

Properties	Gastrointestinal Relief: Licorice root can soothe gastrointestinal issues due to its anti-inflammatory and mucosal protective properties, making it effective for conditions like acid reflux, gastritis, and ulcers. Adrenal Support: Contains compounds that may support adrenal gland function, which is crucial for producing hormones that respond to stress. Antiviral and Antimicrobial: Exhibits antiviral and antimicrobial activities, potentially effective against certain pathogens. Anti-inflammatory: Its anti-inflammatory properties can help relieve pain and discomfort associated with various conditions.
What disease it fights	Gastrointestinal Disorders: Including peptic ulcers, heartburn, and gastritis. Respiratory Conditions: Used to treat coughs and sore throats by acting as an expectorant. Adrenal Insufficiency: May help in managing conditions related to adrenal fatigue by supporting cortisol production. Skin Conditions: Applied topically, licorice can treat eczema, acne, and other inflammatory skin conditions.
How it works	The primary active component of licorice root, glycyrrhizin, is responsible for most of its therapeutic effects. Glycyrrhizin can inhibit the breakdown of adrenal hormones like cortisol, helping to manage stress and reduce inflammation. It also enhances mucous production in the gastrointestinal tract, providing a protective effect and aiding in the healing of ulcers.
How to use	Tea: Licorice root can be steeped in hot water to make a tea, often used for gastrointestinal and respiratory relief. Capsules/Supplements: For those who prefer not to drink the tea, licorice is available in capsule or tablet form. Tincture: A liquid extract of licorice can be taken orally or added to water. Topical Applications: Licorice extract is used in various skincare products to treat eczema, acne, and other skin conditions.
Dosage	Tea: Use 1 teaspoon of dried licorice root per cup of boiling water, steeped for 5-10 minutes. Drink 1-3 cups daily. Capsules/Supplements: Typically, 200-600 mg of licorice root extract is taken daily, divided into several doses. Products should be standardized to glycyrrhizin content. Tincture: 1-2 ml three times daily, but it's essential to follow specific product instructions.
How long to use	Licorice root is generally used for short-term treatment, up to 4-6 weeks, due to potential side effects from long-term use, such as increased blood pressure and potassium loss. For chronic conditions or extended use, it's crucial to monitor health effects and consult with a healthcare provider.

Linden Flower

Linden flower (Tilia spp.) has been traditionally used in herbal medicine for its calming, sedative, and anti-inflammatory properties. It's often turned to for relief from anxiety, tension, and to help with sleep disturbances. Additionally, linden flower has benefits for digestive health and can help alleviate cold and flu symptoms due to its diaphoretic (sweat-inducing) action.

Properties	Sedative and Anxiolytic: Linden flower is renowned for its calming effects, helping to reduce anxiety and promote relaxation. Diaphoretic: Can induce sweating and is useful in managing fevers associated with the cold and flu. Anti-inflammatory: Offers anti-inflammatory benefits, which can help with conditions such as arthritis and other inflammatory disorders. Digestive Aid: Soothes the digestive tract, alleviating symptoms of indigestion and bloating.
What disease it fights	Anxiety and Stress: Helps to calm the nervous system, reducing symptoms of anxiety and stress. Insomnia and Sleep Disorders: Its sedative properties can aid in improving sleep quality. Colds and Flu: The diaphoretic action can help manage fever and alleviate symptoms of colds and flu. Inflammatory Conditions: May provide relief from inflammation-related discomfort.
How it works	The calming effects of linden flower are attributed to its flavonoids and other phytochemicals that have sedative properties, which can help soothe the nervous system. Its diaphoretic action helps in managing fevers by promoting sweating and thereby reducing body temperature.
How to use	Tea: Linden flower tea is a popular way to enjoy its benefits, particularly for relaxation and managing cold symptoms. Tincture: A concentrated liquid form can be taken for more precise dosing. Bath: Adding linden flowers to bathwater can provide a soothing and relaxing experience.
Dosage	Tea: Use 1-2 teaspoons of dried linden flowers per cup of boiling water, steeped for 10-15 minutes. Drink 2-3 cups daily as needed for relaxation or cold symptoms. Tincture: Typically, 1-2 ml three times daily, but follow specific product instructions or consult a healthcare provider for guidance. Bath: A handful of dried flowers can be added directly to bathwater or used in a muslin bag.
How long to use	Linden flower can be used safely for short-term relief of symptoms like anxiety, stress, and colds, generally up to a few weeks. For ongoing use, especially for chronic conditions or regular sleep aid, it's wise to consult a healthcare provider to monitor effectiveness and ensure no adverse effects arise, particularly given concerns about potential heart damage with prolonged and excessive use.

Lotus

Lotus (Nelumbo nucifera), also known as the sacred lotus, is a plant that holds significant cultural and medicinal value, particularly in Asia. It's used in traditional medicine to treat a variety of conditions thanks to its multiple beneficial properties, encompassing every part of the plant—from leaves to seeds to roots.

Properties	Antioxidant: Lotus parts contain compounds that help protect cells from oxidative stress. Anti-inflammatory: Reduces inflammation, beneficial for conditions like arthritis and skin inflammation. Sedative: Some components have calming effects, which can help in reducing stress and improving sleep quality. Digestive Health: Lotus seeds are used to improve digestion and alleviate diarrhea. Heart Health: The plant contains compounds that can help regulate blood pressure and lipid levels, supporting cardiovascular health.
What disease it fights	Digestive Disorders: Lotus seeds are traditionally used to treat digestive issues, including diarrhea and bloating. Stress and Anxiety: Its sedative properties can aid in relaxation and managing stress and anxiety. Skin Conditions: Applied topically, lotus can help in treating inflammation and improving skin health. Heart Disease: Components of the lotus may help in managing blood pressure and cholesterol, contributing to heart health.
How it works	The lotus plant's health benefits are attributed to its rich content of phytochemicals, including flavonoids, alkaloids, and saponins. These compounds collectively contribute to its antioxidant, anti-inflammatory, and sedative effects. Flavonoids and alkaloids, for example, can improve cardiovascular health by regulating blood pressure and cholesterol levels.
How to use	Tea: Lotus leaf tea is commonly consumed for its health benefits, including stress reduction and weight management. Seeds: Lotus seeds can be eaten raw, roasted, or ground into flour and used in traditional dishes for digestive health. Topical Application: Lotus oil or extracts from the flowers and leaves can be applied to the skin for their anti-inflammatory and soothing properties.
Dosage	Tea: Steep 5-10 grams of dried lotus leaves in hot water for 5-10 minutes. Drink 1-2 times daily. Seeds: A typical serving of lotus seeds ranges from 15 to 30 grams, eaten as a snack or incorporated into meals. Topical Application: Use lotus-infused oils or creams as directed, typically applied once or twice daily.
How long to use	Lotus can be used as part of a daily diet or skincare routine for ongoing health benefits. For specific conditions like digestive disorders or acute stress, it might be used for shorter periods (weeks to months) until symptoms improve.

Maca

Maca (Lepidium meyenii) is a root vegetable native to the Andes Mountains of Peru, known for its nutritional richness and its use as a medicinal herb. It's traditionally been used to enhance energy, stamina, and libido. Maca is also noted for its hormone-balancing effects, making it particularly beneficial for managing symptoms of menopause and enhancing fertility.

Properties	Hormonal Balance: Maca can help regulate and support the hormonal system without containing hormones itself. Energy and Stamina: Known for boosting energy and physical stamina, maca is popular among athletes and those seeking an increase in vitality. Libido Enhancer: Often used to increase sexual desire and function in both men and women. Mood Improvement: Contains flavonoids that can improve mood and reduce anxiety and depression symptoms. Nutritional: Rich in vitamins, minerals, and amino acids, providing overall nutritional support.
What disease it fights	Hormonal Imbalances: Useful in alleviating symptoms related to menopause, such as hot flashes and mood swings, and supporting prostate health. Low Libido and Fertility Issues: Can enhance sexual function and fertility in both men and women. Fatigue: Its energizing effects can help combat fatigue and increase overall energy levels. Mood Disorders: May help improve symptoms of depression and anxiety.
How it works	The exact mechanism by which maca affects the endocrine system is not fully understood, but it's believed to act on the hypothalamus and pituitary gland, helping to balance the adrenal, thyroid, pancreas, ovarian, and testicular glands. Its nutritional composition also plays a significant role in its overall health benefits, providing essential vitamins, minerals, and amino acids that support bodily functions.
How to use	Powder: Maca is commonly available in powder form, which can be added to smoothies, juices, or food. Capsules: For those who prefer a more convenient form, maca is also available in capsules. Tincture: A liquid extract form can be used for those looking for rapid absorption.
Dosage	Powder: 1-3 teaspoons (3-9 grams) per day mixed into beverages or food. Capsules: Follow the manufacturer's recommendations, typically around 500-1000 mg taken three times daily. Tincture: Follow specific product instructions, usually 1-2 ml, three times a day.
How long to use	Maca can be used over extended periods as it is essentially a food product. Some people may experience benefits within a few days, while for others, it might take weeks. Continuous use for up to several months is common, but it's wise to assess its effects on your body periodically.

Mallow

Mallow (Malva sylvestris), also known as common mallow, is a plant with a long history in herbal medicine, valued for its soothing, anti-inflammatory, and emollient properties. It's used to treat a variety of conditions, particularly those involving the skin, respiratory system, and digestive tract.

Properties	Soothing and Demulcent: Mallow is rich in mucilage, which soothes and protects irritated or inflamed tissue, making it excellent for sore throats, coughs, and digestive issues. Anti-inflammatory: Helps to reduce inflammation, beneficial for treating skin conditions and internal inflammation. Emollient: Softens and moisturizes the skin, helpful for dry skin, eczema, and other skin irritations. Diuretic: Promotes the production of urine, aiding in the detoxification process.
What disease it fights	Respiratory Conditions: Effective in relieving symptoms of coughs, colds, and bronchitis by soothing irritated mucous membranes. Skin Disorders: Used topically to soothe and heal eczema, psoriasis, and other inflammatory skin conditions. Digestive Issues: Its demulcent properties can alleviate discomfort associated with gastritis, indigestion, and ulcers. Urinary Tract Infections: The diuretic effect helps flush the urinary system, supporting the treatment of infections.
How it works	The health benefits of mallow largely stem from its high mucilage content, which forms a protective layer over mucous membranes, relieving irritation and inflammation. This action not only helps soothe the digestive and respiratory tracts but also aids in skin health by providing moisture and reducing inflammation.
How to use	Tea: Infusions made from mallow leaves or flowers can be consumed for internal health benefits or used as a gargle for sore throats. Topical Application: A poultice of mallow leaves can be applied to the skin to soothe irritation and inflammation. Bath Additive: Leaves and flowers can be added to bathwater for a soothing and emollient effect on the skin.
Dosage	Tea: Steep 1-2 teaspoons of dried mallow leaves or flowers in boiling water for 10-15 minutes. Drink 2-3 cups daily. Topical Application: Apply the poultice or infused oil to the affected area several times a day as needed. Bath Additive: Add a handful of mallow leaves and flowers to a warm bath and soak to relieve skin irritations.
How long to use	For acute conditions, mallow can be used until symptoms improve, typically within a few days to a week. For chronic issues or ongoing skin care, it may be used as part of a regular regimen, with duration tailored to individual needs and responses.

Marigold

Marigold, particularly Calendula officinalis, is a plant with vibrant yellow and orange flowers known for its healing, anti-inflammatory, and antimicrobial properties.

Properties	Wound Healing: Calendula promotes the healing of wounds, cuts, bruises, and insect bites through its anti-inflammatory and antimicrobial properties. Anti-inflammatory: Effective in reducing inflammation in the skin and body, making it useful for conditions like dermatitis, eczema, and hemorrhoids. Antimicrobial: Exhibits antibacterial and antifungal activities, which help prevent wound infection and treat minor skin infections. Skin Health: Supports skin health by improving blood flow to the skin areas applied, aiding in skin repair and regeneration.
What disease it fights	Skin Disorders: Used topically for treating wounds, burns, eczema, and acne due to its healing properties. Inflammatory Conditions: Can relieve symptoms of inflammation in conditions like dermatitis, varicose veins, and hemorrhoids. Menstrual Pain: Some oral preparations of calendula may help in reducing menstrual cramps, though more research is needed in this area.
How it works	Calendula contains various compounds, including flavonoids, triterpenoids, and carotenoids, which contribute to its healing, anti-inflammatory, and antimicrobial effects. These compounds help to promote tissue repair, reduce inflammation, and fight off infection, supporting the skin's healing process.
How to use	Topical Application: Calendula is commonly used in creams, ointments, and salves applied directly to the skin for healing and reducing inflammation. Tea: Calendula flowers can be steeped in hot water to make a tea, which can be consumed or used as a wash for its healing properties. Tincture: A concentrated liquid form that can be diluted in water and applied to the skin or used as a gargle for oral health issues.
Dosage	Topical Creams/Ointments: Apply to the affected area 2-3 times daily or as needed. Tea: 1-2 teaspoons of dried calendula flowers per cup of boiling water, steeped for 10 minutes. Drink or use as a wash 2-3 times daily. Tincture: For skin applications or mouth rinses, dilute 1-2 ml of tincture in a cup of water. Use 2-3 times daily.
How long to use	Marigold (Calendula) preparations can be used as needed to promote healing of skin conditions or for the duration of symptoms. For chronic conditions, it's wise to consult a healthcare provider for guidance on long-term use. Continuous use on the skin should be monitored for any signs of irritation or allergic reaction.

Marshmallow Root

Marshmallow root (Althaea officinalis) is a perennial herb known for its mucilaginous properties, making it an effective natural remedy for soothing irritation and inflammation in the mucous membranes. It has been traditionally used for digestive issues, respiratory problems, and skin health.

Properties	Mucilaginous: Rich in mucilage, marshmallow root can soothe and protect irritated or inflamed tissue. Anti-inflammatory: Helps reduce inflammation in the digestive tract, respiratory system, and skin. Immune Modulating: May support the immune system through its mucilage content and antioxidant properties. Hydrating: The mucilage can retain water, aiding in hydration and skin moisturization.
What disease it fights	Digestive Disorders: Effective in treating conditions like gastritis, peptic ulcers, and irritable bowel syndrome (IBS) by coating and protecting the digestive tract. Respiratory Ailments: Soothes coughs and sore throats and helps with conditions such as bronchitis and asthma by relieving irritation in the throat and bronchial tubes. Skin Conditions: Used topically to soothe eczema, dermatitis, and burns.
How it works	The high mucilage content of marshmallow root forms a protective layer on mucous membranes, reducing irritation and inflammation. This soothing effect can benefit the digestive system, respiratory tract, and skin. Additionally, its anti-inflammatory properties help to reduce swelling and pain in affected areas.
How to use	Tea: A cold infusion or tea made from marshmallow root is commonly used to maximize its mucilaginous properties. Capsules: For those who prefer a more convenient form, marshmallow root is available in capsules. Topical Application: As a cream or ointment for soothing irritated skin. Mouthwash: A solution made from marshmallow root can be used to soothe sore throats or mouth ulcers.
Dosage	Tea: 1-2 tablespoons of dried root soaked in cold water for several hours or overnight; drink 2-3 cups daily. Capsules: Typically, 400-500 mg taken 3 times daily, but follow the manufacturer's recommendations. Topical Application: Apply as directed on the product label, usually 2-3 times daily as needed. Mouthwash/Gargle: Use the tea or diluted tincture as a mouthwash several times a day.
How long to use	Marshmallow root can be used for short-term relief of acute conditions or symptoms. For chronic issues, it may be incorporated into a daily regimen for several weeks, but its long-term use should be monitored for effectiveness and any potential side effects. As with any herbal remedy, it's wise to consult a healthcare provider for guidance, especially for long-term use or if you have existing health conditions.

Milk Thistle

Milk thistle (Silybum marianum) is a plant known for its active ingredient, silymarin, which has potent hepatoprotective properties, making it a valuable herb for liver health.

Properties	Hepatoprotective: Protects the liver cells from toxins and helps regenerate damaged liver tissue. Antioxidant: Silymarin has strong antioxidant properties that help protect the body from oxidative stress. Anti-inflammatory: Helps reduce inflammation, which is beneficial for liver health and other conditions. Detoxification Support: Aids in the detoxification process by supporting the liver in processing and eliminating toxins.
What disease it fights	Liver Disorders: Including hepatitis, cirrhosis, jaundice, and liver damage caused by toxins (such as alcohol and certain medications). Gallbladder Issues: Can aid in gallbladder function and help prevent or treat gallstones. High Cholesterol: May help lower cholesterol levels by improving liver function.
How it works	Milk thistle's hepatoprotective effects are primarily due to its active compound, silymarin, which acts as an antioxidant and anti-inflammatory agent. Silymarin enhances liver function by preventing the depletion of glutathione (an essential antioxidant in the liver), stimulating liver cell regeneration, and blocking toxins from entering liver cells.
How to use	Capsules/Tablets: Milk thistle is most commonly taken in supplement form for its silymarin content. Tea: Although less potent than extracts, milk thistle tea can be used for general liver support. Tincture: A liquid extract that can be taken directly or added to water.
Dosage	Capsules/Tablets: The standard dosage for milk thistle extract (standardized to 70-80% silymarin) is 140-210 mg taken 2-3 times daily. Tea: 1-2 teaspoons of crushed milk thistle seeds steeped in hot water for 10-15 minutes. Drink 1-2 cups daily. Tincture: Follow the manufacturer's instructions, typically 1-2 ml three times daily.
How long to use	Milk thistle can be used over extended periods for chronic liver conditions, often several months to a year, depending on the condition and response to the herb. For general liver support and detoxification, shorter periods (a few weeks to a couple of months) may be sufficient.

Mint

Mint (Mentha spp.) encompasses a variety of plants, including peppermint (Mentha piperita) and spearmint (Mentha spicata), known for their refreshing flavor and medicinal properties. Mint leaves have been used traditionally to aid digestion, relieve symptoms of irritable bowel syndrome (IBS), reduce nausea, and improve oral health.

Properties	Digestive Aid: Mint is well-known for its ability to soothe digestive issues and promote healthy digestion. Antimicrobial: Exhibits antimicrobial properties against bacteria and fungi, contributing to its use in oral health. Anti-inflammatory: Contains compounds that reduce inflammation, which can help with conditions like arthritis and IBS. Antispasmodic: Relieves spasms in the digestive tract, making it beneficial for treating IBS and nausea.
What disease it fights	Digestive Disorders: Helps relieve symptoms of indigestion, gas, and bloating. It's particularly beneficial for IBS. Nausea and Vomiting: Mint can help reduce feelings of nausea and is often used during pregnancy for morning sickness. Oral Health Issues: Its antimicrobial properties make it effective in combating bad breath and improving oral hygiene. Respiratory Conditions: Mint contains menthol, which is soothing for the throat and helps alleviate symptoms of colds and coughs.
How it works	Mint's beneficial effects are primarily due to its active compound, menthol, which has antispasmodic and cooling effects on the digestive tract and skin. Menthol also relaxes the muscles of the digestive system, easing cramps and spasms, and has a mild anesthetic effect that can soothe sore throats.
How to use	Tea: Fresh or dried mint leaves can be steeped in hot water to make a soothing tea for digestive or respiratory relief. Topical Application: Mint oil (diluted with a carrier oil) can be applied to the skin for muscle pain and headache relief. Inhalation: Inhaling mint essential oil can help clear nasal passages and relieve respiratory symptoms. Culinary Use: Fresh mint leaves can be added to a variety of dishes for flavor and health benefits.
Dosage	Tea: Use 1-2 teaspoons of dried mint leaves (or a small handful of fresh) per cup of boiling water, steeped for 5-10 minutes. Drink up to 3 cups daily. Essential Oil: For topical application, dilute 2-3 drops of mint essential oil in a tablespoon of carrier oil. For inhalation, add 2-3 drops to a bowl of hot water or a diffuser.
How long to use	Mint can be used safely as a culinary herb or in tea form on a daily basis for general health benefits. For specific health issues, such as digestive disorders or nausea, mint can be used for short-term relief or as part of a longer-term health strategy, under the guidance of a healthcare provider.

Mistletoe

Mistletoe (Viscum album) is a parasitic plant known for its traditional use in treating various health conditions, including hypertension, respiratory issues, and even as an adjunct treatment in cancer therapy. Its use spans many cultures and includes applications aimed at improving immune function and overall well-being.

Properties	Immunomodulatory: Mistletoe is noted for its ability to modulate the immune system, potentially beneficial in cancer treatment and for enhancing general immune function. Anticancer: Some components in mistletoe have been studied for their anticancer properties, particularly in the context of integrative cancer therapy. Cardiovascular Health: Traditionally used to treat hypertension and improve heart health due to its vasodilatory effects. Sedative: Can have a calming effect on the nervous system, helpful in reducing anxiety and promoting better sleep.
What disease it fights	Cancer: Research has explored mistletoe's role in cancer treatment, particularly as an adjunct to conventional therapies, aiming to improve quality of life and reduce side effects of chemotherapy and radiation. Hypertension: Its vasodilatory effects may help in managing high blood pressure. Respiratory Conditions: Used in traditional medicine to treat asthma and other respiratory ailments. Anxiety and Insomnia: The sedative properties of mistletoe can aid in reducing anxiety and improving sleep quality.
How it works	Mistletoe contains a variety of biologically active compounds, including lectins and viscotoxins, which are thought to contribute to its immunomodulatory and anticancer effects. These substances can stimulate the immune system, potentially helping to target and destroy cancer cells. Additionally, mistletoe's effects on the cardiovascular system can aid in lowering blood pressure and improving heart health.
How to use	Injectable Forms: Most research on mistletoe's anticancer effects involves injectable forms administered under the guidance of healthcare professionals, especially within integrative cancer treatment protocols. Extracts and Tinctures: For non-cancer-related uses, such as for hypertension or anxiety, mistletoe can be taken in the form of extracts or tinctures.
Dosage	Given the complexity and potential risks associated with mistletoe, especially in injectable form for cancer treatment, dosages should be determined by healthcare providers experienced in its use. For extracts or tinctures used for hypertension or anxiety, follow the manufacturer's instructions or the advice of a healthcare provider.
How long to use	The duration of mistletoe use can vary widely depending on the condition being treated and the form in which it's used. For cancer therapy, its use may be ongoing under medical supervision. For other conditions, short to medium-term use (several weeks to months) is common, with periodic evaluation to assess effectiveness and side effects.

Motherwort

Motherwort (Leonurus cardiaca) is a perennial herb in the mint family, valued for its sedative, heart tonic, and emmenagogue properties. Traditionally, it has been used to treat heart conditions, relieve menstrual and menopausal symptoms, and reduce anxiety and stress.

Properties	Cardiotonic: Supports heart health by improving blood flow and potentially regulating heart rate. Anxiolytic: Offers anxiety-reducing effects, helping to calm the nervous system. Emmenagogue: Can stimulate menstrual flow and help relieve menstrual cramps. Hypotensive: May help in lowering high blood pressure, contributing to cardiovascular health.
What disease it fights	Cardiovascular Issues: Used to treat conditions like heart palpitations, hypertension, and to improve overall heart function. Menstrual and Menopausal Symptoms: Relieves cramps, regulates menstrual flow, and helps with symptoms associated with menopause. Anxiety and Stress: Its calming properties can reduce anxiety and stress levels. Hyperthyroidism: There is anecdotal evidence that motherwort can be beneficial for managing symptoms of hyperthyroidism, though more research is needed.
How it works	Motherwort's benefits are attributed to its bioactive compounds, including alkaloids, flavonoids, and phenolic acids, which collectively contribute to its cardiotonic, anxiolytic, and hypotensive effects. These compounds can help modulate the nervous system, reduce inflammation, and improve cardiovascular health.
How to use	Tea: Dried motherwort can be steeped in hot water to make tea. This method is commonly used for menstrual and menopausal symptoms as well as for anxiety relief. Tincture: A more concentrated form, useful for precise dosing, especially for cardiovascular benefits and anxiety reduction. Capsules: For those who prefer not to taste the herb, capsules offer a convenient alternative.
Dosage	Tea: 1-2 teaspoons of dried herb per cup of boiling water, steeped for 10-15 minutes. Drink 1-3 times daily. Tincture: Generally, 1-2 ml three times a day. However, dosages can vary, so it's important to follow the product's specific recommendations or consult with a healthcare provider. Capsules: Follow the manufacturer's instructions, usually taken 1-3 times daily.
How long to use	Motherwort can be used as needed for acute relief of symptoms like menstrual cramps or anxiety. For chronic conditions like hypertension or ongoing stress management, it may be incorporated into daily routines for several weeks to months. As with any herbal remedy, it's advisable to periodically evaluate its effectiveness and any potential side effects, especially with long-term use.

Mugwort

Mugwort (Artemisia vulgaris) is a plant with a long history of use in herbal medicine, known for its versatile properties including digestive, nervine, and emmenagogue effects. It has been traditionally used for its ability to stimulate digestion, ease menstrual cramps, support dream work, and as a general tonic for the nervous system.

Properties	Digestive Aid: Mugwort is known to stimulate digestion and alleviate gastrointestinal issues such as bloating, gas, and indigestion. Emmenagogue: It has properties that can stimulate menstrual flow and relieve menstrual cramps. Nervine: Offers support for the nervous system, potentially reducing anxiety and promoting relaxation. Dream Enhancement: Traditionally used to enhance dream recall and vividness, often placed under pillows for prophetic dreams.
What disease it fights	Digestive Disorders: Useful in treating a range of digestive complaints, improving overall digestive health. Menstrual Discomfort: Helps in managing painful menstruation and irregular cycles. Anxiety and Stress: Its calming properties can alleviate symptoms of anxiety and stress. Sleep and Dream Issues: May aid in achieving a more restful sleep and enhancing dream work.
How it works	Mugwort's effects are attributed to its diverse array of bioactive compounds, including volatile oils, flavonoids, and sesquiterpenes, which together contribute to its digestive, nervine, and emmenagogue properties. These compounds stimulate the digestive system, soothe the nervous system, and support uterine health.
How to use	Tea: Dried mugwort leaves can be steeped in hot water to make tea, often used for digestive issues and menstrual cramps. Tincture: A concentrated liquid form can be taken for more precise dosing, particularly for its nervine effects. Smudging: Dried mugwort is sometimes burned for purification and relaxation, akin to sage. Dream Pillows: Dried mugwort leaves placed in pillows to promote vivid dreams.
Dosage	Tea: 1-2 teaspoons of dried mugwort per cup of boiling water, steeped for 10-15 minutes. Drink 1-2 cups daily, especially before bedtime for dream enhancement or during menstruation for cramp relief. Tincture: Generally, 1-2 ml taken 2-3 times a day. Follow specific product instructions or consult a healthcare provider.
How long to use	Mugwort can be used as needed for immediate relief of digestive discomfort or menstrual cramps. For ongoing issues like stress management or menstrual irregularities, it might be incorporated into daily routines for several weeks to months. However, due to its powerful effects, especially as an emmenagogue, long-term continuous use should be approached with caution and under the guidance of a healthcare provider.

Mullein

Mullein (Verbascum thapsus) is an herb known for its soft, woolly leaves and tall flower spikes, widely used in herbal medicine for respiratory ailments. Its properties include being a demulcent, expectorant, anti-inflammatory, and antispasmodic, making it particularly effective for coughs, colds, and bronchial issues.

Properties	Demulcent: Mullein's high mucilage content soothes irritated mucous membranes in the respiratory system. Expectorant: Aids in the expulsion of mucus from the lungs and throat, making it beneficial for conditions like bronchitis and asthma. Anti-inflammatory: Helps reduce inflammation in the respiratory tract, soothing symptoms of coughs and sore throats. Antispasmodic: Can relieve spasms in the respiratory system, easing dry coughs and helping in conditions like asthma.
What disease it fights	Respiratory Ailments: Mullein is most commonly used for respiratory conditions, including coughs, colds, bronchitis, and asthma, due to its soothing and expectorant properties. Ear Infections: Mullein oil, often combined with garlic oil, can be used as a remedy for ear infections. Inflammatory Conditions: Its anti-inflammatory properties make it useful for addressing inflammation-related pain and discomfort.
How it works	Mullein works by soothing the respiratory system with its mucilaginous content, which coats the throat and lungs, alleviating irritation. Its expectorant properties help clear mucus, making breathing easier, while its anti-inflammatory compounds reduce swelling in the respiratory tract.
How to use	Tea: Dried mullein leaves and flowers can be steeped in boiling water to make a tea. This method is commonly used for respiratory issues. Tincture: A concentrated liquid form of mullein can be taken orally for internal use. Ear Drops: Mullein oil is used topically as ear drops for ear infections. Ensure it's specifically prepared for this use. Inhalation: Steam inhalation with mullein leaves can also provide relief for respiratory conditions.
Dosage	Tea: Use 1-2 teaspoons of dried mullein per cup of boiling water, steeped for 10-15 minutes. Drink up to 3 cups daily. Tincture: Typically, 1-4 ml of tincture three times a day. Follow specific product instructions. Ear Drops: Use as directed on the product label, usually a few drops in the affected ear.
How long to use	Mullein can be used for the duration of acute respiratory symptoms, usually a few days to a week. For chronic respiratory conditions, it may be used longer, but it's wise to consult a healthcare provider for guidance on long-term use, especially to ensure the underlying condition is appropriately managed.

Nettle

Stinging nettle (Urtica dioica) is a perennial plant widely recognized for its nutritional value and therapeutic properties. Rich in vitamins, minerals, and phytonutrients, nettle is used for its anti-inflammatory, diuretic, and analgesic effects. It has been traditionally employed to treat a variety of conditions, including allergies, arthritis, urinary issues, and eczema.

Properties	Anti-inflammatory: Nettle is known for its ability to reduce inflammation, making it beneficial for conditions like arthritis and allergies. Diuretic: Helps in flushing toxins from the body, supporting kidney health and reducing edema. Nutritional: High in vitamins A, C, and K, minerals like iron, magnesium, and calcium, and rich in chlorophyll. Antihistamine: Nettle can relieve allergy symptoms by acting as a natural antihistamine. Analgesic: Offers pain relief, useful in conditions like arthritis or for general pain management.
What disease it fights	Allergic Rhinitis: Effective in reducing symptoms of hay fever and other allergies. Arthritis and Joint Pain: Its anti-inflammatory and analgesic properties help alleviate joint pain and stiffness. Urinary Tract Health: The diuretic effect aids in treating urinary tract infections (UTIs) and supports prostate health. Anemia: High in iron, nettle can help improve iron levels and overall blood health.
How it works	Nettle's health benefits are attributed to its broad spectrum of vitamins, minerals, and phytonutrients, including flavonoids and phenolic compounds, which contribute to its anti-inflammatory and antioxidant effects. Its diuretic properties are beneficial for removing waste and excess fluid from the body, while the natural antihistamines can reduce allergic reactions.
How to use	Tea: Dried nettle leaves can be steeped in hot water to make a nutritious tea. Capsules/Supplements: Nettle is available in capsule form, offering a convenient way to consume its extract. Topical Applications: Nettle leaf extract can be applied to the skin for conditions like eczema. Cooked Greens: Fresh nettle leaves can be cooked and eaten like spinach, providing a nutritious addition to meals.
Dosage	Tea: Use 1-2 teaspoons of dried nettle leaves per cup of boiling water, steeped for 10 minutes. Drink 2-3 cups daily. Capsules/Supplements: Typically, 300-500 mg of nettle leaf extract taken three times daily. Follow the product's specific recommendations. Topical Applications: Apply as directed on the product label, usually 2-3 times daily.
How long to use	Nettle can be used safely over extended periods for chronic conditions like allergies or arthritis. For acute symptoms, such as during allergy season, it might be used for several weeks to months. As with any supplement, it's wise to periodically evaluate its effectiveness and any potential side effects.

Oat Straw

Oat straw, made from the stems, leaves, and flowers of the oat plant (Avena sativa) before it fully matures, is rich in nutrients and has been cherished in herbal medicine for its soothing and restorative properties. It's especially known for supporting nervous system health, improving sleep, enhancing mood, and boosting cognitive function.

Properties	Nervine: Supports the nervous system, helping to reduce stress and anxiety, and improve sleep quality. Nutritive: High in vitamins and minerals, including magnesium, iron, and B vitamins, which contribute to its overall health benefits. Antidepressant: Some components of oat straw may have a mild antidepressant effect, contributing to mood enhancement. Cognitive Enhancer: Studies suggest oat straw can improve cognitive performance, including attention and focus.
What disease it fights	Anxiety and Stress: Helps alleviate symptoms of stress and anxiety, promoting a sense of calm. Sleep Disorders: Can improve sleep quality and duration, beneficial for those with insomnia. Mild Depression: The mood-enhancing properties may help manage symptoms of mild depression. Cognitive Decline: Its potential cognitive-enhancing effects make it a candidate for preventing or mitigating cognitive decline.
How it works	The beneficial effects of oat straw are attributed to its rich nutritional profile and bioactive compounds, which nourish the body and support brain health. These compounds, including avenanthramides, have antioxidant properties and may enhance blood flow to the brain, contributing to improved cognitive functions and mood regulation.
How to use	Tea: Oat straw can be brewed as a tea, offering a gentle way to ingest its benefits. Tincture: A liquid extract provides a concentrated form, often used for therapeutic purposes. Bath: An oat straw bath can soothe and relax the body, beneficial for skin health and stress relief. Supplements: Available in capsule or powder form for those seeking a more convenient intake method.
Dosage	Tea: Steep 1-2 teaspoons of dried oat straw in a cup of boiling water for 10-15 minutes. Drink 1-3 cups daily. Tincture: Typically, 2-4 ml three times a day. Follow specific product instructions. Bath: Add a handful of oat straw to a cloth bag and place it in bathwater, soaking for at least 15 minutes. Supplements: Follow the manufacturer's instructions, usually around 350-500 mg per day.
How long to use	Oat straw is suitable for long-term use due to its gentle nature and nutritional benefits. For addressing specific conditions like anxiety or cognitive decline, it may be incorporated into daily routines for several weeks to months to observe significant benefits. As with any herbal remedy, it's wise to periodically evaluate its effectiveness and consult a healthcare provider, especially for long-term use.

Olive Leaf

Olive leaf, derived from the olive tree (Olea europaea), is celebrated for its medicinal properties, largely attributed to the compound oleuropein. This natural compound provides olive leaf with its antioxidant, anti-inflammatory, antimicrobial, and cardioprotective effects.

Properties	Antioxidant: Olive leaf is rich in antioxidants, helping to protect the body from oxidative damage caused by free radicals. Antimicrobial: Exhibits broad-spectrum antimicrobial activity against bacteria, viruses, and fungi. Anti-inflammatory: Can reduce inflammation in the body, which is beneficial for conditions associated with chronic inflammation. Cardioprotective: Supports heart health by lowering blood pressure and cholesterol levels.
What disease it fights	Infections: Its antimicrobial properties make it effective in fighting various microbial infections. Hypertension: Olive leaf can help lower high blood pressure, contributing to cardiovascular health. Diabetes: May improve insulin sensitivity and help regulate blood sugar levels. Chronic Inflammation: Useful in managing conditions related to inflammation, such as arthritis.
How it works	The health benefits of olive leaf are primarily due to oleuropein and other phenolic compounds. Oleuropein has been shown to have a powerful antioxidant effect, which protects cells from oxidative damage. Additionally, it can inhibit the growth of a wide range of pathogens, reduce inflammation, and improve cardiovascular health by affecting the pathways involved in blood pressure regulation and lipid metabolism.
How to use	Supplements: Olive leaf is commonly taken in capsule or tablet form for its convenience and concentrated dose. Tea: Dried olive leaves can be steeped in hot water to make a tea, offering a gentler dosage. Extract: Liquid olive leaf extract can be used for a more potent and flexible dosing option.
Dosage	Supplements: The typical dosage for olive leaf extract supplements is 500-1000 mg daily, standardized to contain a specific percentage of oleuropein. Tea: Use 1-2 teaspoons of dried olive leaves per cup of boiling water, steeped for 10-15 minutes. Drink 1-3 cups daily. Extract: Dosage can vary depending on the concentration of the extract; follow the product's specific recommendations or consult with a healthcare provider.
How long to use	Olive leaf can be used as a short-term remedy for acute conditions or as part of a long-term wellness regimen, particularly for chronic diseases like hypertension or diabetes. It's advisable to periodically assess the effects and consult with a healthcare professional, especially when used over extended periods, to ensure continued safety and effectiveness.

Oregano

Oregano, particularly its oil form known as oil of oregano (derived from the leaves of the Origanum vulgare plant), is celebrated for its potent antimicrobial, antioxidant, anti-inflammatory, and antifungal properties. This herb is widely used in holistic health practices for treating various conditions, especially infections and digestive issues.

Properties	Antimicrobial: Oil of oregano is known for its ability to fight bacteria, viruses, and fungi, making it a natural antibiotic. Antioxidant: Contains powerful antioxidants that can protect the body from oxidative stress and free radical damage. Anti-inflammatory: Offers anti-inflammatory benefits that can help reduce inflammation throughout the body. Antifungal: Effective in treating fungal infections, including candida overgrowth.
What disease it fights	Respiratory Infections: Used to treat and prevent illnesses like the common cold, flu, and bronchitis due to its antimicrobial properties. Digestive Problems: Helps in relieving digestive issues, including bloating, gas, and indigestion, and can combat gastrointestinal infections. Skin Conditions: Applied topically (in a diluted form) to treat fungal and bacterial skin infections. Candida Overgrowth: Its antifungal action is beneficial in managing candida-related issues.
How it works	The primary active components in oregano, carvacrol, and thymol, are responsible for its antimicrobial and antifungal effects. These compounds disrupt the cell membranes of bacteria and fungi, leading to their destruction. The anti-inflammatory and antioxidant effects of oregano further support the body's healing processes.
How to use	Oil of Oregano Supplements: Available in capsules or liquid form, taken orally for internal infections or digestive health. Dried Oregano: Can be used in cooking or made into a tea for a milder health support. Topical Application: Diluted oil of oregano can be applied to the skin for fungal infections, but it must be diluted to avoid irritation.
Dosage	Oil of Oregano Supplements: For the oil, a common dose is 1-3 drops taken 2-3 times daily, mixed with water or under the tongue, for short-term use. Capsule dosages depend on the concentration and should follow the manufacturer's instructions. Dried Oregano for Tea: Steep 1-2 teaspoons of dried oregano in a cup of boiling water for 5-10 minutes. Drink 1-2 cups daily. Topical Application: Mix 1 drop of oil of oregano with a teaspoon of a carrier oil (like coconut or olive oil) before application.
How long to use	Oil of oregano is typically used for short-term treatment, not exceeding two to three weeks, due to its potent nature. For chronic conditions or ongoing support, such as digestive health, using dried oregano in cooking or tea may be more appropriate for long-term use.

Parsley

Parsley (Petroselinum crispum) is not only a popular culinary herb but also a powerful medicinal plant, known for its diuretic, antioxidant, anti-inflammatory, and nutritive properties. It's rich in vitamins A, C, and K, iron, and flavonoids, making it beneficial for supporting kidney health, enhancing detoxification, boosting immunity, and promoting cardiovascular health.

Properties	Diuretic: Helps increase urine production, supporting kidney function and the body's natural detoxification processes. Antioxidant: Rich in vitamins C and A, parsley can help protect the body from oxidative stress and free radical damage. Anti-inflammatory: Contains compounds that reduce inflammation, potentially benefiting conditions like arthritis. Nutritive: A great source of vitamins and minerals, supporting overall health and well-being.
What disease it fights	Urinary Tract Infections (UTIs): The diuretic effect helps flush out bacteria from the urinary tract. Hypertension: By promoting increased urine output, parsley can help lower blood pressure. Digestive Disorders: Aids in digestion and helps reduce bloating and gas. Anemia: High in iron, parsley can help improve iron levels and combat anemia.
How it works	Parsley's diuretic effect is attributed to its high potassium content, which helps balance fluid levels in the body without causing potassium depletion, unlike some synthetic diuretics. Its antioxidants, particularly vitamin C and flavonoids, protect cells from damage and support immune function. The anti-inflammatory effects are likely due to its volatile oil content, including eugenol.
How to use	Fresh Leaves: Incorporating fresh parsley into your diet, either as a garnish or in salads, soups, and smoothies, is an easy way to enjoy its health benefits. Tea: Parsley tea can be made from fresh or dried leaves and is particularly useful for its diuretic properties. Juice: Parsley can be juiced, often combined with other vegetables, for a concentrated nutritive boost. Supplements: Available in capsules for those seeking a more concentrated dose of parsley's beneficial compounds.
Dosage	Fresh Leaves: There are no specific dosage recommendations; incorporating parsley into meals as desired is generally considered safe. Tea: Steep 1-2 teaspoons of dried parsley or a small handful of fresh parsley in a cup of boiling water for 10 minutes. Drink 1-2 cups daily. Juice: Can be consumed in small amounts daily, typically not exceeding one-half cup (4 ounces or 118 ml). Supplements: Follow the manufacturer's instructions, typically involving taking 1-2 capsules daily.
How long to use	Parsley can be safely consumed daily in culinary amounts. For medicinal purposes, such as using parsley tea or juice for its diuretic effects, it's typically used on a short-term basis, ranging from a few days to a few weeks. Long-term use of high doses should be monitored for potential side effects, particularly for those with kidney disease or those taking blood thinners due to its high vitamin K content.

Passionflower

Passionflower (Passiflora incarnata) is widely recognized for its calming and sedative properties, making it a popular herb for treating anxiety, insomnia, and stress-related disorders. This climbing vine, characterized by its beautiful flowers, has been used in traditional medicine for centuries.

Properties	Anxiolytic: Passionflower is known for its ability to reduce anxiety without the side effects commonly associated with synthetic sedatives. Sedative: Helps promote relaxation and improve sleep quality, making it beneficial for those with insomnia. Antispasmodic: Can relieve muscle spasms and help with conditions like seizures or hysteria. Hypotensive: Some studies suggest passionflower may help lower blood pressure due to its calming effects.
What disease it fights	Anxiety and Stress: Effective in managing general anxiety and reducing stress levels. Sleep Disorders: Helps improve sleep quality and duration, beneficial for people experiencing insomnia. Menopausal Symptoms: May alleviate hot flashes and mood swings associated with menopause. Hypertension: Its calming properties can indirectly help in managing high blood pressure.
How it works	The calming effects of passionflower are attributed to a variety of phytochemicals it contains, including flavonoids and alkaloids. These compounds interact with the central nervous system, enhancing the efficacy of gamma-aminobutyric acid (GABA), a neurotransmitter that reduces the activity of nerve cells, promoting relaxation and reducing anxiety.
How to use	Tea: Dried passionflower can be steeped in hot water to make a soothing tea. Capsules/Extracts: Available in capsule or liquid extract form for those who prefer a more concentrated or convenient option. Tincture: A liquid form that can be used to precisely control dosage according to individual needs.
Dosage	Tea: Use 1 teaspoon of dried passionflower per cup of boiling water, steeped for 10 minutes. Drink 1-3 cups daily, especially before bedtime for sleep disorders. Capsules/Extracts: Typically, 400-800 mg of extract is taken daily, divided into 2-3 doses. Follow the product's specific recommendations. Tincture: 0.5-2 ml three times a day, although dosages can vary based on the concentration of the tincture.
How long to use	Passionflower is generally used for short to medium-term management of conditions like anxiety and insomnia, ranging from a few weeks to a couple of months. Long-term use should be approached with caution, and it's wise to consult a healthcare provider to monitor effectiveness and adjust the treatment as necessary.

Patchouli

Patchouli (Pogostemon cablin) is a fragrant herb from the mint family, known for its distinctive scent and versatile use in perfumery, skincare, and traditional medicine. The essential oil extracted from its leaves is valued for its grounding, mood-enhancing, and skin-healing properties.

Properties	Antidepressant: Patchouli oil can help uplift the mood, alleviate symptoms of depression, and reduce anxiety. Antimicrobial: Exhibits antibacterial and antifungal properties, making it beneficial for skin health and wound healing. Anti-inflammatory: Useful in reducing inflammation, especially in skin conditions like eczema or dermatitis. Astringent: Helps tighten the skin, which can be beneficial for acne and skin irritation.
What disease it fights	Skin Conditions: Effective in treating acne, eczema, and dandruff due to its antimicrobial and anti-inflammatory properties. Stress and Anxiety: The grounding aroma of patchouli oil is used in aromatherapy to reduce stress and anxiety levels. Fungal Infections: Its antifungal properties make it useful in treating athlete's foot and other fungal infections.
How it works	Patchouli oil's health benefits are primarily attributed to its chemical composition, including patchoulol, alpha-guaiene, and beta-caryophyllene, which contribute to its distinctive aroma and therapeutic effects. These compounds interact with the brain's limbic system through olfaction, influencing mood and stress levels. Additionally, they provide antimicrobial and anti-inflammatory effects when applied topically.
How to use	Aromatherapy: Used in diffusers, inhalers, or added to bathwater to harness its mood-enhancing and stress-relieving effects. Topical Application: Diluted in a carrier oil and applied to the skin to treat acne, eczema, or fungal infections. Always dilute patchouli essential oil to a safe concentration (usually 2-3% for most adults). Perfumery and Skincare: Incorporated into lotions, creams, and perfumes for its scent and skin-healing properties.
Dosage	Aromatherapy: There's no strict dosage for inhalation. Use as needed or preferred in a diffuser, following the device's guidelines. Topical Application: When diluted, patchouli oil can be applied 1-2 times daily to the affected area. For a 2% dilution, mix 12 drops of patchouli oil with 1 ounce (30 ml) of carrier oil.
How long to use	For acute conditions like skin irritation or fungal infections, patchouli oil can be used until symptoms improve. As part of aromatherapy for stress or anxiety, it can be used as needed over an extended period. Long-term topical use should be monitored for any skin reactions or sensitivities.

Peppermint

Peppermint (Mentha piperita) is a popular herb known for its refreshing flavor and a wide array of medicinal properties. It's highly valued for its digestive, analgesic, and antimicrobial benefits.

Properties	Digestive Aid: Peppermint is well-known for its ability to soothe digestive issues, such as indigestion, gas, and irritable bowel syndrome (IBS). Analgesic: Offers pain relief, especially useful for headaches and muscle pain. Antimicrobial: Exhibits antimicrobial properties that can help fight certain types of bacteria and viruses. Antispasmodic: Can relieve spasms in the gastrointestinal tract, making it effective for IBS and nausea.
What disease it fights	Digestive Disorders: Particularly effective in managing symptoms of IBS, nausea, and indigestion. Headaches and Migraines: Topical application of peppermint oil can alleviate headache pain. Common Colds and Flu: The menthol in peppermint acts as a decongestant, helping to clear nasal passageways. Dental Issues: Its antimicrobial properties contribute to oral health, reducing bad breath and preventing dental plaque.
How it works	Peppermint's primary active ingredient, menthol, is responsible for many of its therapeutic effects. Menthol has a cooling effect on the skin and mucous membranes, helps relax the muscles of the digestive tract, and can inhibit the growth of certain bacteria and fungi. Its ability to alleviate headaches is partly due to its muscle-relaxing properties and its capability to improve blood flow.
How to use	Tea: Drinking peppermint tea is a common way to soothe digestive discomforts. Essential Oil: Peppermint oil can be used topically for headaches or muscle pain and inhaled for respiratory relief. Always dilute with a carrier oil for topical use. Capsules: Enteric-coated peppermint oil capsules are specifically used for treating IBS, as they pass through the stomach intact and dissolve in the intestines.
Dosage	Tea: Use 1-2 teaspoons of dried peppermint leaves per cup of boiling water, steeped for 10 minutes. Drink up to 3-4 cups daily. Essential Oil: For headache relief, apply a 10% dilution (about 2 drops of essential oil per teaspoon of carrier oil) to the temples and forehead, avoiding the eye area. Capsules: Typically, 0.2-0.4 ml of peppermint oil in enteric-coated capsules taken three times daily.
How long to use	Peppermint tea can be consumed regularly as part of a daily diet. For specific conditions like IBS, enteric-coated capsules are often used for a few weeks to months under medical guidance. Essential oil applications for acute issues like headaches should be used as needed, monitoring for any skin irritation or adverse reactions.

Plantain

Plantain (Plantago major for broadleaf plantain or Plantago lanceolata for narrowleaf plantain) is a common herb often found in yards and along roadsides, known for its medicinal properties. It's utilized in traditional medicine for wound healing, as an anti-inflammatory, for respiratory conditions, and for its antimicrobial effects.

Properties	Wound Healing: Plantain leaves have a high mucilage content, which can soothe and protect wounds, promoting healing. Anti-inflammatory: Contains compounds that reduce inflammation, helpful in treating skin conditions, and gastrointestinal inflammation. Antimicrobial: Exhibits antibacterial and antiviral properties, making it useful in preventing infection in wounds and treating respiratory infections. Respiratory Aid: Acts as an expectorant, helping to clear mucus from the respiratory tract, which is beneficial for coughs, colds, and bronchitis.
What disease it fights	Skin Injuries and Conditions: Effective in treating cuts, scrapes, insect bites, and eczema. Respiratory Disorders: Used to alleviate symptoms of colds, coughs, and bronchitis. Digestive Issues: Can relieve inflammation in the gastrointestinal tract, aiding in the treatment of ulcers and irritable bowel syndrome (IBS). Oral Health: The antimicrobial properties help in treating mouth ulcers and gum infections.
How it works	Plantain works through several mechanisms depending on the condition being treated. The mucilage provides a protective layer over wounds and inflamed tissues, promoting healing and reducing pain. The anti-inflammatory effect is attributed to flavonoids and other phytochemicals, which also contribute to its antimicrobial activity against bacteria and viruses. Additionally, certain compounds in plantain can help thin and expel mucus, supporting respiratory health.
How to use	Fresh Leaves: Crushed or chewed leaves can be applied directly to the skin for wounds or used as a poultice for inflammation. Tea: Dried leaves can be steeped in hot water to make a tea for respiratory or digestive issues. Tincture: A concentrated liquid form can be used internally for respiratory health or diluted and used as a mouth rinse for oral health. Ointment: Plantain-infused oils can be made into ointments for skin conditions.
Dosage	Tea: Use 1-2 teaspoons of dried plantain leaves per cup of boiling water, steeped for 10 minutes. Drink up to 3 cups daily. Tincture: Typically, 1-2 ml three times a day. Adjust based on the strength of the tincture and the condition being treated. Topical: Apply fresh leaves or ointment to the affected area several times a day as needed.
How long to use	For acute conditions like wounds or respiratory infections, plantain can be used until symptoms improve, typically for a few days to a week. For chronic conditions or ongoing support, such as digestive health, use might extend for several weeks to months, monitoring for effectiveness and any adverse reactions.

Pomegranate

Pomegranate (Punica granatum) is celebrated not only for its delicious fruit but also for its numerous health benefits, stemming from its rich antioxidant content. This fruit, along with its juice, seeds, and even the peel, has been used traditionally and in modern times for its anti-inflammatory, cardioprotective, and anticancer properties.

Properties	Antioxidant: Pomegranates are loaded with antioxidants, particularly punicalagins and tannins, which help protect the body from oxidative stress and inflammation. Cardioprotective: Regular consumption can improve heart health by reducing blood pressure, decreasing cholesterol levels, and increasing blood flow. Anticancer: Some studies suggest pomegranate may inhibit cancer cell growth and promote cancer cell death, particularly in prostate and breast cancer. Anti-inflammatory: Its compounds can reduce inflammation in the body, potentially benefiting conditions like arthritis and chronic inflammatory diseases.
What disease it fights	Cardiovascular Diseases: Helps lower risk factors for heart disease, including high blood pressure and high cholesterol. Cancer: May help prevent and slow the progression of certain types of cancer. Diabetes: Antioxidants in pomegranate can help improve insulin sensitivity and blood glucose levels. Digestive Health: Pomegranate juice and peel extract can support gut health and reduce inflammation in the gut.
How it works	The health benefits of pomegranate are primarily due to its high concentration of antioxidants, which scavenge free radicals, reducing oxidative damage and inflammation. These effects can contribute to its protective properties against various diseases, including supporting cardiovascular health, potentially preventing cancer, and managing blood sugar levels.
How to use	Fresh Fruit and Juice: Consuming the fruit directly or drinking pomegranate juice is the most common way to enjoy its health benefits. Extract Supplements: Pomegranate extract, available in capsules or liquid, can provide a concentrated dose of its beneficial compounds. Peel Powder: The dried, powdered peel can be used in teas or as a supplement, offering additional antioxidants and fiber.
Dosage	Fresh Fruit and Juice: There is no specific dosage but consuming 1-2 cups of pomegranate juice daily or eating the seeds from one pomegranate can offer health benefits. Extract Supplements: Dosages vary by product; typically, 500-1000 mg of pomegranate extract is taken daily. Always follow the product's specific recommendations. Peel Powder: If using for digestive health, a small amount (around 1 teaspoon) can be added to teas or smoothies.
How long to use	Pomegranate can be incorporated into the daily diet as a regular part of a healthy eating pattern. For specific health conditions or when using concentrated supplements or peel powder, it might be used for several weeks to months, monitoring for effectiveness and any potential side effects.

Prickly Pear

Prickly pear, or Opuntia, is a genus of flowering plants in the cactus family. It's known for its edible fruit, which is rich in vitamins, minerals, antioxidants, and fiber. Prickly pear has been traditionally used to treat diabetes, high cholesterol, obesity, and hangovers. It's also applied topically for wounds and inflammation.

Properties	Antioxidant: High in vitamin C and flavonoids, prickly pear can help protect the body against oxidative stress. Anti-inflammatory: Contains compounds that reduce inflammation, beneficial for conditions like arthritis. Blood Glucose Regulation: Can lower blood sugar levels by decreasing the absorption of sugar in the stomach and intestines. Cholesterol-lowering: Its fiber content can help reduce cholesterol levels.
What disease it fights	Diabetes: Prickly pear can help manage blood sugar levels, making it beneficial for those with diabetes. Obesity: The high fiber content can promote satiety and reduce overall calorie intake. High Cholesterol: Can aid in lowering LDL cholesterol and triglycerides. Hangovers: Some studies suggest it can reduce symptoms by reducing inflammation.
How it works	Prickly pear cactus lowers blood sugar by blocking the absorption of sugar in the intestines. Its fiber content helps in controlling appetite and reducing cholesterol levels. The antioxidants and anti-inflammatory compounds can neutralize free radicals and reduce inflammation in the body.
How to use	Fresh Fruit: The fruit can be eaten raw or used in juices, smoothies, and desserts. Supplements: Prickly pear is available in capsule or powder form for those who prefer a concentrated dose. Topical Application: The juice or pulp can be applied directly to the skin for cuts, wounds, and inflammation.
Dosage	Fresh Fruit: There's no specific dosage; consuming the fruit as part of a balanced diet is generally considered safe. Supplements: For blood sugar regulation, dosages of 500-1000 mg of prickly pear extract before meals have been used in studies. Always follow the product's specific recommendations. Topical Application: Apply as needed directly to the affected area.
How long to use	As a dietary supplement for conditions like diabetes or high cholesterol, prickly pear might be used over an extended period, under the guidance of a healthcare professional. Continuous use should be monitored for effectiveness and any potential side effects. For acute conditions like hangovers, it might be used as needed.

Psyllium

Psyllium (Plantago ovata), specifically the husk derived from its seeds, is renowned for its high soluble fiber content, making it a powerful tool in managing digestive health. It's used extensively as a dietary supplement to improve bowel regularity, lower cholesterol levels, manage blood sugar, and aid in weight management.

Properties	Laxative: Psyllium husk absorbs water in the gut, making bowel movements easier by increasing stool bulk. Cholesterol-lowering: Can help reduce LDL ("bad") cholesterol levels, contributing to heart health. Blood Sugar Regulation: The soluble fiber helps slow down the digestion of food, which can help control blood sugar levels. Appetite Suppressant: Its bulking properties can promote a feeling of fullness, aiding in weight management.
What disease it fights	Constipation: Effectively relieves constipation by increasing stool bulk and softening it, making it easier to pass. High Cholesterol: Regular intake can contribute to lowering high cholesterol levels, potentially reducing the risk of heart disease. Diabetes: Helps manage blood sugar levels, making it beneficial for people with diabetes. Obesity: By promoting satiety, it can help reduce overall calorie intake, supporting weight loss efforts.
How it works	Psyllium husk is rich in soluble fiber, which absorbs water and expands in the colon, forming a gel-like substance. This process helps soften the stool and increases its volume, facilitating smoother passage through the digestive tract. Additionally, the presence of this soluble fiber in the digestive system can bind to fats and sugars, slowing their absorption and aiding in cholesterol and blood sugar management.
How to use	Powder or Husks: Psyllium is most commonly available in powder or whole husk form, which can be mixed with water, juice, or smoothies. Capsules: For those who prefer not to consume it in powder form, psyllium is also available in capsules.
Dosage	Powder or Husks: The typical dosage is 1-2 teaspoons (5-10 grams) mixed with at least 8 ounces (about 240 milliliters) of water or another liquid, taken 1-3 times daily. Capsules: Dosage varies by product, but generally ranges from 2-6 capsules taken with a full glass of water, 1-3 times daily.
How long to use	Psyllium can be used daily as part of a long-term strategy for managing constipation, high cholesterol, blood sugar levels, or for weight management. It's important to start with a lower dose to assess your tolerance and gradually increase as needed, ensuring adequate fluid intake to prevent digestive discomfort.

Raspberry Leaf

Raspberry leaf (Rubus idaeus) has been traditionally esteemed for its use in women's health, particularly during pregnancy, childbirth, and menstruation. Rich in vitamins and minerals, including magnesium, potassium, iron, and B vitamins, raspberry leaf supports uterine health and can ease menstrual discomfort.

Properties	Uterine Tonic: Strengthens and tones the uterine muscles, which can help prepare the body for a more efficient labor. Menstrual Relief: Eases menstrual cramps and regulates heavy menstrual flow due to its antispasmodic properties. Nutritive: High in essential nutrients that support overall health and wellness. Digestive Aid: The leaves also contain tannins, which can aid in relieving nausea, diarrhea, and gastrointestinal upset.
What disease it fights	Pregnancy-Related Issues: Used to support uterine health, ease labor, and assist in postpartum recovery. Menstrual Discomfort: Relieves symptoms of PMS and menstrual cramps, promoting a more regular menstrual cycle. Digestive Problems: Can help in managing diarrhea and gastrointestinal inflammation.
How it works	Raspberry leaf's effectiveness is attributed to its high content of vitamins, minerals, and phytochemicals, which together contribute to its uterine-toning, anti-inflammatory, and antispasmodic effects. These components work synergistically to strengthen uterine muscles, potentially making childbirth more efficient, and to relieve menstrual cramps by relaxing uterine muscles.
How to use	Tea: The most common form of consumption is tea made from dried raspberry leaves. Capsules: For those who prefer not to drink tea, raspberry leaf is also available in capsule form.
Dosage	Tea: 1-2 teaspoons of dried raspberry leaves steeped in boiling water for 10-15 minutes. Pregnant women often start with one cup a day in the second trimester and increase to two or three cups as they approach their due date. Capsules: Follow the manufacturer's instructions, but typically, the dosage is around 400-500 mg taken 1-3 times daily.
How long to use	For menstrual relief, raspberry leaf can be used a few days before and during menstruation each month. In pregnancy, it's commonly used from the second trimester onward under the guidance of a healthcare provider. As with any herbal remedy, especially during pregnancy, it's important to consult with a healthcare professional to determine the appropriate dosage and duration of use based on individual health needs and circumstances.

Red Clover

Red clover (Trifolium pratense) is a perennial herb that has been traditionally used for various health conditions, particularly those related to menopause, skin health, and cardiovascular wellness. It's rich in isoflavones, a type of phytoestrogen, which can mimic estrogen in the body, making it particularly beneficial for menopausal symptoms.

Properties	Phytoestrogenic: Red clover isoflavones can act similarly to estrogen, helpful in balancing hormone levels, especially during menopause. Blood Purifier: Traditionally used to support detoxification and improve circulation. Anti-inflammatory: Can help reduce inflammation throughout the body, beneficial for skin conditions and general health. Cardioprotective: May improve cardiovascular health by improving arterial elasticity and reducing cholesterol levels.
What disease it fights	Menopausal Symptoms: Helps alleviate hot flashes, night sweats, and hormonal imbalances. Skin Conditions: Used to treat eczema, psoriasis, and acne due to its anti-inflammatory and detoxifying properties. Osteoporosis: The phytoestrogens in red clover can help improve bone density. Cardiovascular Health: Can assist in lowering LDL cholesterol and improving arterial flexibility.
How it works	The isoflavones in red clover act as phytoestrogens, which can bind to estrogen receptors in the body, helping to alleviate symptoms associated with estrogen deficiency. Its anti-inflammatory properties are beneficial for skin health and overall inflammation reduction. Additionally, red clover has been shown to have a positive effect on cardiovascular health by improving arterial flexibility and potentially lowering cholesterol levels.
How to use	Tea: Dried flowers can be steeped in hot water to make a herbal tea. Capsules/Supplements: For those who prefer a more convenient form, red clover is available in capsules or as a liquid extract. Topical Applications: Some products are designed for external use, particularly for skin conditions.
Dosage	Tea: 1-2 teaspoons of dried red clover flowers steeped in 8 ounces of boiling water for 15-30 minutes. Drink 2-3 cups daily. Capsules/Supplements: Typically, 40-80 mg of red clover isoflavones per day, divided into 2 doses. Follow the manufacturer's recommendations. Topical Applications: Use as directed on the product label.
How long to use	Red clover can be used for several months to manage menopausal symptoms or support skin health. However, due to its phytoestrogen content, long-term use should be approached with caution. It's advisable to take breaks from use and consult a healthcare professional, especially for individuals with hormone-sensitive conditions.

Rhodiola

Rhodiola rosea, often referred to simply as Rhodiola, is an herb renowned for its adaptogenic properties, meaning it helps the body resist various stressors, both physical and emotional. It grows in cold regions of the world, including the Arctic and mountains of Central Asia.

Properties	Adaptogenic: Rhodiola supports the body's ability to cope with stress. Antifatigue: It has been shown to reduce symptoms of fatigue and improve mental performance, especially during periods of stress or intense work. Antidepressant: Rhodiola may help alleviate mild to moderate depression, promoting emotional well-being. Cardioprotective: Offers benefits for heart health by reducing stress-induced damage and regulating heart rate.
What disease it fights	Stress and Anxiety: Helps manage stress levels and reduces anxiety, enhancing mental clarity and focus. Fatigue: Effective in combating physical and mental fatigue, including chronic fatigue syndrome. Depression: May offer relief from mild to moderate depression without the side effects of conventional antidepressants. Physical Performance: Can improve endurance and physical performance, making it popular among athletes.
How it works	Rhodiola works by influencing key neurotransmitters in the brain, including serotonin, dopamine, and norepinephrine, which play essential roles in mood regulation and response to stress. It also affects the stress-response system by helping to balance the hormones involved in the body's reaction to stress, such as cortisol.
How to use	Capsules/Tablets: Rhodiola is commonly taken in supplement form for convenience and precise dosing. Tea: While less common, Rhodiola can be brewed as a tea, although this may not provide as strong a dose as supplements. Tincture: A liquid extract offers another way to consume Rhodiola, allowing for adjustable dosing.
Dosage	Capsules/Tablets: The recommended dosage can vary, but a common range is 200-600 mg daily, usually taken in the morning to avoid potential interference with sleep. It's often advised to start with a lower dose to assess tolerance. Tea/Tincture: Due to variation in strength and concentration, follow manufacturer or practitioner guidelines.
How long to use	Rhodiola is generally considered safe for short-term use, ranging from a few weeks to several months. Long-term effects are less well understood, so it's wise to consult with a healthcare provider for guidance on extended use, particularly for managing chronic conditions.

Rose Hips

Rose hips, the fruit of the rose plant, are rich in vitamin C, antioxidants, and bioflavonoids, making them an excellent natural remedy for boosting the immune system, promoting skin health, and reducing inflammation.

Properties	Immune Boosting: High vitamin C content supports the immune system, helping to prevent and fight off infections. Anti-inflammatory: Contains anti-inflammatory compounds that can help with arthritis and other inflammatory conditions. Antioxidant: Rich in antioxidants that protect cells from oxidative stress and reduce the risk of chronic diseases. Skin Health: Vitamin C and antioxidants promote collagen production, aiding in skin repair and reducing signs of aging.
What disease it fights	Common Colds and Flu: The high vitamin C content can help reduce the severity and duration of colds. Arthritis: Anti-inflammatory properties may reduce symptoms of arthritis and joint pain. Cardiovascular Health: Antioxidants in rose hips can improve heart health by lowering cholesterol levels and blood pressure. Skin Conditions: Supports skin regeneration and may help in treating conditions like eczema and acne.
How it works	The health benefits of rose hips are attributed primarily to their high concentration of vitamin C, which is essential for immune function, skin health, and collagen production. Additionally, the bioflavonoids and other antioxidants present in rose hips work synergistically with vitamin C to enhance its absorption and effectiveness, combat free radicals, and reduce inflammation.
How to use	Tea: Dried rose hips can be steeped in boiling water to make a tea, often consumed for its immune-boosting and anti-inflammatory benefits. Capsules/Supplements: For those seeking a more concentrated form, rose hips are available in capsules or as powdered supplements. Topical Application: Rose hip oil, extracted from the seeds, is used in skincare for its moisturizing and healing properties.
Dosage	Tea: Use about 1-2 tablespoons of dried rose hips per cup of boiling water, steeped for 10-15 minutes. Drink 1-3 cups daily. Capsules/Supplements: Dosages can vary; typically, 500-1000 mg of rose hip extract is taken daily. Follow the manufacturer's instructions. Topical Application: Rose hip oil can be applied directly to the skin, usually a few drops once or twice daily.
How long to use	Rose hips can be used regularly as part of a daily diet or supplement regimen for ongoing support of immune health, skin health, and inflammation reduction. For acute conditions like colds or flare-ups of arthritis, they might be used for the duration of symptoms. As with any supplement, it's advisable to periodically evaluate the effectiveness and any potential side effects, especially with long-term use.

Rosemary

Rosemary (Rosmarinus officinalis) is a fragrant herb known for its culinary, medicinal, and aromatic properties. It's rich in antioxidants and anti-inflammatory compounds, making it beneficial for cognitive health, digestion, and potentially for hair growth and circulatory improvement.

Properties	Cognitive Enhancer: Rosemary is reputed to improve memory and concentration, partly due to its antioxidant properties. Digestive Aid: It can help relieve digestive discomfort, such as bloating or indigestion. Antimicrobial: Exhibits antimicrobial activity, making it useful in treating infections and preserving food. Anti-inflammatory: Contains compounds that reduce inflammation, potentially benefiting conditions like arthritis.
What disease it fights	Cognitive Decline: May protect against cognitive impairment and support brain health. Digestive Issues: Helps in managing digestive disorders and improving liver function. Hair Loss: Rosemary oil is often used topically to stimulate hair growth and improve scalp health. Respiratory Conditions: Its antimicrobial and anti-inflammatory effects can help treat respiratory infections.
How it works	The active compounds in rosemary, such as rosmarinic acid, carnosic acid, and essential oils, contribute to its health benefits. These compounds have antioxidant effects that protect neural cells from damage, improve blood circulation to the brain, and reduce inflammation. Additionally, rosemary can aid in the production of digestive enzymes, improving digestion and liver function.
How to use	Culinary: Fresh or dried rosemary can be used in cooking to flavor dishes. Tea: Steeping the leaves in hot water to make tea can help with digestion and provide antioxidant benefits. Essential Oil: Applied topically (diluted) for hair growth, or inhaled for cognitive benefits and respiratory health. Supplements: Available in capsules or extracts for those seeking more concentrated forms of rosemary's active compounds.
Dosage	Tea: 1-2 teaspoons of dried rosemary per cup of boiling water, steeped for about 10 minutes. Drink up to 2 cups daily. Essential Oil: For hair treatment, mix a few drops with a carrier oil and apply to the scalp. For inhalation, use in a diffuser according to the manufacturer's instructions. Supplements: Dosage varies by product; follow the manufacturer's recommendations, typically ranging from 400-600 mg daily for extracts.
How long to use	Rosemary can be consumed regularly in culinary amounts with no specific duration. For therapeutic uses, such as tea or supplements, it might be used for specific periods depending on the health issue being addressed, ranging from a few weeks to several months. Essential oils or topical applications should be monitored for skin reactions and effectiveness.

Sage

Sage (Salvia officinalis) is a perennial, evergreen herb with a long history of medicinal use. It's known for its aromatic leaves, which are rich in essential oils, antioxidants, and anti-inflammatory compounds. Sage has been used traditionally to enhance cognitive function, treat digestive problems, relieve sore throats, and reduce menopausal symptoms.

Properties	Cognitive Enhancer: Sage is believed to improve memory and cognitive function, making it a subject of interest for Alzheimer's research. Antimicrobial: Its essential oils can fight bacterial and viral infections, especially in the mouth and throat. Anti-inflammatory: Contains compounds that reduce inflammation, which can help with digestive issues and sore throats. Antioxidant: High in antioxidants, sage can protect the body from oxidative stress and support overall health. Menopausal Symptom Relief: Some studies suggest sage can reduce hot flashes and night sweats in menopausal women.
What disease it fights	Cognitive Decline: May protect against memory loss and cognitive impairment. Digestive Problems: Helps relieve indigestion, bloating, and flatulence. Oral Health Issues: Used in mouthwashes and gargles to treat sore throats, gum disease, and mouth ulcers. Menopausal Symptoms: Can alleviate hot flashes, sweating, and mood swings.
How it works	The beneficial effects of sage are attributed to its various active compounds, including rosmarinic acid, carnosic acid, and flavonoids. These substances enhance cognitive function, have antimicrobial and anti-inflammatory properties, and help protect cells from oxidative damage.
How to use	Tea: Dried or fresh sage leaves can be steeped in hot water to make a tea, often used for sore throats or digestive health. Essential Oil: Used in aromatherapy or diluted for topical application, but it must be used cautiously due to its potency. Culinary: Sage is commonly used as a spice in cooking, which can also impart some of its health benefits. Supplements: Available in capsule form for those seeking a more concentrated dose for specific health concerns like menopausal symptoms.
Dosage	Tea: Use 1-2 teaspoons of dried sage or a small handful of fresh leaves per cup of boiling water, steeped for 5-10 minutes. Drink up to 3 cups daily. Essential Oil: Always dilute with a carrier oil (a few drops of sage oil per tablespoon of carrier oil) for topical use. For aromatherapy, follow diffuser instructions. Supplements: Follow the manufacturer's instructions; doses can vary, typically ranging from 300-600 mg daily for menopausal symptoms.
How long to use	Sage can be used daily in culinary amounts indefinitely. For medicinal uses, such as teas or supplements, it's generally safe for short to medium-term use (several weeks to a few months). Long-term use should be monitored for potential side effects, especially when using concentrated forms like essential oils or supplements.

Sandalwood

Sandalwood (Santalum album) is a highly valued wood and oil known for its aromatic properties and extensive use in cosmetics, fragrances, and traditional medicine across various cultures. With its soothing, anti-inflammatory, and antimicrobial characteristics.

Properties	Antimicrobial: Sandalwood oil can inhibit the growth of various bacteria and fungi, making it beneficial for treating skin infections. Anti-inflammatory: Its compounds help reduce inflammation, offering relief in skin conditions and other inflammatory diseases. Sedative: The scent of sandalwood has a calming effect, which can reduce stress and promote relaxation. Astringent: Can tighten the skin, aiding in the healing of minor cuts and providing a clean, smooth complexion.
What disease it fights	Skin Conditions: Effective in treating acne, eczema, psoriasis, and other skin infections due to its antimicrobial and anti-inflammatory properties. Anxiety and Stress: The soothing aroma of sandalwood can help alleviate anxiety, stress, and promote mental clarity and relaxation. Respiratory Conditions: In traditional medicine, it's used to treat coughs and other respiratory issues due to its anti-inflammatory properties.
How it works	Sandalwood oil contains alpha-santalol, a compound that contributes to its antimicrobial and anti-inflammatory effects. These properties make it effective in treating skin conditions and infections. Additionally, the soothing fragrance of sandalwood is believed to impact the limbic system of the brain, which helps in reducing stress and anxiety, promoting a sense of calmness.
How to use	Topical Application: Sandalwood oil can be diluted with a carrier oil and applied to the skin to treat acne, inflammation, or for general skincare. Aromatherapy: Using sandalwood in a diffuser or as part of massage oil can help in reducing stress and improving relaxation. Inhalation: For respiratory benefits, inhaling sandalwood oil vapor can help ease coughs and sore throats.
Dosage	Topical Application: Dilute sandalwood essential oil with a carrier oil (such as almond or jojoba oil) at a ratio of 2-3 drops of essential oil to 1 tablespoon of carrier oil before applying to the skin. Aromatherapy: Use 3-5 drops in a diffuser filled with water, following the manufacturer's instructions.
How long to use	For acute conditions like skin infections or stress, sandalwood can be used until symptoms improve, typically a few days to a week. For ongoing conditions or for general wellness and skincare, sandalwood can be incorporated into daily routines over the longer term, monitoring for any skin sensitivity or adverse reactions.

Sarsaparilla

Sarsaparilla (Smilax spp.) is a tropical plant known for its use in traditional medicine across various cultures. It's famed for its potential to purify the blood, reduce inflammation, and treat skin conditions.

Properties	Detoxifying: Traditionally used to purify the blood and remove toxins from the body. Anti-inflammatory: May help reduce inflammation, beneficial for joint pain and other inflammatory conditions. Antimicrobial: Contains compounds that have been shown to fight certain types of bacteria and fungi. Skin Health: Often used for treating psoriasis, eczema, and acne due to its purported blood purifying and anti-inflammatory properties.
What disease it fights	Skin Conditions: Used to alleviate symptoms of psoriasis, eczema, and acne. Rheumatoid Arthritis: The anti-inflammatory effects can help relieve joint pain associated with arthritis. Syphilis: Historically, sarsaparilla was used to treat syphilis, though modern treatments are more effective. Digestive Health: May aid in improving overall digestive function and relieving related disorders.
How it works	Sarsaparilla's beneficial effects are attributed to its saponins, flavonoids, and phytosterols. These compounds are thought to have detoxifying, anti-inflammatory, and antimicrobial properties. Saponins, in particular, may help in binding endotoxins in the gut, facilitating their removal from the body, which supports the traditional use of sarsaparilla in blood purification and detoxification processes.
How to use	Tea: The root of sarsaparilla can be boiled and simmered to make tea, often consumed for its health benefits. Capsules/Supplements: Sarsaparilla is available in capsule form or as an extract, providing a more concentrated dose of its active compounds. Topical Applications: Though less common, some topical products contain sarsaparilla for its skin health benefits.
Dosage	Tea: Use about 1-2 teaspoons of dried sarsaparilla root per cup of boiling water, simmer for 15-20 minutes, and drink 1-3 cups daily. Capsules/Supplements: Follow the manufacturer's instructions, typically ranging from 100-500 mg of sarsaparilla extract taken up to three times daily.
How long to use	Sarsaparilla can be used for short to medium-term periods, such as a few weeks to a couple of months, especially for addressing specific conditions like skin issues or joint pain. Long-term use should be approached with caution, as excessive consumption could lead to side effects due to its potent active ingredients.

Saw Palmetto

Saw palmetto (Serenoa repens) is a small palm native to the southeastern United States, renowned for its use in treating benign prostatic hyperplasia (BPH), a noncancerous enlargement of the prostate gland, and for its potential benefits in hair loss and urinary tract function.

Properties	Anti-androgenic: Saw palmetto can block 5-alpha-reductase, an enzyme that converts testosterone to dihydrotestosterone (DHT), a hormone associated with hair loss and prostate enlargement. Anti-inflammatory: Helps reduce inflammation in the prostate and other tissues. Urinary Tonic: Improves urinary flow and reduces nighttime urination in men with BPH.
What disease it fights	Benign Prostatic Hyperplasia (BPH): Saw palmetto is most commonly used to treat symptoms of BPH, such as urinary retention and frequent urination. Hair Loss: Its ability to inhibit DHT production can help prevent hair loss in men and women. Urinary Tract Symptoms: May relieve urinary symptoms by improving bladder function and reducing inflammation.
How it works	Saw palmetto's mechanism of action is primarily through its ability to inhibit the enzyme 5-alpha-reductase, reducing the conversion of testosterone to DHT, which is involved in the development of BPH and hair loss. Additionally, its anti-inflammatory properties can alleviate symptoms associated with prostate enlargement and urinary tract issues.
How to use	Capsules/Softgels: Saw palmetto is commonly taken in capsule or softgel form, offering a concentrated dose of its active components. Tea: While less common, saw palmetto berries can be brewed into a tea, though this method may not provide a sufficient dose for therapeutic effects. Tincture: A liquid extract of saw palmetto can also be used, allowing for flexible dosing.
Dosage	Capsules/Softgels: The typical dosage ranges from 160 to 320 mg per day, often divided into two doses, taken with meals to enhance absorption. Tea: If opting for tea, boiling a handful of dried berries in water for about 10-15 minutes is suggested, though efficacy may vary. Tincture: Follow the manufacturer's instructions for dosage, usually a few milliliters per day.
How long to use	For BPH and hair loss, saw palmetto may need to be taken for several weeks to months before improvements are noticed. Continual use under the guidance of a healthcare provider is recommended to monitor effectiveness and adjust dosage as needed.

Schisandra

Schisandra (Schisandra chinensis) is a berry known for its unique flavor profile and adaptogenic properties, meaning it helps the body resist stressors of all kinds, including physical, chemical, and biological. This berry is used in traditional Chinese medicine to promote longevity, stimulate the immune system, and increase energy levels.

Properties	Adaptogenic: Schisandra helps the body adapt to stress and exerts a normalizing effect on overall bodily functions. Liver Protection: Supports liver function and promotes liver health through its hepatoprotective properties. Antioxidant: Contains powerful antioxidants that protect cells from oxidative stress and damage. Immune Boosting: Can enhance immune system performance, making the body more resistant to diseases.
What disease it fights	Stress and Anxiety: By reducing stress hormones in the blood, Schisandra can help manage stress and reduce anxiety. Liver Disorders: Its hepatoprotective effects make it beneficial for people with liver diseases, such as hepatitis. Fatigue: Can increase energy levels and endurance, combating both physical and mental fatigue. Respiratory Conditions: Traditionally used to treat coughs and other respiratory ailments due to its astringent properties.
How it works	Schisandra's adaptogenic effects are attributed to its bioactive compounds, including lignans, which help modulate stress hormones and improve stress response. Its antioxidants and anti-inflammatory compounds protect the liver and other organs from oxidative stress and inflammation, enhancing overall health and resilience.
How to use	Tea: Dried Schisandra berries can be steeped in hot water to make a tea, often consumed for its health benefits. Capsules/Supplements: Schisandra is available in capsule form, providing a convenient way to consume a concentrated dose. Tincture: A liquid extract of Schisandra offers an easy method for dosage adjustment and fast absorption.
Dosage	Tea: Use 1-2 teaspoons of dried Schisandra berries per cup of boiling water, steeped for about 10 minutes. Drink 1-2 cups daily. Capsules/Supplements: Typically, the dosage ranges from 500-2000 mg daily, divided into two doses. Always follow the product's specific recommendations. Tincture: Follow manufacturer guidelines, generally a few milliliters taken 1-3 times daily.
How long to use	Schisandra can be used both for short-term relief from acute conditions like stress and for long-term health support, including liver health and immune function. For ongoing use, it's generally considered safe for several months, but it's advisable to monitor for any side effects and consult with a healthcare provider to assess its effectiveness and safety over time.

Senna

Senna (from the plant genus Senna) is well-known for its potent laxative properties, making it a commonly used remedy for constipation. It contains compounds called sennosides, which irritate the lining of the bowel, inducing a laxative effect.

Properties	Laxative: Senna's sennosides increase gastrointestinal motility, helping to stimulate bowel movements. Detoxifying: Often used in detox teas and regimens to cleanse the colon and eliminate toxins. Anti-parasitic: Some traditional medicine practices use senna to expel intestinal parasites.
What disease it fights	Constipation: Primarily used to relieve occasional constipation and restore regular bowel movements. Hemorrhoids: By facilitating easier bowel movements, senna can help reduce strain and discomfort associated with hemorrhoids.
How it works	Sennosides in senna irritate the bowel lining, which leads to increased intestinal movement and water secretion into the colon, softening stool and promoting its passage. This effect typically occurs within 6 to 12 hours after ingestion.
How to use	Tea: Senna leaves can be steeped in hot water to make a tea. This form allows for easier dosage adjustment. Capsules/Tablets: Senna is also available in capsules or tablets for oral consumption, providing a controlled dose. Liquid Extracts: Liquid forms of senna are available for those who prefer not to take pills or capsules.
Dosage	Tea: Typically, 1-2 teaspoons of dried senna leaves are used per cup of boiling water, steeped for no longer than 10 minutes. It's recommended to drink at bedtime for relief by morning. Capsules/Tablets: The dosage can vary, but generally, it's recommended to start with the lowest possible dose. For adults, this might be 15-30 mg of sennosides. Follow the product's specific instructions. Liquid Extracts: Dosage instructions vary by product; it's important to adhere to the manufacturer's guidelines.
How long to use	Senna should be used for the short-term relief of constipation, typically not longer than 7-10 days, unless under medical supervision. Prolonged use can lead to dependency or loss of normal bowel function, along with other potential side effects like electrolyte imbalances.

Shepherd's Purse

Shepherd's purse (Capsella bursa-pastoris) is a plant known for its unique, purse-shaped seed pods and its use in traditional medicine to treat bleeding and urinary tract issues. It contains compounds that can constrict blood vessels, making it effective for reducing bleeding.

Properties	Hemostatic: Shepherd's purse is best known for its ability to stop bleeding, both internally and externally. Diuretic: Can increase urine output, helping to manage urinary tract conditions and reduce bloating from water retention. Antimicrobial: Exhibits some resistance against bacterial and fungal infections. Anti-inflammatory: May help reduce inflammation, contributing to its use in wound healing and urinary tract support.
What disease it fights	Menorrhagia (Heavy Menstrual Bleeding): Used to reduce heavy menstrual flow. Postpartum Hemorrhage: Traditionally utilized to control bleeding after childbirth. Urinary Tract Infections (UTIs): Its diuretic and antimicrobial effects can support the treatment of UTIs. Nosebleeds and Minor Wounds: Applied topically to stop bleeding from small cuts and nosebleeds.
How it works	The hemostatic effect of shepherd's purse is primarily attributed to its amines (such as histamine, acetylcholine, and tyramine), which induce vasoconstriction, leading to reduced blood flow to the affected area. Additionally, its diuretic properties help promote the elimination of excess fluids from the body, supporting kidney and urinary tract health.
How to use	Tea: Dried shepherd's purse can be steeped in hot water to make tea, often consumed for its diuretic and hemostatic benefits. Tincture: A more concentrated form, used for precise dosing, especially for managing menstrual bleeding or postpartum hemorrhage. Topical Application: Fresh plant material or a prepared poultice can be applied directly to wounds to stop bleeding.
Dosage	Tea: Use 1-2 teaspoons of dried herb per cup of boiling water, steeped for 10-15 minutes. Drink 2-3 cups daily. Tincture: Follow the product's specific instructions, but a general guideline is 1-4 ml three times daily. Topical Application: As needed, based on the size and severity of the wound. Ensure cleanliness to prevent infection.
How long to use	Shepherd's purse should be used on an as-needed basis for acute conditions like heavy menstrual bleeding or to stop bleeding from wounds. For chronic issues like recurring UTIs or to manage menorrhagia, it may be used under the guidance of a healthcare provider for several cycles or as part of a broader treatment plan. Long-term internal use is generally not recommended without medical supervision due to potential side effects and interactions.

Skullcap

Skullcap (Scutellaria lateriflora) is a perennial herb known for its calming and neuroprotective properties, making it a valuable plant in herbal medicine for reducing anxiety, promoting sleep, and supporting overall nervous system health.

Properties	Anxiolytic: Skullcap has a calming effect, helping to reduce anxiety without the sedative effects associated with stronger pharmaceuticals. Nervine: Supports nerve health, potentially beneficial for conditions like insomnia, nervous tension, and even some neurological disorders. Antispasmodic: Can relieve muscle spasms and cramps, contributing to its use in treating conditions such as menstrual cramps and gastrointestinal discomfort. Antioxidant: Contains compounds that protect cells from oxidative stress, supporting overall health.
What disease it fights	Anxiety and Stress: Helps to manage anxiety levels and reduce stress without causing drowsiness. Sleep Disorders: Promotes relaxation and can aid in improving sleep quality. Nervous System Disorders: Its neuroprotective effects may benefit certain neurological conditions by supporting nerve health. Muscle Tension and Spasms: Relieves physical symptoms of stress and tension, including muscle spasms.
How it works	The calming effects of skullcap are attributed to its bioactive compounds, including flavonoids and scutellarin, which modulate neurotransmitter activity in the brain, promoting a sense of relaxation and well-being. These compounds also offer antioxidant protection, reducing cellular damage caused by stress and environmental factors.
How to use	Tea: Dried skullcap leaves can be steeped in hot water to make a soothing tea, often consumed for its anxiolytic and sedative effects. Tincture: A liquid extract of skullcap provides a more concentrated form, allowing for easy dosage adjustment and rapid absorption. Capsules: For those who prefer standardized dosages, skullcap is available in capsule form.
Dosage	Tea: Use 1-2 teaspoons of dried skullcap per cup of boiling water, steeped for 10-15 minutes. Drink up to 3 cups daily. Tincture: Typically, 1-2 ml three times a day. However, dosages can vary, so follow the product's specific recommendations or consult a healthcare provider. Capsules: Follow the manufacturer's instructions; a common dosage is 300-600 mg daily, divided into 2-3 doses.
How long to use	Skullcap can be used for short-term relief of acute symptoms like anxiety and insomnia. For chronic conditions or ongoing stress management, it may be used for several weeks to months, monitoring for effectiveness and any potential side effects. As with any herbal remedy, it's wise to take breaks or reevaluate its use over time.

Slippery Elm

Slippery elm (Ulmus rubra) is valued for its soothing and healing properties, particularly for the digestive tract. Its inner bark contains mucilage, a gel-like substance that swells upon contact with water, forming a protective layer on mucous membranes. This action makes slippery elm an effective natural remedy for various gastrointestinal issues.

Properties	Gastrointestinal Soother: Slippery elm can relieve inflammation and irritation in the digestive tract, making it beneficial for conditions like gastritis, acid reflux, and irritable bowel syndrome (IBS). Demulcent: Its mucilage content coats and protects irritated tissues, helping to heal sore throats, coughs, and ulcers. Nutritive: Provides nutrients that can be easily digested, offering support during convalescence or for individuals with digestive weakness.
What disease it fights	Digestive Disorders: Effective in treating gastritis, peptic ulcers, and IBS by soothing the digestive tract. Respiratory Conditions: Can relieve coughs and sore throats due to its soothing mucilage. Skin Conditions: Applied topically, it can help heal wounds, burns, and skin inflammations.
How it works	When mixed with water, slippery elm's mucilage becomes a slick gel that coats and soothes mucous membranes in the digestive system and throat. This action provides a protective barrier against acidity and irritation, promoting healing of affected tissues. Additionally, the mucilage can aid in the reduction of inflammation and may stimulate nerve endings in the gastrointestinal tract to increase mucus secretion, further protecting the digestive tract.
How to use	Tea: The powdered bark can be mixed with hot water to form a tea or gruel, soothing to the digestive system and throat. Capsules/Tablets: For those who prefer not to taste the herb, slippery elm is available in capsule or tablet form. Topical Application: A poultice made from slippery elm powder can be applied to the skin to heal burns, boils, and other skin conditions.
Dosage	Tea/Gruel: Mix 1 tablespoon of slippery elm powder with hot water to form a paste, then slowly add more water to achieve the desired consistency. Drink 2-3 times daily. Capsules/Tablets: Typically, 400-500 mg capsules are taken 3-4 times daily with a glass of water. Always follow the product's specific recommendations. Topical Application: Prepare a poultice by mixing the powder with enough water to form a paste and apply it directly to the affected area, covering it with a cloth.
How long to use	Slippery elm can be used as needed for acute conditions like sore throats or digestive discomfort. For chronic issues, it may be incorporated into a daily regimen for several weeks to months. However, it's essential to monitor for any potential allergic reactions or side effects and to consult a healthcare provider for long-term use, especially for serious conditions.

Spearmint

Spearmint (Mentha spicata) is a pleasantly aromatic herb known for its culinary and medicinal uses. Similar to other members of the mint family, spearmint offers digestive, anti-inflammatory, and antimicrobial benefits. It's often recommended for gastrointestinal issues, hormonal imbalances, and for its calming effects.

Properties	Digestive Aid: Spearmint can help alleviate symptoms of indigestion, gas, and nausea, making it beneficial for overall digestive health. Antioxidant: Contains antioxidants that protect the body from oxidative stress and inflammation. Hormonal Balance: Some research suggests spearmint tea may reduce androgen levels in women with hormonal imbalances, such as those seen in polycystic ovary syndrome (PCOS). Antimicrobial: Exhibits antibacterial and antifungal properties, which can help in managing oral health and preventing infections.
What disease it fights	Digestive Disorders: Effective in treating indigestion, gas, and nausea. Hormonal Imbalances: May help manage symptoms associated with PCOS and other hormonal conditions. Stress and Anxiety: The aroma of spearmint has a calming effect, which can reduce stress levels. Oral Health Issues: Can improve oral health due to its antimicrobial properties.
How it works	Spearmint aids digestion by relaxing the muscles of the stomach and intestines, which can help relieve symptoms of indigestion and bloating. Its potential effect on hormonal balance is attributed to its antioxidant content, which may influence hormone metabolism. Additionally, the menthol in spearmint provides a soothing effect, beneficial for both digestive and respiratory health.
How to use	Tea: Spearmint leaves can be steeped in hot water to make a soothing tea. This is a common method for enjoying its digestive and hormonal benefits. Culinary: Fresh or dried spearmint leaves are widely used in cooking and as a flavoring agent in food and beverages. Aromatherapy: The essential oil of spearmint can be used in aromatherapy for its calming effects.
Dosage	Tea: Use 1-2 teaspoons of dried spearmint leaves or a small handful of fresh leaves per cup of boiling water, steeped for 5-10 minutes. Drink 2-3 cups daily. Culinary: There's no specific dosage for culinary use; spearmint can be added to dishes according to personal taste preferences. Aromatherapy: Use spearmint essential oil according to the diffuser's instructions or dilute with a carrier oil for topical application.
How long to use	Spearmint tea can be consumed daily as part of a regular diet for ongoing support of digestive health and hormonal balance. For acute issues like indigestion or stress, it may be used as needed. Long-term use is generally considered safe, but it's wise to listen to your body and consult with a healthcare provider if using spearmint for specific health concerns, especially in high doses.

St. John's Wort

St. John's Wort (Hypericum perforatum) is widely known for its antidepressant and anti-inflammatory properties, making it a popular natural remedy for depression, anxiety, and wound healing.

Properties	Antidepressant: St. John's Wort is best known for its potential to alleviate symptoms of mild to moderate depression. Antiviral and Antibacterial: Exhibits antiviral and antibacterial properties, which can help in treating certain infections. Anti-inflammatory: Can reduce inflammation, aiding in the treatment of conditions like arthritis and muscle pain. Wound Healing: Applied topically, it can promote the healing of cuts, bruises, and minor burns.
What disease it fights	Depression and Anxiety: Used to treat mild to moderate depression and alleviate anxiety symptoms. Neuropathic Pain: May offer relief from pain caused by nerve damage. Skin Conditions: Effective in healing wounds and reducing symptoms of skin conditions like eczema and psoriasis. Menopausal Symptoms: Some women find relief from hot flashes and mood swings with St. John's Wort.
How it works	The antidepressant effects of St. John's Wort are attributed to its ability to increase the levels of neurotransmitters like serotonin, dopamine, and norepinephrine in the brain, which are involved in regulating mood. Its anti-inflammatory and antibacterial properties are due to the presence of compounds like hyperforin and hypericin.
How to use	Capsules/Tablets: St. John's Wort is commonly taken in capsule or tablet form for depression and anxiety. Tea: Dried herb can be used to make tea, offering a milder effect. Topical Application: Oils and tinctures can be applied to the skin for wound healing and treating skin conditions.
Dosage	Capsules/Tablets: The typical dosage for treating depression is 300 mg of St. John's Wort extract (standardized to 0.3% hypericin content), taken three times a day. Tea: Use 1-2 teaspoons of dried herb per cup of boiling water, steeped for about 10 minutes. Drink up to 3 cups daily. Topical Application: Follow product instructions for creams, oils, or tinctures.
How long to use	St. John's Wort may take several weeks to show effects for depression and anxiety, with typical use ranging from several weeks to months. It's important to monitor for any side effects, especially if taking other medications, as St. John's Wort can interact with them. For skin conditions, use until improvement is noticed.

Stevia

Stevia (Stevia rebaudiana) is a natural sweetener and sugar substitute extracted from the leaves of the plant species Stevia rebaudiana, native to Brazil and Paraguay. Known for its zero-calorie content, stevia has become popular among those looking to reduce sugar intake without sacrificing sweetness.

Properties	Zero-Calorie Sweetener: Stevia contains no calories, making it an attractive alternative for weight management and people with diabetes. Blood Sugar Management: Unlike regular sugar, stevia does not cause spikes in blood glucose levels, making it suitable for people with diabetes or those looking to manage their blood sugar levels. Antioxidant: Contains compounds with antioxidant properties, contributing to the reduction of oxidative stress in the body. Antibacterial: Some studies suggest stevia may have antibacterial properties, particularly in oral health applications.
What disease it fights	Diabetes: Stevia's non-glycemic nature makes it an ideal sweetener for people with diabetes or those looking to prevent the disease. Obesity and Weight Management: Being calorie-free, it can aid in weight loss or maintenance without sacrificing sweetness in the diet. Dental Health: Its antibacterial properties may help prevent cavities and plaque when used in place of sugar.
How it works	The sweetness of stevia comes from its steviol glycosides, including stevioside and rebaudioside A, which are many times sweeter than sugar but do not affect blood glucose levels. This makes it a beneficial sweetener for blood sugar management. Additionally, its antioxidant properties help to neutralize harmful free radicals in the body.
How to use	As a Sweetener: Stevia can be used in both hot and cold beverages, as well as in cooking and baking as a substitute for sugar. The conversion rate varies by product, so it's important to check packaging for equivalent sweetness levels. In Oral Care: Available in some toothpaste and mouthwash products for its antibacterial benefits.
Dosage	General Use: The amount of stevia used depends on the form (liquid, powder, granulated) and the desired level of sweetness, which can vary greatly among different stevia products. Generally, a small amount is sufficient to achieve a similar level of sweetness to sugar. Supplements: Some stevia products are sold as dietary supplements; follow the manufacturer's instructions regarding dosage.
How long to use	Stevia can be used indefinitely as a part of a daily diet for those looking to reduce sugar intake or manage blood sugar levels. Its long-term use as a sugar substitute is considered safe for the general population, including those with diabetes.

Tarragon

Tarragon (Artemisia dracunculus) is a perennial herb in the sunflower family, renowned for its aromatic leaves which are used both in culinary and medicinal applications. It's rich in antioxidants and possesses mild sedative properties, making it beneficial for sleep and digestion.

Properties	Digestive Aid: Tarragon can stimulate the production of digestive enzymes, aiding in digestion and relieving common digestive issues like flatulence and stomach cramps. Appetite Stimulant: It's known to help improve appetite, beneficial for those needing to increase their food intake. Sedative: Contains compounds that may have a mild sedative effect, promoting relaxation and aiding sleep. Antioxidant: Offers antioxidant properties that can help neutralize free radicals in the body.
What disease it fights	Digestive Disorders: Effective in managing indigestion, flatulence, and various forms of stomach discomfort. Insomnia and Anxiety: Its mild sedative effect can help improve sleep quality and reduce anxiety. Oral Health: Tarragon's antimicrobial properties may contribute to better oral health by reducing bacteria that cause tooth decay and gum disease.
How it works	Tarragon works primarily through its active compounds, including flavonoids and phenolic acids, which contribute to its digestive and sedative effects. These compounds stimulate the digestive system, promote the secretion of digestive enzymes, and can help relax the nervous system, thereby aiding digestion and promoting sleep.
How to use	Culinary Uses: Fresh or dried tarragon leaves are widely used in cooking to flavor a variety of dishes, including sauces, soups, and poultry. Tea: Tarragon leaves can be steeped in hot water to make a tea, which is beneficial for digestion and promoting relaxation. Infused Oil: Tarragon can be infused into oils, which are then used as a dressing or for cooking, incorporating its health benefits into daily meals.
Dosage	Tea: Use 1-2 teaspoons of dried tarragon leaves per cup of boiling water, steeped for about 10 minutes. Drink 1-2 cups daily, especially after meals or before bed to aid digestion or promote sleep. Culinary: There is no specific dosage for culinary use; it can be added to taste in various recipes.
How long to use	Tarragon can be used regularly as part of a balanced diet for its digestive benefits and to promote overall well-being. For addressing specific issues like indigestion or sleep difficulties, it might be used for a shorter duration, depending on individual response and improvement of symptoms.

Tea Tree

Tea tree oil, derived from the leaves of the tea tree (Melaleuca alternifolia), is celebrated for its potent antimicrobial and anti-inflammatory properties. It's widely used in skincare and wound care due to its ability to fight infections and reduce inflammation.

Properties	Antimicrobial: Effective against bacteria, viruses, and fungi, making it useful for treating various infections. Anti-inflammatory: Can reduce inflammation and alleviate symptoms of conditions like acne, psoriasis, and eczema. Antiseptic: Widely used for wound care, helping to prevent infection in cuts, burns, and abrasions. Acne Treatment: Its ability to kill bacteria and reduce inflammation makes it effective in treating acne.
What disease it fights	Skin Infections: Including acne, fungal nail infections, athlete's foot, and dermatitis. Wound Healing: Helps clean wounds and prevent bacterial infections. Oral Health: Used in low concentrations, it can combat bad breath and dental plaque. Respiratory Conditions: Inhalation of tea tree oil vapors can relieve congestion and respiratory tract infections.
How it works	The therapeutic effects of tea tree oil are mainly attributed to its compound terpinen-4-ol, which has been shown to kill certain bacteria, viruses, and fungi, and reduce inflammation. This makes it particularly effective for topical applications to treat skin conditions and wounds.
How to use	Topical Application: For skin conditions or wound care, dilute tea tree oil with a carrier oil (such as coconut or almond oil) before application. A general guideline is to use a 5% concentration, which equates to 5 drops of tea tree oil per teaspoon of carrier oil. Inhalation: Add a few drops of tea tree oil to hot water for steam inhalation or use in a diffuser to relieve respiratory conditions. Oral Care: Used in very low concentrations in homemade mouthwash recipes to combat bad breath and dental plaque. Direct ingestion is not recommended.
Dosage	Topical Application: Apply the diluted oil directly to the affected area 1-2 times daily, depending on the condition being treated. Inhalation: Use for 5-10 minutes, up to three times a day for respiratory relief. Oral Care: If using in a mouthwash, ensure the concentration is very low (usually a drop in a glass of water) to avoid toxicity.
How long to use	Tea tree oil can be used until symptoms improve, which may vary from a few days to several weeks, depending on the condition. For chronic conditions, or when used as part of a daily skincare routine, it's important to monitor for any adverse reactions over time.

Thyme

Thyme (Thymus vulgaris) is a culinary herb also recognized for its medicinal properties, particularly its ability to fight respiratory infections, improve digestion, and act as an antimicrobial agent.

Properties	Antimicrobial: Thyme contains thymol, an essential oil with potent antibacterial and antifungal properties. Expectorant: Helps in relieving coughs and expelling mucus from the respiratory tract. Antioxidant: Offers antioxidant benefits that protect cells from oxidative stress. Digestive Aid: Can improve digestion and reduce gas and bloating.
What disease it fights	Respiratory Infections: Effective against coughs, bronchitis, and sore throats. Gastrointestinal Issues: Aids in relieving indigestion, gas, and bloating. Oral Health: Thymol's antimicrobial action can combat bad breath and oral pathogens. Skin Conditions: Applied topically, it can treat fungal infections and minor wounds.
How it works	The primary active component in thyme, thymol, contributes to its antimicrobial and expectorant properties. Thymol helps inhibit the growth of bacteria and fungi, making it effective for both internal and topical use against infections. Its expectorant action aids in clearing mucus from the airways, while its carminative effects help reduce digestive discomfort.
How to use	Tea: Steep dried thyme in hot water to make a tea beneficial for respiratory and digestive health. Essential Oil: Thyme oil can be used in aromatherapy or diluted for topical application. Always dilute with a carrier oil for skin applications or inhalation. Culinary: Incorporating thyme into your diet through cooking can offer mild health benefits and enhance flavor.
Dosage	Tea: Use 1-2 teaspoons of dried thyme per cup of boiling water, steeped for 10 minutes. Drink up to 3 cups daily. Essential Oil: For topical use, dilute 2-3 drops in a tablespoon of carrier oil. For inhalation, add a few drops to hot water or a diffuser. Culinary: No specific dosage; use according to personal taste preferences and culinary guidelines.
How long to use	Thyme can be used as a culinary herb on a regular basis without specific time constraints. For medicinal uses like teas or essential oil applications, it can be used for the duration of symptoms, typically up to 1-2 weeks. If symptoms persist or worsen, consult a healthcare professional.

Tribulus Terrestris

Tribulus terrestris is a plant that has been used traditionally in Ayurvedic and Chinese medicine for various health benefits, including enhancing libido, supporting urinary tract health, and improving athletic performance. Its fruits, leaves, and roots contain active compounds like saponins, which are believed to contribute to its health effects.

Properties	Libido Enhancer: Tribulus is best known for its potential to increase sexual desire and improve sexual function in both men and women. Urinary Tract Health: May support healthy urinary function and reduce the risk of urinary tract infections. Athletic Performance: Some evidence suggests it can enhance strength and muscle mass, contributing to better athletic performance. Cardiovascular Health: Tribulus has been studied for its effects on blood pressure and cholesterol levels, indicating potential heart health benefits.
What disease it fights	Sexual Dysfunction: Used to treat low libido and other sexual health issues. Urinary Disorders: May be beneficial for kidney stones and urinary tract health. Heart Health: Can have a positive impact on blood pressure and cholesterol, supporting overall cardiovascular wellness.
How it works	The active compounds in Tribulus terrestris, particularly the saponins, are thought to stimulate the release of nitric oxide in the endothelium and improve blood flow, which can enhance libido and sexual function. Its potential benefits for athletic performance are attributed to its effects on increasing testosterone levels, though research findings have been mixed.
How to use	Capsules/Tablets: The most common form of supplementation, providing a controlled dose of Tribulus extract. Tea: Leaves or fruit can be steeped in hot water to make tea, though this is less common. Powder: The powdered form can be added to smoothies or beverages for an easy intake.
Dosage	Capsules/Tablets: Dosages can vary widely depending on the concentration of the extract, but a typical range is 250-750 mg per day, taken in divided doses. Tea: Use 1 teaspoon of dried leaves or fruit per cup of boiling water, steeped for 10-15 minutes. Drink 1-2 cups daily. Powder: Follow manufacturer guidelines, typically starting with a small dose such as ¼ to ½ teaspoon.
How long to use	Tribulus terrestris can be used for several weeks to months, depending on the health objective. For sexual dysfunction and athletic performance, it may be used cyclically or as needed. Continuous use beyond 3 months is generally not recommended without consulting a healthcare professional to monitor effects and adjust dosage as necessary.

Turmeric

Turmeric (Curcuma longa) is a spice that has been used for thousands of years in Ayurvedic and Chinese medicine for its medicinal properties. It's highly praised for its anti-inflammatory, antioxidant, and anticancer effects, largely attributed to curcumin, its active compound.

Properties	Anti-inflammatory: Turmeric is renowned for its potent anti-inflammatory properties, making it effective in managing conditions like arthritis, gastrointestinal inflammation, and skin issues. Antioxidant: Curcumin in turmeric neutralizes free radicals, contributing to its antioxidant capacity that supports overall cellular health. Anticancer: Some studies suggest that turmeric can reduce the growth of cancer cells and inhibit the development of tumors. Neuroprotective: Turmeric has shown potential in protecting brain health, including reducing the risk of Alzheimer's disease and improving mood disorders.
What disease it fights	Chronic Inflammation and Pain: Effective in reducing symptoms of arthritis and other inflammatory conditions. Digestive Disorders: Aids in relieving symptoms of indigestion, ulcerative colitis, and Crohn's disease. Cardiovascular Health: May help lower cholesterol and prevent blood clots. Mental Health: Its anti-inflammatory and antioxidant effects contribute to improved mood and cognitive function.
How it works	Curcumin's ability to modulate numerous molecular targets is behind turmeric's wide-ranging health benefits. It inhibits enzymes and proteins involved in inflammation, offers antioxidant protection by neutralizing free radicals, and can influence cell signaling pathways to promote health and prevent disease.
How to use	Dietary Use: Turmeric can be incorporated into meals and beverages, like curries, teas, and smoothies, to enhance flavor and nutritional value. Supplements: For those seeking higher doses of curcumin, turmeric supplements are available in capsules, tablets, and liquid extracts. Topical Applications: Turmeric paste can be applied to the skin for its anti-inflammatory and antimicrobial benefits.
Dosage	Dietary Use: There's no specific dosage; using turmeric in cooking is generally safe and beneficial. Supplements: The typical dosage for curcumin supplements is 500-2,000 mg per day, often divided into smaller doses. Look for supplements containing piperine (black pepper extract), which significantly enhances absorption. Topical Applications: Apply as needed, mixing turmeric powder with water or a carrier oil to form a paste.
How long to use	Turmeric can be used indefinitely as part of a regular diet. For supplements, especially at higher doses, they can be taken for specific periods depending on health goals, usually ranging from a few weeks to several months. Continuous use of high-dose supplements should be under the guidance of a healthcare professional to monitor for any adverse effects and ensure ongoing efficacy.

Uva Ursi

Uva Ursi (Arctostaphylos uva-ursi), also known as bearberry, is a small shrub with a long history of use in traditional medicine, primarily for urinary tract infections (UTIs) and related conditions. Its leaves contain arbutin, a compound that converts into hydroquinone—a potent antimicrobial agent—when metabolized by the body.

Properties	Antimicrobial: Uva ursi's primary compound, arbutin, has strong antimicrobial properties effective against bacteria responsible for UTIs. Anti-inflammatory: Helps reduce inflammation in the urinary tract, aiding in the relief of discomfort and promoting healing. Astringent: The tannins in uva ursi have astringent effects, helping to tighten mucous membranes and reduce bleeding and irritation.
What disease it fights	Urinary Tract Infections (UTIs): Used to prevent and treat infections by inhibiting bacterial growth. Inflammation of the Urinary Tract: Reduces inflammation and irritation associated with UTIs and other urinary disorders. Kidney Stones: May assist in preventing the formation of kidney stones by reducing uric acid levels.
How it works	When ingested, arbutin is converted into hydroquinone, which exerts antimicrobial effects, particularly in the alkaline urine. This action helps to cleanse the urinary tract, reduce bacterial adherence to the bladder walls, and alleviate symptoms of infection and irritation.
How to use	Tea: Dried uva ursi leaves can be steeped in boiling water to make a tea. This method allows for gentle effects and can be used for maintenance or mild conditions. Capsules/Extracts: For more acute conditions, uva ursi is available in capsules or liquid extracts, offering a concentrated dose that should be used under the guidance of a healthcare provider.
Dosage	Tea: Use 1-2 teaspoons of dried leaves per cup of boiling water, steeped for 10-15 minutes. Drink up to 3 cups daily for a short duration. Capsules/Extracts: Dosage varies by product, but a typical range is 250-500 mg of uva ursi extract taken three times daily. Due to potential toxicity, it's recommended for short-term use only (no longer than one week).
How long to use	Uva ursi should be used with caution due to the potential toxicity of hydroquinone. For treating UTIs or other acute urinary conditions, it's typically recommended for short-term use only, such as 5-7 days. Long-term use is not advised without consulting a healthcare professional, as it can lead to liver damage, increased eye pressure, and other side effects.

Valerian

Valerian (Valeriana officinalis) is a perennial plant known for its sedative and anxiolytic properties, making it a popular natural remedy for insomnia, anxiety, and stress-related conditions. Its roots and rhizomes contain compounds that contribute to its calming effects.

Properties	Sedative: Promotes relaxation and improves sleep quality, making it beneficial for those with insomnia. Anxiolytic: Helps reduce anxiety and stress, aiding in the management of stress-related conditions. Muscle Relaxant: Can alleviate physical tension and spasms, contributing to its overall calming effect.
What disease it fights	Insomnia and Sleep Disorders: Valerian is most commonly used to improve sleep quality and reduce the time it takes to fall asleep. Anxiety: Its anxiolytic properties help to calm the mind and reduce symptoms of anxiety. Menstrual and Stomach Cramps: The muscle relaxant effects can help ease cramps and discomfort.
How it works	The calming effects of valerian are thought to be primarily due to its interaction with the gamma-aminobutyric acid (GABA) system in the brain, a key neurotransmitter involved in regulating nervous system activity. Valerian increases GABA levels, which helps reduce nerve activity and promote relaxation.
How to use	Tea: Dried valerian root can be steeped in hot water to make tea. This method allows for a gentle effect, suitable for relaxation. Capsules/Extracts: For more pronounced effects, particularly for sleep, valerian is available in capsules or liquid extracts, providing a more concentrated dose. Aromatherapy: Valerian essential oil can be used in aromatherapy, though it's less common due to its strong odor.
Dosage	Tea: Use 1 teaspoon of dried valerian root per cup of boiling water, steeped for 10-15 minutes. Drink 30 minutes to 2 hours before bedtime. Capsules/Extracts: The typical dosage is 300-600 mg of valerian root extract 30 minutes to 2 hours before bedtime for sleep issues. For anxiety, smaller doses (100-200 mg) may be taken three times daily. Aromatherapy: Use according to diffuser instructions or personal tolerance for the odor.
How long to use	Valerian can be used in the short term to address acute sleep issues or anxiety, typically for a few weeks to a month. Long-term use should be approached with caution, as the effects of prolonged usage are not well-documented, and dependence or withdrawal symptoms have not been thoroughly studied.

Vanilla

Vanilla, derived from the orchids of the genus Vanilla, especially Vanilla planifolia, is cherished not only for its delightful aroma and flavor but also for its therapeutic properties. While primarily used in culinary applications, vanilla also offers mild sedative, antioxidant, and antidepressant effects.

Properties	Antioxidant: Vanilla contains vanillin, a compound with antioxidant properties that can help protect the body from oxidative stress and support overall health. Sedative: The scent of vanilla has a calming effect on the brain, which can reduce anxiety and promote relaxation. Antidepressant: The pleasant aroma of vanilla can uplift mood and has been studied for its potential antidepressant effects.
What disease it fights	Stress and Anxiety: The soothing aroma of vanilla can help alleviate stress and reduce anxiety levels. Depression: Vanilla's pleasant scent might contribute to mood improvement and has been explored for its potential to aid in the treatment of depression. Insomnia: Due to its calming effects, vanilla can be used to promote better sleep-in people experiencing insomnia.
How it works	The primary mechanism through which vanilla exerts its effects is related to its impact on the brain when inhaled. The scent of vanilla can influence the limbic system, which plays a crucial role in emotion and mood regulation. Antioxidant compounds in vanilla, such as vanillin, help neutralize free radicals, contributing to cellular health and disease prevention.
How to use	Culinary Use: Vanilla pods, extract, or powder can be used to flavor a wide range of dishes and beverages, contributing to both the enjoyment of food and intake of antioxidants. Aromatherapy: Vanilla essential oil or natural extract can be used in diffusers or added to bathwater for stress relief and relaxation. Dietary Supplements: Vanilla-flavored dietary supplements, including protein powders and meal replacements, can make healthful eating more enjoyable.
Dosage	Culinary Use: There is no specific dosage for culinary use; it can be added according to taste preferences. Aromatherapy: For diffusing, use a few drops of vanilla essential oil or extract in a diffuser. Follow the manufacturer's instructions for the diffuser. Dietary Supplements: Follow the manufacturer's instructions for any vanilla-flavored supplement products.
How long to use	Vanilla can be used regularly in culinary and aromatherapy applications without specific time constraints, as it's generally considered safe and lacks the potent active ingredients that might warrant caution. However, the enjoyment and potential health benefits can be ongoing.

Vervain

Vervain (Verbena officinalis), also known as verbena, is an herb that has been used historically in various traditional medicines for its numerous health benefits. It's particularly noted for its calming, digestive, and anti-inflammatory properties.

Properties	Nervine: Vervain is known for its calming effects, which can help reduce anxiety and stress, promoting a sense of well-being. Digestive Aid: It stimulates the digestive system, aiding in the relief of indigestion, bloating, and gas. Anti-inflammatory: Has anti-inflammatory properties that can help reduce inflammation throughout the body. Galactagogue: Some traditional uses include promoting lactation in breastfeeding mothers. Antipyretic: Used historically to reduce fever and treat minor illnesses.
What disease it fights	Stress and Anxiety: Helps in managing stress levels and reducing symptoms of anxiety. Digestive Issues: Aids in the relief of various digestive complaints, including indigestion and bloating. Mild Infections: Its antipyretic and immune-boosting properties may help in combating mild fevers and infections. Inflammation-Related Conditions: May provide relief for conditions associated with inflammation, such as arthritis.
How it works	The calming effects of vervain are likely due to its impact on the nervous system, helping to relieve stress and anxiety. Its digestive benefits stem from its ability to stimulate digestive enzymes and improve gut motility. The anti-inflammatory properties may be attributed to the presence of iridoid glycosides, among other compounds, which help modulate the body's inflammatory response.
How to use	Tea: Dried vervain leaves can be steeped in hot water to make an herbal tea. This is a common method for enjoying its health benefits, particularly for relaxation and digestive support. Tincture: A vervain tincture offers a more concentrated form, which may be preferred for therapeutic purposes. Topical Application: For external inflammations, a poultice made from vervain leaves can be applied to the affected area.
Dosage	Tea: Use 1-2 teaspoons of dried vervain per cup of boiling water, steeped for about 10 minutes. Drink up to three times daily. Tincture: Follow the product's specific recommendations, typically 1-2 ml three times a day. Topical Application: There's no specific dosage; apply as needed, ensuring the skin is clean to avoid irritation.
How long to use	Vervain can be used as needed to address specific symptoms, such as stress or digestive issues. For chronic conditions or ongoing support, it might be used for several weeks to months. As with any herbal remedy, it's wise to periodically evaluate its effectiveness and any potential side effects.

Vetiver

Vetiver (Chrysopogon zizanioides), known for its deep, earthy fragrance, is a perennial grass native to India. In traditional medicine, vetiver is celebrated for its calming, grounding, and stabilizing properties. It's also recognized for its antioxidant, anti-inflammatory, and possibly antimicrobial benefits.

Properties	Calming and Relaxing: Vetiver oil is widely used in aromatherapy for its ability to calm the mind, reduce stress, and alleviate anxiety. Antioxidant: The oil has antioxidant properties that can help neutralize free radicals and support overall health. Anti-inflammatory: May reduce inflammation, offering benefits for conditions such as arthritis and muscular pain. Skin Health: Its moisturizing and regenerative properties make it beneficial for skin care, especially in healing scars and marks.
What disease it fights	Stress and Anxiety: The sedative properties of vetiver help in managing stress, anxiety, and sleep disorders like insomnia. Inflammatory Conditions: Can be used to alleviate symptoms of inflammation, including those affecting the joints and muscles. Skin Conditions: Supports the healing of acne, scars, and promotes a healthy complexion.
How it works	Vetiver's calming effects are primarily attributed to its complex composition of sesquiterpenes, which have a grounding effect on the central nervous system. These compounds can help modulate stress responses and promote relaxation. The anti-inflammatory and antioxidant properties contribute to its therapeutic benefits in skin care and inflammation management.
How to use	Aromatherapy: Vetiver essential oil can be used in diffusers, inhalers, or added to bathwater for stress relief and relaxation. Topical Application: Dilute vetiver oil with a carrier oil (like coconut or almond oil) for direct application to the skin, aiding in moisturization and the treatment of skin conditions. Perfumery: Its rich scent makes it a popular choice in natural perfumery and personal care products.
Dosage	Aromatherapy: A few drops in a diffuser or inhaler according to personal preference and device instructions. Topical Application: For skin application, a 2-5% dilution is generally recommended, which equates to about 4-10 drops of vetiver oil per tablespoon of carrier oil.
How long to use	Vetiver can be used as needed for aromatherapy and stress relief, without specific time constraints. For topical applications, particularly for skin conditions, it may be used until improvement is observed. Regular reevaluation is recommended to assess benefits and any skin reactions, especially for long-term use.

Violet

Violet (Viola odorata) is a small plant with fragrant flowers and heart-shaped leaves, known for its gentle soothing, anti-inflammatory, and expectorant properties. In traditional medicine, it's been used to treat a variety of conditions, including respiratory issues, skin disorders, and as a means to soothe the nervous system.

Properties	Soothing and Anti-inflammatory: Effective in soothing irritated skin and mucous membranes, and reducing inflammation. Expectorant: Helps in relieving respiratory conditions by loosening phlegm and facilitating its expulsion. Diuretic: Promotes the production of urine, aiding in the detoxification process. Antiseptic: The presence of salicylic acid in violets provides mild antiseptic properties.
What disease it fights	Respiratory Issues: Useful in treating colds, coughs, and bronchitis by acting as an expectorant. Skin Conditions: Can be applied topically to soothe and treat eczema, acne, and other inflammatory skin conditions. Mild Pain Relief: The salicylic acid content can provide relief from minor pains and headaches. Anxiety and Sleep Disorders: Its gentle soothing effects can help reduce anxiety and promote better sleep.
How it works	The beneficial effects of violet are due to its various compounds, including flavonoids, mucilage, and salicylic acid. Flavonoids and mucilage provide soothing and anti-inflammatory benefits, making it useful for skin and respiratory health. Salicylic acid contributes to its pain-relieving and antiseptic properties.
How to use	Tea: Dried leaves and flowers can be steeped in hot water to make a tea that benefits respiratory health and provides a calming effect. Topical Applications: Infused oils, salves, or compresses made from violet leaves and flowers can be applied to the skin to address inflammation and skin conditions. Tincture: Violet tincture can be used for its expectorant and soothing effects.
Dosage	Tea: Use 1-2 teaspoons of dried violet per cup of boiling water, steeped for 10-15 minutes. Drink 2-3 cups daily. Topical Applications: Apply as needed, depending on the condition being treated. For infused oils and salves, a small amount can be applied to the affected area 2-3 times a day. Tincture: Follow the manufacturer's instructions or consult a healthcare provider for appropriate dosages.
How long to use	Violet can be used as needed for acute conditions like colds or skin inflammation. For chronic issues or ongoing support, such as anxiety or respiratory health, it may be used over a longer period, typically several weeks to months. Always monitor for any adverse reactions, especially with prolonged use.

Vitex

Vitex, also known as Chasteberry (Vitex agnus-castus), is an herb renowned for its ability to regulate hormonal imbalances, particularly in women. It has been traditionally used for centuries to address various gynecological conditions.

Properties	Hormonal Regulation: Vitex works on the pituitary gland to balance levels of progesterone and estrogen, making it beneficial for premenstrual syndrome (PMS), menopause symptoms, and other menstrual irregularities. Promotes Fertility: By normalizing ovulation and improving progesterone levels, vitex can enhance fertility in women experiencing difficulty conceiving due to hormonal issues. Acne Treatment: For some women, balancing hormones can lead to improvements in hormonal acne. Mood Enhancement: Its hormonal regulation may also help in alleviating mood swings and depression associated with PMS and menopause.
What disease it fights	Premenstrual Syndrome (PMS): Vitex can reduce symptoms such as mood swings, breast tenderness, and headaches. Menstrual Disorders: Helps in regulating menstrual cycles and alleviating symptoms of polycystic ovary syndrome (PCOS). Fertility Issues: Assists in correcting hormonal imbalances that affect ovulation and fertility. Menopausal Symptoms: May alleviate hot flashes, night sweats, and mood changes.
How it works	Vitex influences the hypothalamus and pituitary gland, leading to an increase in luteinizing hormone (LH) production and a slight decrease in follicle-stimulating hormone (FSH) levels. This shift promotes ovulation and supports the production of progesterone, helping to balance the estrogen-progesterone ratio in the body.
How to use	Capsules/Tablets: The most common form of vitex supplement, offering precise dosage and convenience. Tincture: Liquid extracts provide flexibility in dosing and are quickly absorbed by the body. Tea: Less common, but dried vitex berries can be used to make tea. This method may offer a gentler effect.
Dosage	Capsules/Tablets: A common dosage is 160-240 mg of standardized extract, taken once daily in the morning on an empty stomach. Tincture: Dosage can vary, but typically 20-40 drops of the tincture are taken in water, 1-3 times daily. Tea: Boil 1 teaspoon of dried berries in a cup of water for 10 minutes. Drink once daily.
How long to use	Vitex is often taken for a minimum of three menstrual cycles to experience noticeable benefits, with some women taking it for up to 18 months. For fertility purposes, it may be used until pregnancy is achieved. It's important to evaluate the effects periodically and consult with a healthcare provider, especially for long-term use.

White Oak Bark

White oak bark (Quercus alba) is derived from the white oak tree and has been used traditionally for its astringent, antiseptic, and anti-inflammatory properties. It's particularly noted for its ability to tighten tissues and reduce inflammation, making it useful in treating wounds, skin conditions, and digestive issues.

Properties	Astringent: The high tannin content provides strong astringent properties, making it effective in tightening tissues and reducing bleeding and inflammation. Antiseptic: Can help prevent infection in wounds and soothe irritated skin. Anti-inflammatory: Useful in reducing inflammation in the gastrointestinal tract and externally on skin conditions. Hemostatic: Helps to stop bleeding, beneficial for treating cuts, bruises, and hemorrhoids.
What disease it fights	Diarrhea and Digestive Issues: The astringent properties can help reduce intestinal inflammation and treat diarrhea. Skin Conditions: Applied topically, it can help heal wounds, eczema, burns, and rashes. Throat Infections: Gargling with white oak bark tea can relieve sore throats and inflammation in the oral mucosa. Varicose Veins and Hemorrhoids: Its ability to tighten tissues can reduce swelling and discomfort associated with varicose veins and hemorrhoids.
How it works	White oak bark's effectiveness is largely due to its high tannin content, which has astringent effects that can tighten and constrict tissues, reduce secretion and bleeding, and help form a protective barrier on the skin or mucous membranes. Its anti-inflammatory and antiseptic properties further support healing and infection prevention.
How to use	Tea: Boil 1-2 teaspoons of dried white oak bark in water for about 15 minutes to make a strong tea. This can be used for gargling, as a wash for skin conditions, or consumed for digestive health. Tincture: A concentrated liquid form can be diluted in water and used for topical applications or taken orally for internal issues. Powder: The powdered form can be used to make a poultice for external application on wounds or skin conditions.
Dosage	Tea: For internal use, drink 1-2 cups of tea per day. For external use or gargling, use as needed. Tincture: Follow the manufacturer's instructions, typically 1-2 ml three times a day for internal use. Powder: For poultices, mix with water to create a paste and apply to the affected area as needed.
How long to use	White oak bark can be used for short-term relief of acute conditions, such as diarrhea or sore throats, typically for a few days up to a week. For chronic issues or ongoing support, such as skin conditions or digestive health maintenance, it may be used for several weeks. It's important to monitor for any signs of tannin overconsumption, such as liver stress or digestive discomfort, especially with prolonged internal use.

White Willow Bark

White willow bark (Salix alba) has been used for centuries for its pain-relieving and anti-inflammatory properties, mainly due to the presence of salicin, a compound like aspirin (acetylsalicylic acid). It's often used in natural medicine as an alternative to conventional non-steroidal anti-inflammatory drugs (NSAIDs) for treating headaches, low back pain, osteoarthritis, and other conditions associated with pain and inflammation.

Properties	Pain Relief: Acts similarly to aspirin, providing relief from headaches, muscle pain, and menstrual cramps. Anti-inflammatory: Helps reduce inflammation, beneficial for conditions such as arthritis and tendinitis. Antipyretic: Can lower fever and ease symptoms of cold and flu. Anticoagulant: Salicin may have mild blood-thinning effects, contributing to improved circulation.
What disease it fights	Chronic Pain Conditions: Effective for managing osteoarthritis, rheumatoid arthritis, and low back pain. Headaches and Migraines: Provides a natural alternative to aspirin for reducing pain and inflammation associated with headaches. Menstrual Cramps: Can alleviate the discomfort of menstrual cramps through its analgesic properties. Fever: Used traditionally to reduce fever and relieve symptoms of the common cold and flu.
How it works	The body converts salicin into salicylic acid, which is responsible for white willow bark's pain-relieving and anti-inflammatory effects. Unlike synthetic aspirin, white willow bark does not irritate the stomach lining to the same extent, making it a gentler alternative for long-term use.
How to use	Tea: Simmer 1-2 teaspoons of dried white willow bark in water for 10-15 minutes. Strain and drink 2-3 times daily. Capsules/Extracts: Available in capsule or liquid extract form for those who prefer not to consume the tea. These forms allow for more precise dosing and convenience.
Dosage	Tea: Drink 2-3 cups daily, depending on the severity of symptoms. Capsules/Extracts: Typical dosages range from 120 to 240 mg of salicin per day. Always follow the product's specific dosage recommendations.
How long to use	White willow bark can be used for short-term relief of acute pain and inflammation, such as headaches or menstrual cramps, over several days. For chronic conditions like arthritis, it may be used for longer periods, but it's wise to consult a healthcare provider for guidance, especially when used for more than a few weeks, to monitor any potential side effects and interactions with other medications.

Wild Yam

Wild yam (Dioscorea villosa) has been traditionally used in herbal medicine for a variety of health issues, particularly for its benefits in balancing hormones and managing menopausal symptoms. It contains diosgenin, a compound that can be chemically converted into various steroids, such as estrogen and dehydroepiandrosterone (DHEA).

Properties	Hormonal Balance: Wild yam is believed to influence hormone levels, making it popular for managing PMS, menstrual irregularities, and menopausal symptoms. Anti-inflammatory: Offers anti-inflammatory properties that may help with arthritis and rheumatic pain. Antispasmodic: Can relieve muscle spasms, including those related to digestive issues and menstrual cramps.
What disease it fights	Menopausal Symptoms: Helps alleviate hot flashes, night sweats, and mood swings. Premenstrual Syndrome (PMS) and Menstrual Irregularities: May reduce symptoms of PMS and regulate menstrual cycles. Digestive Issues: Its antispasmodic properties can aid in relieving colic and intestinal cramps. Arthritis and Rheumatic Pain: The anti-inflammatory effects may help reduce pain and inflammation associated with arthritis.
How it works	The presence of diosgenin in wild yam is thought to be the key to its effects on hormonal balance, though the body cannot directly convert diosgenin into hormones without laboratory processing. However, wild yam may influence hormone production through other mechanisms or provide plant-based sterols that support the body's hormone balance. Its anti-inflammatory and antispasmodic effects help alleviate pain and discomfort in conditions like arthritis and menstrual cramps.
How to use	Capsules/Supplements: Wild yam is commonly taken in capsule or tablet form for ease of dosing and convenience. Creams and Gels: For symptoms of menopause or PMS, wild yam creams can be applied topically to the skin. Tea: While less common, wild yam can be brewed into a tea.
Dosage	Capsules/Supplements: Dosages can vary widely depending on the product, but a general guideline is 400-600 mg of wild yam extract taken daily. Creams and Gels: Follow the manufacturer's instructions for application, usually applied once or twice daily. Tea: Steep 1 teaspoon of dried wild yam in a cup of boiling water for 10-15 minutes. Drink 2-3 cups daily.
How long to use	Wild yam can be used over the short to medium term for relieving specific symptoms, such as during menopausal transition or for menstrual discomfort, typically for a few months. For ongoing issues, it's wise to consult a healthcare provider for guidance and monitoring, especially for long-term use, to ensure safety and effectiveness.

Witch Hazel

Witch hazel (Hamamelis virginiana) is a shrub native to North America, renowned for its astringent, anti-inflammatory, and hemostatic properties. It's extracted from the bark and leaves of the plant and is commonly used in skin care and natural health remedies.

Properties	Astringent: The tannins in witch hazel provide powerful astringent properties, making it effective in tightening skin and reducing inflammation. Anti-inflammatory: Helps to soothe irritated skin, reduce redness, and alleviate inflammation. Hemostatic: Can stop minor bleeding, useful in treating cuts and abrasions. Antimicrobial: Exhibits mild antibacterial and antifungal effects, contributing to its use in acne treatment and preventing infection in wounds.
What disease it fights	Skin Conditions: Including acne, eczema, and psoriasis. Witch hazel can reduce inflammation and soothe irritated skin. Hemorrhoids: Its astringent and anti-inflammatory properties make it effective in relieving discomfort and reducing inflammation. Minor Cuts and Bruises: Helps in the healing process by reducing inflammation and stopping bleeding. Varicose Veins: Can temporarily reduce the appearance of varicose veins by tightening the skin.
How it works	Witch hazel works primarily through its high content of tannins, which have astringent effects that tighten skin and mucous membranes, reduce leakage of fluids, and help soothe irritated tissues. Its anti-inflammatory action is beneficial for treating skin conditions and hemorrhoids, while its hemostatic and antimicrobial properties support wound healing and prevent infection.
How to use	Topical Application: Witch hazel is most commonly used in a liquid form, applied directly to the skin with a cotton ball or pad. Compresses: Soaked in witch hazel and applied to affected areas to soothe and reduce inflammation. Creams and Gels: Some products contain witch hazel for treating specific conditions like hemorrhoids and varicose veins.
Dosage	Topical Application: Apply as needed to the affected area. For acne, it can be used 1-2 times daily after washing the face. For hemorrhoids, apply several times a day or as needed to relieve symptoms. Compresses: Use 2-3 times daily by soaking a clean cloth in witch hazel and applying it to the affected area. Creams and Gels: Follow the manufacturer's instructions, typically applied 2-3 times daily.
How long to use	Witch hazel can be used as needed to provide relief from symptoms. For acute conditions like cuts or hemorrhoids, it may be used until symptoms improve. For ongoing skin care or chronic conditions, it can be incorporated into daily routines indefinitely, as it is generally safe for long-term use. However, individuals with sensitive skin should monitor for any adverse reactions over time.

Wormwood

Wormwood (Artemisia absinthium) is an herb known for its bitter properties, which stimulate the digestive system, making it useful for treating various gastrointestinal issues. It has been used traditionally as a component in absinthe, a potent alcoholic beverage.

Properties	Digestive Stimulant: Wormwood can increase stomach acid and bile production, aiding in digestion and the absorption of nutrients. Antiparasitic: Traditionally used to expel intestinal worms and other parasites. Antimicrobial: Contains compounds with antimicrobial properties that can inhibit the growth of bacteria and fungi. Anti-inflammatory: Offers anti-inflammatory benefits that can help in managing inflammation in the digestive tract.
What disease it fights	Digestive Disorders: Helps in treating indigestion, bloating, and gas. It can also be beneficial for gallbladder issues and to stimulate appetite. Intestinal Parasites: Used to eliminate worms and other parasitic infections in the gut. Mild Infections: The antimicrobial properties may be helpful in addressing certain bacterial and fungal infections.
How it works	The bitter compounds in wormwood, particularly thujone and absinthin, stimulate digestive secretions and bile flow, improving digestion and nutrient absorption. These compounds also possess antimicrobial and antiparasitic properties, making wormwood effective against infections and intestinal parasites.
How to use	Tea: Wormwood can be steeped in hot water to make a bitter tea, which is taken before meals to stimulate digestion. Tincture: A more concentrated form used for specific therapeutic purposes, such as treating parasitic infections. Capsules: Available for those who prefer not to taste the bitterness but wish to benefit from its digestive and antimicrobial effects.
Dosage	Tea: Use 1/2 to 1 teaspoon of dried wormwood per cup of boiling water, steeped for 5-10 minutes. It's recommended to drink this tea 15-30 minutes before meals, not exceeding 3 cups daily. Tincture: Follow the manufacturer's instructions, typically 2-3 ml taken up to three times a day. Capsules: Dosage can vary by product; follow the package instructions, usually taken before meals.
How long to use	Wormwood should be used with caution and typically for short periods—no longer than 4-6 weeks—due to potential side effects from thujone, a neurotoxic compound found in the herb. Long-term use or high doses can lead to neurotoxicity and other adverse effects.

Yarrow

Yarrow (Achillea millefolium) is a perennial herb with a wide range of medicinal properties, celebrated for its ability to stop bleeding, heal wounds, and support the digestive and circulatory systems. It has been utilized in traditional medicine across many cultures for centuries.

Properties	Hemostatic and Wound Healing: Yarrow is well-known for its ability to quickly stop bleeding and promote the healing of wounds. Anti-inflammatory: Offers anti-inflammatory benefits that can help reduce swelling and support the healing of various conditions. Digestive Aid: Stimulates the appetite and aids in the digestion process by improving bile secretion. Antimicrobial: Possesses antimicrobial properties that can help prevent infection in wounds and treat minor internal infections. Diaphoretic: Can induce sweating and help reduce fever.
What disease it fights	Wounds and Bleeding: Effective in treating cuts, abrasions, and internal bleeding. Digestive Issues: Used to improve digestive health, including treating indigestion, cramps, and bloating. Infections: Its antimicrobial action makes it useful for treating colds, flu, and urinary tract infections. Inflammatory Conditions: Can be used to alleviate inflammation in conditions like arthritis and eczema.
How it works	Yarrow's healing properties are attributed to its diverse range of active constituents, including flavonoids, tannins, and salicylic acid. These compounds contribute to its hemostatic, anti-inflammatory, and antimicrobial effects. Yarrow's ability to stimulate the digestive system is beneficial for overall gut health, while its diaphoretic action helps in reducing fevers and detoxifying the body.
How to use	Tea: Yarrow tea can be made by steeping dried leaves and flowers in boiling water, ideal for digestive issues or as a diaphoretic. Topical Application: A poultice or infused oil with yarrow can be applied to wounds or inflamed skin areas. Tincture: Yarrow tincture is used for its concentrated benefits, particularly for internal use to boost digestion or treat colds.
Dosage	Tea: Use 1-2 teaspoons of dried yarrow per cup of boiling water, steep for 5-10 minutes. Drink up to 3 cups daily. Topical Application: Apply as needed to the affected area, ensuring the skin is clean to prevent infection. Tincture: Follow the manufacturer's instructions, typically 1-4 ml three times a day.
How long to use	Yarrow can be used as needed for acute conditions, such as wounds or digestive upset. For chronic issues or general health maintenance, it may be used for longer periods, up to a few weeks. Long-term internal use should be approached with caution due to potential side effects, such as increased photosensitivity and allergic reactions in sensitive individuals.

Yellow Dock

Yellow dock (Rumex crispus) is a perennial herb known for its detoxifying, digestive, and anti-inflammatory properties. It has been traditionally used to support liver function, improve digestion, and treat skin conditions. The roots of yellow dock contain anthraquinones, which contribute to its mild laxative effect, as well as a wealth of other beneficial compounds like tannins and flavonoids.

Properties	Digestive Aid: Stimulates bile production, aiding in digestion and the absorption of nutrients. Detoxifying: Supports liver function and the elimination of toxins from the body. Mild Laxative: The anthraquinones present have a mild laxative effect, helpful in relieving constipation. Anti-inflammatory: Beneficial for reducing inflammation, particularly in skin conditions such as eczema and psoriasis. Iron-rich: The high iron content can help in addressing anemia and improving overall energy levels.
What disease it fights	Digestive Disorders: Including constipation, indigestion, and liver detoxification. Skin Conditions: Used to treat eczema, psoriasis, and acne due to its anti-inflammatory and detoxifying effects. Anemia: The iron content in yellow dock can contribute to the treatment of anemia when used as part of a balanced approach to nutrition.
How it works	Yellow dock works by enhancing bile production, which is essential for the digestion of fats and the detoxification of the liver. Its mild laxative effect aids in relieving constipation by stimulating bowel movements. Additionally, its anti-inflammatory properties can soothe skin conditions, while its nutritional content supports blood health.
How to use	Tea: Dried root can be boiled and simmered to make a tea, consumed before meals to aid digestion. Tincture: A concentrated liquid form that can be used for more precise dosing, particularly for detoxification and skin conditions. Capsules: Powdered yellow dock root is available in capsules for those who prefer not to taste the herb.
Dosage	Tea: Boil 1 teaspoon of dried root in a cup of water for about 10 minutes. Drink 1-2 cups daily. Tincture: Typically, 2-4 ml of tincture is taken three times a day. Capsules: Follow the manufacturer's recommendations, usually 500-2000 mg daily, divided into two or three doses.
How long to use	Yellow dock can be used for short-term interventions, such as during periods of digestive upset or when addressing acute skin conditions, typically for a few weeks. For ongoing liver support or chronic skin conditions, it may be used for longer periods under the guidance of a healthcare professional. Due to its laxative effect, long-term use should be monitored to avoid dependency or disruption of normal bowel function.

Yerba Mate

Yerba Mate (Ilex paraguariensis) is a traditional South American beverage known for its unique combination of caffeine, antioxidants, vitamins, and minerals. It's consumed widely in countries like Argentina, Uruguay, and Brazil for its energizing effects and health benefits.

Properties	Stimulant: Contains caffeine, which can increase energy levels, improve mental focus, and enhance physical performance. Antioxidant: Rich in polyphenols, yerba mate has strong antioxidant properties that can protect against oxidative stress and reduce the risk of chronic diseases. Immune Booster: The presence of saponins and vitamins (C and E) helps strengthen the immune system. Digestive Aid: Yerba mate can stimulate the production of bile and other digestive acids, aiding in digestion and improving gut health. Anti-inflammatory: Contains compounds that may help reduce inflammation in the body.
What disease it fights	Fatigue and Mental Fog: The caffeine and nutrients in yerba mate can help improve energy levels and cognitive function. Cardiovascular Diseases: Antioxidants in yerba mate may contribute to heart health by lowering bad cholesterol levels and improving blood vessel health. Weight Management: Can increase metabolism and fat oxidation, supporting weight loss efforts. Digestive Disorders: Its digestive stimulant properties can aid in the treatment of digestive issues.
How it works	Yerba mate's stimulating effects are primarily due to its caffeine content, which increases alertness and reduces fatigue. The antioxidants and anti-inflammatory compounds in yerba mate help combat oxidative stress and inflammation, supporting overall health and disease prevention. Additionally, its digestive and immune-boosting properties further contribute to its health benefits.
How to use	Traditional: Steeped in hot water and consumed from a gourd (calabash) with a metal straw (bombilla) that filters out the leaf fragments. Tea: Brewed like tea and consumed hot or cold, depending on preference. Supplements: Available in capsule or powder form for those who prefer not to drink the beverage.
Dosage	Traditional/Tea: For traditional preparation, about 1-2 tablespoons of yerba mate leaves are used per serving. It can be refilled with hot water several times before the flavor weakens. Drink 1-3 cups daily, based on caffeine tolerance. Supplements: Follow the manufacturer's instructions, typically ranging from 500-1000 mg of yerba mate extract per day.
How long to use	Yerba mate can be consumed daily as part of a healthy lifestyle. However, due to its caffeine content, individuals with sensitivity to caffeine should monitor their intake. Long-term, excessive consumption should be approached with caution, as it may increase the risk of certain health issues related to high caffeine intake.

Yerba Santa

Yerba Santa (Eriodictyon californicum) is a perennial shrub native to the western United States, known for its medicinal properties, particularly in treating respiratory conditions. It has been used traditionally by Native Americans for a range of health issues, including coughs, colds, asthma, and allergies.

Properties	Expectorant: Helps clear mucus from the respiratory tract, making it beneficial for coughs, colds, and bronchial infections. Anti-inflammatory: Reduces inflammation in the respiratory system, aiding in the treatment of asthma and allergic reactions. Antimicrobial: Contains compounds that can fight off bacterial and viral infections. Antioxidant: Offers protection against oxidative stress, contributing to overall health and well-being.
What disease it fights	Respiratory Conditions: Including asthma, bronchitis, coughs, and colds by easing congestion and reducing inflammation. Allergic Reactions: Helps manage symptoms of allergies, such as hay fever, by reducing nasal inflammation and irritation. Mild Infections: The antimicrobial properties make it useful in combating and preventing infections.
How it works	The active compounds in yerba santa, including flavonoids and saponins, contribute to its expectorant, anti-inflammatory, and antimicrobial effects. These compounds help loosen phlegm, reduce inflammation in the respiratory tract, and combat pathogens that can cause respiratory illnesses.
How to use	Tea: Dried leaves can be steeped in hot water to make tea, which can be drunk several times a day to relieve respiratory symptoms. Tincture: A concentrated form that can be taken orally or added to water. Topical Applications: In some traditional practices, yerba santa leaves are applied topically as poultices for minor wounds or muscle pain.
Dosage	Tea: Use 1-2 teaspoons of dried yerba santa leaves per cup of boiling water, steep for 10-15 minutes. Drink 2-3 cups daily. Tincture: Typically, 2-4 ml of tincture three times a day. Follow specific product recommendations. Topical Applications: As needed, based on the specific condition being treated.
How long to use	Yerba santa can be used for the duration of respiratory symptoms or until relief is achieved. For chronic conditions like asthma or allergies, it may be used as part of a longer-term management strategy under the guidance of a healthcare provider. Continuous use should be monitored for any potential side effects or interactions with other medications.

Chapter 10: The O'Neill Lifestyle

Daily Routines for Optimal Health

Dr. Barbara O'Neill, with her holistic approach to health and wellness, likely advocates for establishing daily routines that support optimal health across all dimensions of well-being: physical, mental, emotional, and spiritual. Such routines are designed to harmonize the body's natural rhythms, reinforce healthy habits, and promote a state of balance and vitality. Here's an overview of how she might suggest structuring daily routines for optimal health:

Morning
- Wake Up with the Sun: Starting the day early, in sync with natural light cycles, can help regulate the body's internal clock, improving energy levels and mood throughout the day.
- Hydrate: Drinking a glass of water upon waking helps rehydrate the body after sleep, kickstart metabolism, and flush out toxins.
- Mindful Movement: Engaging in gentle exercise, such as yoga, stretching, or a morning walk, can increase circulation, enhance mood, and prepare the body and mind for the day ahead.
- Mindfulness Practice: Spending a few minutes in meditation or deep breathing exercises can center the mind, reduce stress, and set a positive tone for the day.
- Nourishing Breakfast: Consuming a healthy breakfast that includes a balance of proteins, fats, and carbohydrates provides the energy and nutrients needed for the morning.

Midday
- Mindful Eating: Taking the time to eat lunch mindfully, away from work or distractions, allows for better digestion and provides a mental break.
- Short Breaks: Incorporating short breaks throughout the day to stand, stretch, or take a brief walk can reduce the negative effects of prolonged sitting and help maintain focus and energy levels.
- Hydration: Continuing to drink water or herbal teas throughout the day ensures ongoing hydration and supports detoxification processes.

Afternoon/Evening
- Outdoor Time: Spending time outdoors, especially in natural settings, can improve mental well-being, reduce stress, and support vitamin D synthesis.
- Wind-Down Activities: Engaging in relaxing activities in the evening, such as reading, taking a warm bath, or practicing relaxation techniques, can help ease the transition to sleep.
- Digital Detox: Limiting exposure to screens and electronic devices at least an hour before bedtime reduces blue light exposure, supporting melatonin production and improving sleep quality.
- Reflective Journaling: Reflecting on the day through journaling can provide emotional release and foster a sense of gratitude and accomplishment.

Night
- Consistent Sleep Schedule: Going to bed and waking up at the same times each day, even on weekends, reinforces the body's sleep-wake cycle, enhancing sleep quality.
- Sleep-Inducing Environment: Creating a sleep-conducive environment — cool, dark, and quiet — can significantly improve the quality of rest.

In advocating for these daily routines, Dr. O'Neill emphasizes the importance of consistency and personalization. Recognizing individual differences in lifestyles, preferences, and bodies, she likely encourages adapting these suggestions to fit personal needs and circumstances. The goal of such routines is not rigid adherence to a set of rules but the cultivation of practices that nourish and sustain the body, mind, and spirit, leading to improved health, vitality, and well-being.

Tips for Sustainable Living

Dr. Barbara O'Neill, with her holistic perspective on health, likely emphasizes the importance of sustainable living as an integral part of maintaining personal and environmental well-being. Sustainable living practices not only benefit the planet by reducing waste and conserving resources but also support individual health by encouraging mindful consumption and interaction with the natural world. Here are some tips for sustainable living that align with Dr. O'Neill's approach to health and wellness:

Reduce, Reuse, Recycle
- Mindful Consumption: Before making a purchase, consider the necessity of the item, its environmental impact, and whether there's a more sustainable alternative.
- Reuse and Repurpose: Find new uses for items that might otherwise be discarded, reducing waste and the demand for new products.
- Recycling: Properly recycle materials like paper, glass, and plastic to minimize waste and reduce the need for virgin materials in new products.

Sustainable Eating Habits
- Organic and Locally Sourced Foods: Choose organic produce to avoid pesticides and support local farmers to reduce carbon footprint associated with transportation.
- Plant-Based Diet: Incorporating more plant-based foods can reduce environmental impact compared to diets high in animal products.
- Minimize Food Waste: Plan meals, store food properly, and use leftovers creatively to reduce the amount of food that goes to waste.

Energy Conservation
- Energy-Efficient Appliances: Use appliances rated for energy efficiency to reduce electricity consumption and lower bills.
- Reduce Energy Use: Turn off lights and electronics when not in use, and consider using natural light during the day.
- Renewable Energy Sources: If possible, invest in renewable energy solutions like solar panels for your home.

Water Conservation
- Mindful Water Use: Fix leaks, take shorter showers, and use water-saving appliances to reduce unnecessary water consumption.
- Rainwater Harvesting: Collect rainwater for gardening and outdoor cleaning to decrease dependence on treated water supplies.

Sustainable Transportation
- Alternative Transport: Use public transportation, carpool, bike, or walk when possible to reduce carbon emissions and improve physical health.
- Fuel-Efficient Vehicles: If driving is necessary, choose a fuel-efficient or electric vehicle to minimize environmental impact.

Reducing Chemical Exposure
- Natural Cleaning Products: Opt for natural, non-toxic cleaning products to reduce exposure to harmful chemicals in the home and their release into the environment.
- Organic Personal Care Products: Choose personal care products made with natural ingredients to avoid synthetic chemicals and reduce environmental pollution.

Support Sustainable Practices
- Advocate and Educate: Share knowledge about sustainable living practices with friends, family, and community to inspire collective action towards environmental conservation.

- Support Eco-Friendly Businesses: Purchase from companies committed to sustainable practices and ethical production methods.

Dr. O'Neill's approach likely advocates for an integrated view of health that encompasses not just the individual but also the broader ecosystem. By adopting sustainable living practices, individuals can contribute to a healthier planet while also promoting their own well-being, highlighting the interconnectedness of human health and environmental health.

Glossary of Terms

1. Antioxidants: Substances that protect the body from damage caused by harmful molecules called free radicals. Commonly found in fruits, vegetables, and certain herbs, antioxidants support the body's natural defense systems.
2. Deep Breathing Exercises: Techniques that involve conscious deepening of breaths to enhance lung capacity, reduce stress, and improve oxygen supply to the body. These exercises are often recommended for their calming effects and support of the mind-body connection.
3. Detoxification: The physiological or medicinal removal of toxic substances from the human body, primarily performed by the liver. Dr. O'Neill emphasizes natural methods to support the body's detox processes.
4. Digestive Health: A crucial aspect of overall wellness that involves the proper functioning of the digestive system. Dr. O'Neill often highlights the importance of a fiber-rich diet and hydration for maintaining digestive health.
5. Emotional Well-being: The aspect of holistic health that involves understanding and respecting your feelings and managing stress effectively. Techniques such as mindfulness and meditation are recommended to enhance emotional well-being.
6. Environmental Toxins: Harmful chemicals and pollutants found in the environment that can affect human health. Reducing exposure to these toxins through choices in diet, lifestyle, and household products is a key aspect of Dr. O'Neill's holistic health approach.
7. Fiber-Rich Foods: Foods high in dietary fiber, such as vegetables, fruits, legumes, and whole grains, which support digestive health and detoxification.
8. Functional Foods: Foods that have a potentially positive effect on health beyond basic nutrition. Dr. O'Neill may highlight the role of functional foods, such as probiotics and omega-3 fatty acids, in promoting health and preventing disease.
9. Herbal Supplements: Supplements made from plants, used for their therapeutic properties. They play a significant role in Dr. O'Neill's natural health recommendations for supporting bodily functions and enhancing wellness.
10. Holistic Health: An approach to life that considers multiple factors of well-being, including physical, mental, emotional, and spiritual health, emphasizing the connection between these aspects.
11. Immune Function: The body's natural defense mechanism against infection and disease. Nutrition, sleep, and stress management are key factors that Dr. O'Neill focuses on to support immune function.
12. Meditative Movement: Activities such as yoga, tai chi, and qigong that combine movement with elements of meditation and mindfulness to enhance physical and mental well-being.
13. Mind-Body Connection: The interrelationship between mental and physical health, where psychological well-being can affect physical health and vice versa. Dr. O'Neill incorporates practices that nurture this connection for overall health.
14. Mindfulness: A mental state achieved by focusing one's awareness on the present moment, while calmly acknowledging and accepting one's feelings, thoughts, and bodily sensations. Used as a therapeutic technique.
15. Natural Remedies: Treatments that use natural ingredients, including herbs, foods, and teas, to heal and support the body's health. Dr. O'Neill often advocates for using natural remedies as part of a holistic health approach.
16. Nutritional Deficiencies: Conditions that occur when the body doesn't get enough essential nutrients. Addressing nutritional deficiencies through a balanced diet is a key part of Dr. O'Neill's method.
17. Organic Foods: Foods that are produced without the use of synthetic pesticides, chemical fertilizers, or genetically modified organisms (GMOs). Dr. O'Neill recommends organic foods to reduce toxin intake.
18. Physical Activity: Regular bodily movement that is conducted to enhance or maintain physical fitness and overall health. Dr. O'Neill emphasizes the importance of incorporating physical activity into daily routines for health benefits.

19. Plant-Based Proteins: Proteins derived from plants rather than animal products. Incorporating plant-based proteins into the diet is often recommended for health and environmental reasons, aligning with Dr. O'Neill's advocacy for a plant-based diet.
20. Sleep Hygiene: Practices and habits that are conducive to sleeping well on a regular basis. Dr. O'Neill emphasizes the importance of good sleep hygiene for overall health, including consistent sleep schedules and creating a restful environment.
21. Spiritual Wellness: An aspect of holistic health that involves having a set of beliefs, principles, or values that give meaning and purpose to life. Dr. O'Neill might encourage practices that foster spiritual wellness, such as meditation, prayer, or spending time in nature, for comprehensive well-being.
22. Sustainable Living: Making lifestyle choices that aim to reduce an individual's or society's use of the Earth's natural resources. Dr. O'Neill advocates for practices that promote sustainability in diet and lifestyle.
23. Stress Management: Techniques and practices that help reduce or manage stress levels. Dr. O'Neill recommends various strategies, including exercise, meditation, and time in nature, for effective stress management.
24. Water Filtration: The process of purifying water to remove impurities and contaminants. Given the importance of hydration and reducing toxin intake, Dr. O'Neill may recommend using water filtration systems to ensure clean drinking water.
25. Whole Foods: Foods that are consumed in their natural, unprocessed form. Dr. O'Neill emphasizes the health benefits of a diet based on whole foods for optimal nutrition and detoxification.

Dr. Barbara O'Neill Herbal Remedies for a Disease-Free Life

Say Goodbye to Any Kind of Illness and Step Into a Life of Vibrant Health and Vitality Without Relying on Conventional Medicine

Janet Moore

Foreword

In an era increasingly dominated by quick fixes and a reliance on pharmaceutical solutions, the teachings of Dr. Barbara O'Neill shine as a beacon for those seeking a different path. This book aims to illuminate that path, offering readers an in-depth exploration of Dr. O'Neill's philosophy, methods, and the profound impact they have had on natural healing and holistic health practices.

Dr. O'Neill, a respected naturopath, nutritionist, and educator, has dedicated her life to the study and dissemination of knowledge on how to achieve wellness through natural means. Her approach is both revolutionary and deeply rooted in the timeless wisdom of nature's own capacity for healing. By focusing on the body's inherent ability to heal itself, given the right conditions and nutrients, Dr. O'Neill's work challenges conventional health paradigms and opens up new avenues for wellness and vitality.

The teachings of Dr. O'Neill are not just about avoiding or treating disease; they are about a comprehensive lifestyle approach that encompasses diet, exercise, mental health, and spiritual well-being. This holistic view is crucial in an age where health is often compartmentalized, and the connections between physical health, emotional balance, and environmental factors are frequently overlooked.

This foreword invites you on a journey to explore the profound and life-changing teachings of Dr. O'Neill. The chapters that follow delve into her methodology, providing practical advice, insights, and case studies that showcase the effectiveness of her natural healing approach. From overcoming digestive disorders to managing chronic conditions such as diabetes and heart disease, the book covers a wide range of topics that are at the forefront of health concerns today.

Moreover, this book is a testament to the power of natural healing and the potential for each individual to take control of their health. It is a guide, a resource, and an inspiration for those who wish to live in harmony with nature's laws, advocating for a health-conscious lifestyle that prioritizes wellness over merely the absence of disease.

As you turn these pages, we hope you find not only valuable information but also motivation and encouragement to embark on your own journey toward holistic health. Whether you are new to the concepts of natural healing or have been following Dr. O'Neill's work for years, this book offers something for everyone—a chance to transform your health, your life, and perhaps even your perspective on what it means to truly thrive.

Welcome to the world of natural healing through the teachings of Dr. Barbara O'Neill. Let this foreword be the first step on a path to a healthier, happier, and more harmonious life.

A Short Biography of Dr. O'Neill: Her Journey and Achievements

D r. Barbara O'Neill, a figure synonymous with natural healing and holistic health, embarked on her journey with a simple yet profound conviction: the body is designed to heal itself, provided it is given the right conditions. This belief, rooted in the principles of naturopathy and nurtured by years of study, research, and practice, has guided her career and shaped her contributions to the field of natural health.

Born into a family that valued the principles of healthy living, Dr. O'Neill's early life was marked by an exposure to natural remedies and the healing power of nutrition. However, it was her personal health challenges and those of her close family members that truly catalyzed her interest in natural therapies. Faced with health conditions that conventional medicine struggled to address effectively, she turned to nature for answers, embarking on what would become a lifelong quest for knowledge and healing.

Dr. O'Neill pursued formal education in naturopathy, nutrition, and herbal medicine, acquiring a comprehensive foundation that would underpin her future work. Her academic journey was characterized by an insatiable curiosity and a relentless drive to understand the intricate ways in which diet, lifestyle, and natural remedies could influence health and well-being.

After completing her studies, Dr. O'Neill began her practice with a focus on educating her clients about the importance of diet and lifestyle in preventing and treating disease. Her approach, holistic and patient-centered, quickly gained recognition for its effectiveness. She advocated for the use of whole foods, herbal remedies, and lifestyle modifications, not just as interventions for health issues but as foundational elements of a healthy life.

Dr. O'Neill's impact extended far beyond her clinical practice. She became a sought-after speaker, educator, and author, dedicating a significant part of her career to sharing her knowledge and experiences. Through workshops, seminars, and online platforms, she reached a global audience, spreading her message of natural healing and empowering individuals to take control of their health.

Her contributions to the field of natural health have been widely recognized, earning her accolades and respect from peers and followers alike. However, perhaps her most significant achievement is the legacy of health transformation she has facilitated for countless individuals. Through her teachings, Dr. O'Neill has ignited a passion for natural health in others, fostering a community of informed, health-conscious individuals committed to living in harmony with nature's principles.

Dr. O'Neill's journey is a testament to the power of natural healing and the potential for each person to achieve optimal health through a holistic approach. Her achievements not only reflect her dedication and expertise but also her deep compassion and desire to see others thrive. As her teachings continue to inspire and guide, Dr. O'Neill's legacy in the world of natural health is both profound and enduring.

Introduction to Natural Healing: Understanding Dr. O'Neill's Approach

At the heart of Dr. Barbara O'Neill's philosophy lies a profound respect for the natural world and an unwavering belief in the body's innate capacity for self-healing. Her approach to natural healing is not merely a set of techniques or remedies but a holistic lifestyle that encompasses the physical, mental, emotional, and spiritual aspects of wellbeing. This chapter delves into the core principles and practices that define Dr. O'Neill's approach to natural healing, offering insight into a methodology that seeks to harmonize the individual with the natural laws of life and health.

The Foundation of Natural Healing

Dr. O'Neill's methodology is grounded in the principle that health is the natural state of the body. Disease, she argues, arises when there are obstacles to the body's inherent healing processes. These obstacles can be physical, such as toxins or nutritional deficiencies, emotional, such as stress and unresolved trauma, or environmental, like exposure to harmful chemicals. Her approach seeks to identify and remove these obstacles, thereby allowing the body to heal itself.

The Pillars of Health

Dr. O'Neill identifies several key pillars of health that are essential to her natural healing approach:

- **Nutrition**: At the forefront is the role of nutrition. Dr. O'Neill emphasizes the importance of a whole-foods diet, rich in fruits, vegetables, whole grains, and lean proteins, as foundational to health. She advocates for foods that are as close to their natural state as possible, minimally processed, and free from additives and chemicals.
- **Detoxification**: Recognizing the burden that toxins place on the body, detoxification is another cornerstone of her approach. This includes practices such as fasting, herbal detoxes, and the consumption of foods that support the body's natural detoxification pathways.
- **Exercise and Fresh Air**: Physical activity and exposure to fresh air are viewed as essential for stimulating circulation, enhancing oxygenation, and promoting overall vitality. Dr. O'Neill encourages regular, moderate exercise and spending time in nature as key components of a healthy lifestyle.
- **Rest and Relaxation**: Understanding the critical role of rest in the healing process, Dr. O'Neill advocates for sufficient sleep and relaxation practices. These practices are crucial for reducing stress, supporting immune function, and allowing the body to repair and rejuvenate.
- **Positive Mindset and Emotional Wellbeing**: Emphasizing the mind-body connection, Dr. O'Neill highlights the importance of a positive outlook, stress management techniques, and addressing emotional health as integral to natural healing.

The Role of Herbal Medicine

Herbal medicine plays a significant role in Dr. O'Neill's approach. She utilizes a wide range of herbs for their therapeutic properties, tailoring herbal remedies to support the body's healing processes and address specific health concerns. Her expertise in herbal medicine complements her nutritional and lifestyle recommendations, providing a comprehensive toolkit for natural healing.

Personalized Healing

A key aspect of Dr. O'Neill's methodology is its personalized nature. She acknowledges the unique biological and psychological makeup of each individual, advocating for personalized assessments and treatments. This bespoke approach ensures that the strategies and remedies recommended are optimally aligned with the individual's specific health needs and goals.

Education and Empowerment

Above all, Dr. O'Neill's approach is characterized by an emphasis on education and empowerment. She believes that informed individuals are better equipped to make choices that support their health and wellbeing. Through her teachings, she aims to demystify the principles of natural healing, making them accessible and actionable for everyone.

In summary, Dr. O'Neill's approach to natural healing is a comprehensive, holistic methodology that seeks to align individuals with the natural laws of health and vitality. By addressing the root causes of disease, advocating for a return to natural, life-supporting habits, and empowering individuals with the knowledge to take control of their health, Dr. O'Neill's work stands as a powerful testament to the healing potential of the natural world.

Philosophy Behind Natural Healing

The philosophy behind natural healing, as advocated by Dr. Barbara O'Neill, is deeply rooted in the belief that the body possesses an inherent wisdom and capacity for self-regulation and healing. This perspective stands in contrast to conventional medicine's often symptom-focused approach, advocating instead for addressing the underlying causes of disease through holistic means. At the core of this philosophy are several key principles that not only guide natural healing practices but also encourage a profound reconnection with the natural world and our place within it.

Holism

The holistic approach is fundamental to natural healing. It posits that an individual is more than the sum of their parts, emphasizing the interconnectedness of the body, mind, and spirit. This principle asserts that health and wellness depend on the harmonious balance of these components. Dr. O'Neill's teachings stress that disturbances in any one area can affect the whole organism, thereby advocating for healing strategies that encompass physical, mental, emotional, and spiritual dimensions.

The Healing Power of Nature

Central to natural healing is the "vis medicatrix naturae," or the healing power of nature. This concept suggests that the body naturally seeks to restore itself to health when given the proper support. Dr. O'Neill's philosophy embraces this idea, promoting practices that align with natural processes and rhythms. This includes the use of natural remedies, such as herbs and foods, that the body can easily assimilate and utilize in its healing efforts.

Prevention Is Primary

Preventative care is a cornerstone of the natural healing philosophy. Instead of waiting for disease to manifest, Dr. O'Neill emphasizes the importance of proactive measures to maintain health and prevent illness. This involves a lifestyle that supports health through nutrition, exercise, stress management, and avoidance of toxins—measures that not only ward off disease but also promote vitality and longevity.

The Root Cause Approach

Rather than merely addressing symptoms, natural healing seeks to identify and treat the root causes of illness. This diagnostic principle is crucial to Dr. O'Neill's philosophy, which looks beyond the immediate manifestations of disease to understand the underlying imbalances or dysfunctions. By correcting these foundational issues, natural healing aims for lasting wellness rather than temporary relief.

The Individual as an Active Participant

Empowerment and education are key in Dr. O'Neill's approach to healing. This philosophy champions the individual's role as an active participant in their health journey. By equipping people with knowledge and understanding about how their bodies work and how various lifestyle factors affect health, Dr. O'Neill encourages personal responsibility and informed decision-making in health care.

Integration with Nature

A reverence for and integration with the natural environment is also intrinsic to this philosophy. Recognizing that humans are part of the broader ecosystem, natural healing promotes living in a way that is sustainable and in harmony with the Earth. This includes practices that respect the cycles of nature, such as seasonal eating and herbal medicine, and an awareness of the impact of environmental factors on health.

Education for Empowerment

Finally, the philosophy behind natural healing is deeply educational. Dr. O'Neill believes in empowering individuals through education, providing them with the tools and knowledge necessary to make informed decisions about their health. This aspect of her philosophy seeks to demystify health and healing, making it accessible to all and encouraging a proactive, preventative approach to wellness.

In essence, the philosophy of natural healing as championed by Dr. O'Neill is a call to return to the basics of health care. It emphasizes the body's innate wisdom, the importance of a holistic approach, and the power of nature in the healing process. It advocates for prevention, addresses the root causes of disease, and empowers individuals to take charge of their health. Through this lens, health is seen not just as the absence of disease, but as a state of complete physical, mental, and social well-being.

Core Principles of Dr. O'Neill's Methodology

The core principles of Dr. Barbara O'Neill's methodology are deeply embedded in the philosophy of natural healing, emphasizing the body's inherent ability to heal itself when supported by a conducive environment. Her approach is holistic, addressing not only the physical aspects of health but also the mental, emotional, and spiritual dimensions. These principles serve as the foundation for her teachings and practices, guiding individuals towards achieving optimal health and wellness naturally. Let's delve into these core principles in detail:

1. The Body as an Integrated Whole

Dr. O'Neill emphasizes the interconnectedness of the body's systems, advocating for a holistic approach to health. She teaches that the body should be viewed as an integrated whole, where physical symptoms are often manifestations of imbalances or disharmonies within the system. This principle underlines the importance of addressing health concerns holistically rather than isolating symptoms.

2. The Healing Power of Nature

A fundamental tenet of Dr. O'Neill's methodology is the healing power of nature, or "Vis Medicatrix Naturae." She believes that the body has an inherent ability to heal itself and that natural remedies and practices can support and facilitate this healing process. This respect for nature's wisdom informs her use of herbal medicines, whole foods, and natural therapies.

3. Prevention is Better than Cure

Preventative health is a cornerstone of Dr. O'Neill's approach. She advocates for lifestyle choices and habits that support health and prevent disease, arguing that it is more effective and beneficial to maintain health than to treat disease after it has developed. This includes dietary recommendations, exercise, stress management, and avoidance of toxins.

4. The Importance of Nutrition

Dr. O'Neill places a strong emphasis on the role of nutrition in health and healing. She promotes a diet rich in whole, unprocessed foods that provide the nutrients the body needs to function optimally. Her nutritional guidelines focus on the quality of food, the importance of dietary diversity, and the role of specific nutrients in supporting health.

5. Education and Self-Responsibility

Empowering individuals through education is a critical aspect of Dr. O'Neill's methodology. She believes that informed individuals are better equipped to make decisions about their health and well-being. By educating people about the principles of natural health, she encourages self-responsibility and proactive engagement in one's health journey.

6. Tailored and Personalized Care

Recognizing the uniqueness of each individual, Dr. O'Neill's approach is highly personalized. She acknowledges that each person's health needs, lifestyle, and biological makeup are unique, necessitating a tailored approach to diet, herbal medicine, and lifestyle interventions. This personalized care ensures that health recommendations are effective and sustainable for the individual.

7. Balance and Harmony

Balance and harmony are key concepts in Dr. O'Neill's methodology. She teaches that health is a state of balance between the body, mind, and environment. Her recommendations aim to restore balance and harmony, whether through addressing nutritional deficiencies, managing stress, detoxifying the body, or fostering emotional well-being.

8. The Mind-Body Connection

Dr. O'Neill highlights the profound connection between the mind and the body. She emphasizes that emotional and mental health are integral to physical health, advocating for practices that support mental and emotional well-being, such as meditation, stress management techniques, and fostering positive relationships.

In summary, the core principles of Dr. Barbara O'Neill's methodology are rooted in a deep respect for the body's natural healing capabilities and the holistic nature of health. By integrating these principles into one's life, Dr. O'Neill believes individuals can achieve a state of wellness that encompasses not only physical health but emotional, mental, and spiritual well-being.

Overview of Holistic Health

Holistic health is an approach to well-being that considers the whole person, including their physical, mental, emotional, and spiritual health, rather than focusing solely on individual symptoms or diseases. This comprehensive perspective stems from the understanding that all aspects of a person's life are interconnected and contribute to their overall health status. The philosophy behind holistic health emphasizes the body's inherent ability to heal and maintain balance, advocating for natural and preventive measures to support this process. Here's an in-depth look at the principles, practices, and benefits of holistic health:

Principles of Holistic Health

1. **Interconnectedness**: Holistic health recognizes the interplay between the physical, emotional, mental, and spiritual components of an individual. It posits that imbalances in one aspect can affect overall health, necessitating a comprehensive approach to healing and wellness.
2. **Individualized Care**: Given the unique nature of each individual, holistic health stresses personalized care plans that address specific needs, preferences, and circumstances. It respects the individual's health choices and encourages active participation in their health journey.
3. **Preventive Approach**: Prevention is a key tenet of holistic health. By addressing potential health issues before they arise and fostering healthy lifestyle habits, holistic health aims to minimize the risk of disease and promote long-term wellness.
4. **Natural Remedies and Therapies**: Holistic health often incorporates natural remedies and therapies, including herbal medicine, nutrition, acupuncture, massage, and mindfulness practices, among others. These are chosen for their ability to support the body's healing capabilities with minimal side effects.
5. **Mind-Body-Spirit Connection**: Acknowledging the mind-body-spirit connection is fundamental. Holistic health practices often include techniques to calm the mind, nurture the spirit, and support emotional well-being as integral components of physical health.

Practices in Holistic Health
- **Nutritional Counseling**: Emphasizing whole, unprocessed foods to nourish the body and support healing.
- **Physical Activity**: Encouraging regular exercise tailored to the individual's preferences and capabilities to improve physical health and mental well-being.
- **Mindfulness and Stress Reduction**: Utilizing practices such as meditation, yoga, and deep-breathing exercises to reduce stress and enhance mental clarity.
- **Herbal and Natural Supplements**: Recommending herbal remedies and supplements to support the body's health and address specific concerns.
- **Complementary Therapies**: Incorporating therapies like acupuncture, chiropractic care, and massage therapy to address various health issues and promote relaxation.

Benefits of Holistic Health
1. **Comprehensive Health Improvements**: By addressing multiple aspects of well-being, holistic health can lead to comprehensive improvements in health, including better physical condition, mental clarity, emotional resilience, and spiritual fulfillment.
2. **Empowerment and Self-care**: Holistic health empowers individuals to take control of their health by providing them with the knowledge and tools to care for themselves, encouraging a proactive approach to well-being.
3. **Prevention of Disease**: The preventive nature of holistic health can lead to a lower incidence of chronic diseases by addressing risk factors and promoting healthy lifestyles.
4. **Reduced Reliance on Pharmaceuticals**: By focusing on natural remedies and lifestyle adjustments, holistic health can reduce dependence on pharmaceutical interventions and their potential side effects.
5. **Enhanced Quality of Life**: The holistic approach aims not just to treat or prevent disease but to enhance the overall quality of life, leading to greater satisfaction and happiness.

In summary, an overview of holistic health reveals a deep and multifaceted approach to wellness that transcends conventional medical practices. It underscores the importance of viewing the individual as a whole, advocating for natural, preventive, and personalized care strategies to foster true well-being. This paradigm shift towards holistic health reflects a growing recognition of the complex, interconnected nature of health and the value of natural, integrative approaches to healing and wellness.

Chapter 1: Overcoming Digestive Disorders

D igestive disorders encompass a wide range of conditions that affect the gastrointestinal (GI) tract, from common issues like indigestion and irritable bowel syndrome (IBS) to more complex diseases such as Crohn's and celiac disease. Dr. Barbara O'Neill's approach to overcoming these disorders is rooted in natural healing and holistic health principles. This chapter delves into the signs and symptoms of common digestive issues, explores herbal and dietary interventions, and outlines lifestyle changes that can significantly improve gut health.

Signs and Symptoms of Common Digestive Issues

Digestive disorders encompass a wide range of conditions that affect the gastrointestinal (GI) tract. Understanding the signs and symptoms of these issues is the first step toward identifying and addressing underlying health concerns. Common digestive disorders include irritable bowel syndrome (IBS), inflammatory bowel disease (IBD), gastroesophageal reflux disease (GERD), celiac disease, and various food intolerances. Here, we delve into the signs and symptoms characteristic of these conditions, providing a foundational understanding that can guide individuals towards seeking appropriate care and adopting beneficial lifestyle changes.

Irritable Bowel Syndrome (IBS)

IBS is characterized by a combination of symptoms that can include abdominal pain, bloating, and changes in bowel habits (such as diarrhea and/or constipation). Symptoms often worsen during periods of stress or after eating certain foods. Despite its discomfort, IBS does not cause changes in bowel tissue or increase the risk of colorectal cancer.

Inflammatory Bowel Disease (IBD)

IBD primarily refers to two conditions: Crohn's disease and ulcerative colitis. These diseases are marked by chronic inflammation of the GI tract. Symptoms include severe diarrhea, abdominal pain, fatigue, and weight loss. IBD can be debilitating and sometimes leads to life-threatening complications.

Gastroesophageal Reflux Disease (GERD)

GERD occurs when stomach acid frequently flows back into the tube connecting the mouth and stomach (esophagus). This backwash (acid reflux) can irritate the lining of the esophagus, leading to symptoms such as heartburn, regurgitation of food or sour liquid, chest pain, and difficulty swallowing.

Celiac Disease

Celiac disease is an autoimmune disorder in which the ingestion of gluten leads to damage in the small intestine. Symptoms vary widely and may include diarrhea, bloating, gas, fatigue, low blood count (anemia), and osteoporosis. Some individuals may have no symptoms, while others suffer severe malabsorption.

Food Intolerances

Food intolerances, such as lactose intolerance, occur when the digestive system cannot break down certain components of foods. Symptoms can include bloating, abdominal pain, diarrhea, gas, and nausea, often occurring hours after consuming the offending food.

- **Changes in Bowel Habits**: Unexplained and persistent changes in bowel habits, including constipation, diarrhea, or the appearance of blood or mucus in the stool.
- **Abdominal Pain and Discomfort**: Frequent abdominal cramping, pain, or discomfort that may be related to meals or might occur at any time.
- **Bloating and Gas**: Excessive bloating or gas, which might also be accompanied by a feeling of fullness or pressure in the abdomen.
- **Weight Fluctuations**: Unintended weight loss or gain without a clear cause can be a sign of a digestive disorder.
- **Fatigue and Weakness**: Chronic fatigue or weakness that does not improve with rest could be linked to malabsorption of nutrients due to a GI condition.

Recognizing these signs and symptoms is critical in seeking early intervention and management. While some symptoms may be mild and manageable through lifestyle adjustments, others may indicate more serious underlying conditions that require medical attention. It's important for individuals experiencing these symptoms to consult healthcare professionals for a thorough evaluation and to explore both conventional and holistic treatment options tailored to their specific needs.

Herbal and Dietary Interventions for Digestive Disorders

Addressing digestive disorders through herbal and dietary interventions involves a comprehensive approach that not only targets symptoms but also aims to restore the overall balance and health of the gastrointestinal (GI) system. The integration of specific herbs along with dietary adjustments can significantly improve digestion, alleviate discomfort, and support the body's natural healing processes. Below, we explore effective herbal remedies and dietary recommendations for managing digestive issues, accompanied by guidance on preparing these herbs for consumption.

Herbal Remedies for Digestive Health

1. **Ginger (Zingiber officinale)**
   - **Benefits**: Ginger is renowned for its anti-inflammatory and gastrointestinal motility properties. It can help alleviate nausea, vomiting, and indigestion.
   - **Preparation**: Fresh ginger root can be grated and steeped in boiling water for 10-15 minutes to make a soothing tea. Alternatively, ginger can be included in meals or taken as a supplement.
   - **When to Take**: Ginger tea can be consumed 20-30 minutes before meals to stimulate digestion or after meals to alleviate indigestion or nausea.
   - **Quantity**: For tea, use about 1 teaspoon of freshly grated ginger per cup of boiling water. If using supplements, follow the manufacturer's dosage instructions, typically around 250 mg to 1 gram, 3 times daily.
   - **Duration**: Ginger can be used on an as-needed basis. For chronic conditions, it can be consumed daily, with periodic evaluations every few weeks to assess benefits and side effects.

2. **Peppermint (Mentha piperita)**
   - **Benefits**: Peppermint oil is effective in relieving symptoms of IBS, including abdominal pain, bloating, and gas. Its antispasmodic properties help relax the muscles of the digestive tract.
   - **Preparation**: Peppermint tea can be made by steeping dried peppermint leaves in hot water for 5-10 minutes. Peppermint oil capsules are also available for more targeted relief.

- **When to Take**: Peppermint tea is best consumed between meals to avoid affecting the absorption of iron and other minerals. Peppermint oil capsules should be taken as directed, usually 1-2 hours before meals.
- **Quantity**: One cup of peppermint tea can be made with 1-2 teaspoons of dried leaves. Peppermint oil capsules typically contain 0.2 to 0.4 ml of oil per capsule, taken 2-3 times daily.
- **Duration**: Use for 4-6 weeks to assess effectiveness. Some people may experience heartburn or discomfort, in which case, discontinue use.

3. **Chamomile (Matricaria recutita)**
    - **Benefits**: Chamomile is known for its calming effects, which can be beneficial for stress-related digestive complaints. It also possesses anti-inflammatory properties.
    - **Preparation**: Prepare chamomile tea by infusing dried chamomile flowers in boiling water for 5 minutes. It can be consumed 2-3 times daily, especially after meals or before bedtime.
    - **When to Take**: Chamomile tea is beneficial when consumed after meals to aid digestion or before bedtime to promote relaxation.
    - **Quantity**: Use 2-3 teaspoons of dried chamomile flowers per cup of boiling water. Steep for 5-10 minutes.
    - **Duration**: Chamomile can be used daily. Evaluate its effects over a period of a few weeks. It's generally considered safe for long-term use.

4. **Slippery Elm (Ulmus rubra)**
    - **Benefits**: The mucilage content of slippery elm forms a soothing film over the mucous membranes, aiding in the healing of ulcers and reducing irritation in the GI tract.
    - **Preparation**: Mix one tablespoon of powdered slippery elm bark with hot water to create a gel-like substance. This can be taken after meals.
    - **When to Take**: Chamomile tea is beneficial when consumed after meals to aid digestion or before bedtime to promote relaxation.
    - **Quantity**: Use 2-3 teaspoons of dried chamomile flowers per cup of boiling water. Steep for 5-10 minutes.
    - **Duration**: Chamomile can be used daily. Evaluate its effects over a period of a few weeks. It's generally considered safe for long-term use.

5. **Fennel (Foeniculum vulgare)**
    - **Benefits**: Fennel seeds are effective in reducing gas and bloating. They also support digestion by stimulating the secretion of digestive enzymes.
    - **Preparation**: Fennel tea can be made by crushing fennel seeds and steeping them in boiling water for 10 minutes. Alternatively, fennel seeds can be chewed after meals.
    - **When to Take**: Fennel tea or chewed seeds are most effective when taken after meals to aid in digestion and alleviate gas and bloating.
    - **Quantity**: For tea, use 1-2 teaspoons of crushed seeds per cup of boiling water. If chewing seeds, a half teaspoon chewed slowly after meals is sufficient.
    - **Duration**: Fennel can be used as needed for digestive discomfort. For chronic issues, daily use over several weeks can help assess its effectiveness.

Dietary Recommendations
1. **Increase Fiber Intake**
    - Gradually incorporate more soluble and insoluble fibers into your diet to help regulate bowel movements. Sources include fruits, vegetables, whole grains, and legumes.
2. **Stay Hydrated**
    - Drinking sufficient water is essential for digestive health, as it helps dissolve fats and soluble fiber, allowing these substances to pass through more easily.
3. **Limit Inflammatory Foods**

- Reduce the intake of foods known to exacerbate inflammation and digestive discomfort, such as fried foods, processed meats, dairy products (for those lactose intolerant), and refined sugars.
4. **Incorporate Probiotic and Fermented Foods**
   - Foods rich in probiotics, like yogurt, kefir, sauerkraut, and kimchi, can enhance the gut microbiome, improving digestion and immunity.
5. **Mindful Eating Practices**
   - Eating slowly and mindfully, chewing thoroughly, and avoiding overeating can significantly improve digestion and prevent discomfort.

In integrating these herbal and dietary interventions, it's essential to listen to your body and adjust according to your specific needs and responses. Starting with small doses and monitoring effects can help identify what works best for you. For chronic or severe digestive disorders, these interventions should complement, not replace, the guidance and treatment provided by healthcare professionals.

Lifestyle Changes for Gut Health Improvement

Improving gut health is a multifaceted endeavor that extends beyond diet and herbal remedies. Lifestyle changes play a crucial role in enhancing digestive function and overall wellness. Adopting a holistic approach to living can foster a healthier gut microbiome, reduce inflammation, and mitigate many of the symptoms associated with digestive disorders. Below are key lifestyle modifications aimed at boosting gut health:

1. Stress Management

Chronic stress has been shown to negatively impact gut health, exacerbating symptoms of various digestive disorders. Implementing effective stress management techniques is vital for maintaining a healthy digestive system.
- **Mindfulness and Meditation**: Regular practice can reduce stress levels and inflammation, positively affecting gut health.
- **Yoga and Tai Chi**: These practices combine physical movement with breath control and meditation, helping to lower stress and improve digestion.
- **Adequate Sleep**: Ensuring 7-9 hours of quality sleep per night helps regulate stress hormones and supports gut health.

2. Regular Physical Activity

Exercise plays a significant role in promoting a healthy digestive system. It can enhance gut motility, reduce inflammation, and even positively alter the composition of the gut microbiota.
- **Moderate Exercise**: Aim for at least 150 minutes of moderate aerobic activity weekly, such as brisk walking, cycling, or swimming.
- **Strength Training**: Incorporating strength training exercises twice a week can improve overall body composition and gut health.
- **Consistency is Key**: Regular, consistent physical activity is more beneficial than intermittent intense workouts.

3. Adequate Hydration

Water is essential for digestion. It aids in the breakdown of food, allows for smooth passage through the digestive tract, and helps prevent constipation.
- **Water Intake**: Aim to drink at least 8-10 glasses of water a day, more if you're active or live in a hot climate.
- **Limit Caffeinated and Sugary Beverages**: These can disrupt the balance of your gut microbiota and lead to dehydration.

4. Improve Sleep Hygiene

Poor sleep quality and duration can negatively affect gut health. Establishing a regular sleep schedule and creating a restful environment are critical steps toward improving both sleep and digestive health.

- **Consistent Sleep Schedule**: Go to bed and wake up at the same time every day, even on weekends.
- **Sleep Environment**: Ensure your bedroom is quiet, dark, and cool. Consider using white noise machines and blackout curtains if necessary.

5. Limit Alcohol and Stop Smoking

Both excessive alcohol consumption and smoking can harm the gut lining, leading to increased permeability (leaky gut) and inflammation.

- **Moderate Alcohol Consumption**: If you consume alcohol, do so in moderation. Consider limiting intake to one drink per day for women and two drinks per day for men.
- **Seek Help to Quit Smoking**: Smoking cessation is challenging but crucial for gut health. Numerous resources are available to support quitting.

6. Mindful Eating Practices

How you eat can be just as important as what you eat. Mindful eating can enhance digestion and nutrient absorption.

- **Chew Thoroughly**: Take time to chew your food thoroughly to aid in digestion and nutrient extraction.
- **Eat Without Distractions**: Avoid eating while watching TV or working. Focus on your meal to improve digestion and satiety signals.

Chapter 2: Managing Diabetes Naturally

Diabetes, a chronic condition characterized by elevated blood sugar levels, poses significant health challenges worldwide. Traditional medical treatments often focus on medication to control blood sugar levels, but a holistic approach emphasizing natural management strategies can be highly beneficial. This chapter delves into the natural ways to manage diabetes, focusing on dietary interventions, key herbs for blood sugar regulation, incorporating exercise, and the importance of lifestyle changes.

Understanding the Role of Diet in Diabetes

The cornerstone of managing diabetes, whether it's Type 1, Type 2, or gestational diabetes, lies in understanding and implementing a balanced diet. The foods we consume have a direct impact on blood glucose levels, and by making informed dietary choices, individuals with diabetes can significantly improve their blood sugar management, enhance their overall health, and reduce the risk of diabetes-related complications. This section delves into the critical aspects of diet in the context of diabetes management.

The Impact of Carbohydrates

Carbohydrates have the most immediate impact on blood glucose levels. Understanding the different types of carbohydrates and how they affect blood sugar is crucial:

- **Complex Carbohydrates**: These are found in whole grains, legumes, vegetables, and fruits. They are broken down more slowly, providing a steady release of glucose into the bloodstream and thus are preferable for blood sugar control.
- **Simple Carbohydrates**: Often referred to as "sugars," they are found in refined grains, sweets, and sugary beverages. These carbs are rapidly absorbed, causing spikes in blood sugar levels and should be limited.

Glycemic Index and Glycemic Load

- **Glycemic Index (GI)**: This measures how quickly a carbohydrate-containing food raises blood glucose levels. Low-GI foods are beneficial for blood sugar control.
- **Glycemic Load (GL)**: This considers the GI and the amount of carbohydrate in a serving. It provides a more accurate picture of how a food affects blood sugar levels.

Fiber Intake

- Dietary fiber, particularly soluble fiber, can slow the absorption of sugar and help improve blood sugar levels. High-fiber foods include vegetables, fruits, legumes, and whole grains.

Healthy Fats

- Incorporating healthy fats from sources like avocados, nuts, seeds, and olive oil can slow carbohydrate absorption, thereby preventing rapid spikes in blood glucose. Omega-3 fatty acids, found in fatty fish, flaxseeds, and walnuts, are particularly beneficial for heart health, which is crucial since diabetes increases heart disease risk.

Protein

- Adequate protein intake is vital for blood sugar management and overall health. It has a minimal effect on blood glucose levels and can promote satiety, reducing the likelihood of overeating. Choose lean protein sources such as poultry, fish, tofu, legumes, and eggs.

Meal Timing and Portion Control

- Consistency in meal timing helps maintain steady blood sugar levels throughout the day. Portion control is equally important to prevent overeating, which can lead to weight gain and increased insulin resistance.

Monitoring and Adjusting
- Individuals with diabetes should closely monitor their blood sugar responses to different foods and adjust their diets accordingly. What works for one person may not work for another, making personalized dietary planning essential.

Practical Tips for Dietary Management
1. **Plan Meals**: Include a balance of carbohydrates, proteins, and fats in each meal.
2. **Read Labels**: Be mindful of the carbohydrate content in packaged foods.
3. **Choose Whole Foods**: Opt for whole, unprocessed foods for the majority of your diet.
4. **Stay Hydrated**: Choose water or other non-caloric beverages over sugary drinks.
5. **Seek Professional Guidance**: Consult with a registered dietitian who specializes in diabetes for personalized dietary advice.

Understanding the role of diet in diabetes management is the first step toward taking control of the disease. By making informed food choices, individuals with diabetes can significantly improve their quality of life, stabilize blood sugar levels, and reduce the risk of complications. This holistic approach to diabetes management empowers individuals to live healthier, more balanced lives.

Key Herbs for Blood Sugar Regulation

Several herbs have been traditionally used and are supported by modern research for their potential in regulating blood sugar levels. Integrating these herbs into a diabetes management plan can complement dietary and lifestyle interventions. Here, we discuss the best herbs for blood sugar regulation, outlining their benefits, preparation methods, optimal times for consumption, recommended quantities, and duration of use.

1. Cinnamon (Cinnamomum verum)
- **Benefits**: Cinnamon is known for its ability to improve insulin sensitivity and lower blood sugar levels. It may mimic insulin, helping glucose get into cells and be used for energy, thereby reducing blood sugar.
- **Preparation**: Cinnamon can be incorporated into the diet by sprinkling powdered cinnamon on oatmeal, yogurt, or in smoothies. Cinnamon tea is another option, made by steeping cinnamon sticks in boiling water for 10-15 minutes.
- **When to Take**: Consume cinnamon with carbohydrate-containing meals to help manage the post-meal blood sugar spike.
- **Quantity**: 1–2 grams of cinnamon powder per day is generally recommended, equivalent to about half to one teaspoon.
- **Duration**: Continuous use is supported by research, but it's advisable to have periodic evaluations of blood sugar levels to adjust intake as needed.

2. Fenugreek (Trigonella foenum-graecum)
- **Benefits**: Fenugreek seeds are high in soluble fiber, which can help control blood sugar by slowing down digestion and absorption of carbohydrates.
- **Preparation**: The seeds can be soaked in water overnight and consumed on an empty stomach in the morning. Fenugreek powder can also be added to dishes or taken in capsule form.
- **When to Take**: Soaked fenugreek seeds are best taken on an empty stomach in the morning. If using in meals, include it in dishes that are part of your main meals.
- **Quantity**: About 5–10 grams of soaked seeds or 1–2 teaspoons of fenugreek seed powder per day.
- **Duration**: Fenugreek is generally safe for long-term use, but as with any supplement, monitoring and adjustments based on blood sugar readings are recommended.

3. Gymnema Sylvestre
- **Benefits**: Gymnema Sylvestre can help reduce sugar cravings and improve blood sugar control. It appears to enhance insulin production and regeneration of pancreas islet cells.

- **Preparation**: Available in supplement form, as it's difficult to incorporate directly into the diet due to its form and taste.
- **When to Take**: Take Gymnema Sylvestre supplements with meals to aid in blood sugar regulation.
- **Quantity**: The typical dose is 200–400 mg per day of extract, but follow the specific dosing recommendations on the supplement.
- **Duration**: As with other supplements, start with a lower dose to assess tolerance and effect, then adjust based on blood sugar control and under the guidance of a healthcare provider.

4. Bitter Melon (Momordica charantia)
- **Benefits**: Bitter melon contains compounds that act like insulin, helping to reduce blood sugar levels by increasing glucose uptake by cells.
- **Preparation**: Bitter melon can be consumed as a vegetable in cooking, juiced, or taken as a supplement.
- **When to Take**: If eating as part of a meal, it can help with post-meal blood sugar spikes. Supplements should be taken according to package instructions, typically with meals.
- **Quantity**: For cooking or juicing, one small bitter melon per day. As a supplement, follow the manufacturer's instructions.
- **Duration**: Monitor blood sugar levels to determine effectiveness and adjust intake as needed. Long-term use should be discussed with a healthcare provider.

5. Berberine
- **Benefits**: This compound, found in several plants, is known for its ability to lower blood sugar and improve insulin sensitivity. It's believed to work via multiple mechanisms, including improving the breakdown of carbohydrates and reducing sugar production in the liver.
- **Preparation**: Berberine is taken in supplement form.
- **When to Take**: It's recommended to take berberine with meals to maximize its blood sugar-lowering effects.
- **Quantity**: The common dose is 500 mg taken 2–3 times per day.
- **Duration**: Because berberine can interact with medications and is potent, it's essential to use under medical supervision, especially if taking it for an extended period.

General Guidelines for Taking Herbs for Blood Sugar Regulation
- **Consultation**: Before adding any supplements to your regimen, consult with a healthcare provider, especially if you are taking medications for diabetes, as there could be interactions.
- **Start Slow**: Begin with a lower dose to assess your body's response. Gradually increase to the recommended dose if no adverse effects are observed.
- **Monitoring**: Regularly monitor your blood sugar levels to evaluate the effectiveness of the herb and adjust dosages accordingly. This is particularly important for individuals on blood sugar-lowering medications, as there may be a risk of hypoglycemia (low blood sugar).
- **Quality and Purity**: Choose high-quality supplements from reputable manufacturers to ensure purity and potency. The supplement industry varies in quality standards, so selecting products certified by third-party organizations can add an extra layer of trust.
- **Lifestyle Integration**: Remember that these herbs should complement, not replace, conventional diabetes treatments. They work best when integrated into a holistic approach that includes a healthy diet, regular physical activity, and stress management techniques.
- **Duration of Use**: Continuous use of some herbs may be appropriate, but it's crucial to periodically evaluate the necessity and effectiveness of each supplement. This might involve taking breaks or adjusting dosages based on ongoing monitoring and consultation with a healthcare provider.
- **Side Effects and Interactions**: Be aware of potential side effects. For example, berberine can cause digestive disturbances in some individuals. Similarly, interactions between herbs and medications can occur. For instance, taking cinnamon in large quantities can potentially interact with blood thinners.

Herbs can play a significant role in managing blood sugar levels and improving insulin sensitivity, but their inclusion in a diabetes management plan should always be carefully considered and monitored. With the right approach, these natural interventions can significantly contribute to the overall strategy for managing diabetes, enhancing the quality of life, and reducing the risk of complications associated with the condition. Always prioritize a dialogue with healthcare professionals to tailor a comprehensive, effective, and safe management plan for diabetes.

Incorporating Exercise for Diabetes Management

Exercise plays a pivotal role in managing diabetes, with profound benefits that extend beyond mere blood sugar control. Engaging in regular physical activity can improve insulin sensitivity, contribute to weight loss, and reduce the risk of cardiovascular disease. Here, we explore how to effectively incorporate exercise into a diabetes management plan, including types of exercises, scheduling considerations, and safety tips.

Understanding the Benefits

1. **Improves Insulin Sensitivity**: Physical activity helps muscle cells use blood glucose for energy more efficiently, reducing blood sugar levels.
2. **Aids Weight Management**: Regular exercise contributes to weight loss and maintenance, which is particularly beneficial for Type 2 diabetes management.
3. **Lowers Risk of Heart Disease**: Exercise strengthens the heart and improves blood circulation, reducing the risk of heart disease, a common complication of diabetes.
4. **Enhances Mental Well-being**: Engaging in physical activity has been shown to improve mood and reduce stress, factors that can positively influence diabetes management.

Types of Exercise for Diabetes Management

1. **Aerobic Exercise**: Activities such as walking, swimming, cycling, and running increase heart rate and breathing, improving cardiovascular fitness and insulin sensitivity. Aim for at least 150 minutes of moderate to vigorous aerobic activity spread throughout the week.
2. **Resistance Training**: Using weights, resistance bands, or bodyweight exercises to build muscle mass can enhance insulin sensitivity and glucose uptake by the muscles. Try to include resistance training at least two days a week.
3. **Flexibility and Stretching Exercises**: Practices like yoga and Pilates can increase flexibility, reduce stress, and have a positive impact on blood glucose levels.
4. **Balance and Coordination**: Activities that improve balance and coordination, such as tai chi, can reduce the risk of falls, particularly important for older adults with diabetes.

Scheduling Exercise

1. **Consistency is Key**: Regular, daily activity is more beneficial than sporadic intense sessions. Find a routine that fits into your schedule and stick with it.
2. **Monitor Blood Sugar Levels**: Check your blood sugar before and after exercise to understand how different activities affect your glucose levels. This can help you adjust your exercise intensity and duration as needed.
3. **Best Times to Exercise**: The optimal time can vary based on individual blood sugar patterns and medication schedules. Some people find exercising after meals helps control postprandial (after eating) blood sugar spikes.

Safety Tips

1. **Stay Hydrated**: Drink plenty of water before, during, and after exercise to stay hydrated, as dehydration can affect blood sugar levels.
2. **Wear Appropriate Footwear**: Choose well-fitting, comfortable shoes designed for the type of exercise you're doing to prevent blisters and foot injuries.
3. **Carry a Source of Fast-Acting Carbohydrates**: Have a snack or glucose tablets on hand in case of hypoglycemia (low blood sugar) during or after exercise.
4. **Inform Others**: When exercising, especially outside or alone, let someone know your plans and carry identification that notes you have diabetes.

Creating an Exercise Plan

1. **Consult with Healthcare Professionals**: Before starting any new exercise regimen, consult with your doctor or a diabetes educator, particularly if you have any diabetes-related complications.
2. **Start Slowly and Build Up Gradually**: If you're new to exercise or have been inactive, begin with light activities and slowly increase the intensity and duration.
3. **Incorporate Variety**: Mix different types of exercises to keep things interesting and work various muscle groups.

Incorporating exercise into your diabetes management plan can significantly improve your health and quality of life. By understanding the benefits, choosing the right types of activities, scheduling appropriately, and following safety guidelines, you can harness the power of physical activity to control your diabetes more effectively.

Chapter 3: Heart Health and Hypertension

Heart health is paramount for individuals with diabetes, as they are at increased risk of developing cardiovascular complications. This chapter explores strategies for maintaining a healthy heart and managing hypertension, a common comorbidity of diabetes. From dietary considerations to lifestyle modifications, we delve into comprehensive approaches to safeguard cardiovascular well-being.

Essential Heart Health Nutrients and Herbs

Maintaining heart health is crucial for individuals with diabetes, as they are at higher risk of cardiovascular complications. Incorporating specific nutrients and herbs into their daily regimen can support heart function, regulate blood pressure, and reduce the risk of heart disease. Here, we explore some of the best herbs and nutrients for heart health, their benefits, preparation methods, optimal times for consumption, recommended quantities, and duration of use.

Omega-3 Fatty Acids
- **Benefits**: Omega-3 fatty acids, particularly eicosapentaenoic acid (EPA) and docosahexaenoic acid (DHA), have been shown to reduce inflammation, lower triglyceride levels, and decrease the risk of heart disease. They also support overall cardiovascular health by improving blood vessel function and reducing the risk of arrhythmias.
- **Sources**: Fatty fish such as salmon, mackerel, and sardines are rich sources of omega-3s. Plant-based sources include flaxseeds, chia seeds, and walnuts.
- **Preparation**: Incorporate fatty fish into your diet at least twice a week. Plant-based sources can be added to smoothies, salads, oatmeal, or consumed as snacks.

Magnesium and Potassium
- **Benefits**: Magnesium and potassium play essential roles in regulating blood pressure, maintaining proper heart rhythm, and supporting overall cardiovascular function. They also help reduce the risk of stroke and heart attack.
- **Sources**: Magnesium-rich foods include leafy greens (spinach, kale), nuts and seeds (almonds, pumpkin seeds), and whole grains (brown rice, quinoa). Potassium-rich foods include bananas, sweet potatoes, beans, and yogurt.
- **Preparation**: Incorporate magnesium- and potassium-rich foods into your meals and snacks daily. Aim for a variety of sources to ensure adequate intake.

Hawthorn
- **Benefits**: Hawthorn has been used for centuries in traditional medicine to support heart health. It contains compounds that help dilate blood vessels, improve blood flow, and strengthen the heart muscle. Hawthorn may also lower blood pressure and cholesterol levels.
- **Preparation**: Hawthorn supplements are available in various forms, including capsules, tablets, and liquid extracts. Follow the manufacturer's instructions for dosage and administration.

Coenzyme Q10 (CoQ10)
- **Benefits**: CoQ10 is an antioxidant that plays a crucial role in cellular energy production, including in the heart muscle. It helps maintain heart function, reduce inflammation, and protect against oxidative damage.
- **Sources**: While CoQ10 is naturally produced by the body, levels may decline with age or certain medical conditions. Food sources include fatty fish, organ meats (liver, heart), and whole grains.
- **Supplementation**: CoQ10 supplements are available in various strengths and formulations. Consult with a healthcare provider to determine the appropriate dosage based on individual needs.

Garlic
- **Benefits**: Garlic contains compounds like allicin and sulfur, which have antioxidant and anti-inflammatory properties. Garlic supplementation may help lower blood pressure, reduce cholesterol levels, and improve overall heart health.
- **Preparation**: Fresh garlic can be added to cooked dishes or consumed raw. Garlic supplements are also available in various forms, including capsules, tablets, and extracts.

Dosage and Duration
- **Omega-3 Fatty Acids**: Aim for 1-2 servings of fatty fish per week or consider supplementation with fish oil capsules containing 1000-2000 mg of EPA and DHA combined daily.
- **Magnesium and Potassium**: Consume magnesium-rich foods daily and ensure adequate potassium intake through a balanced diet. Consider supplementation if levels are deficient, under the guidance of a healthcare provider.
- **Hawthorn, CoQ10, and Garlic**: Follow the manufacturer's instructions for dosage and administration when using herbal supplements. Start with a lower dose and gradually increase as needed. Monitor for any adverse effects and consult with a healthcare provider if necessary.

Timing and Considerations
- **Omega-3 Fatty Acids**: Consume fatty fish or omega-3 supplements with meals to enhance absorption and minimize digestive discomfort.
- **Herbal Supplements**: Take herbal supplements as directed by the manufacturer, typically with meals to improve absorption and reduce the risk of gastrointestinal upset.

Duration and Monitoring
- **Long-Term Use**: Many of these nutrients and herbs can be safely incorporated into a long-term heart health regimen. Monitor blood pressure, cholesterol levels, and overall cardiovascular health regularly to assess efficacy.
- **Consultation**: Before starting any new supplement regimen, consult with a healthcare provider, particularly if you have underlying health conditions or are taking medications that may interact with these supplements.

Incorporating these essential nutrients and herbs into your daily routine can support heart health, reduce the risk of cardiovascular complications, and complement diabetes management efforts. However, it's essential to prioritize a balanced diet, regular physical activity, and ongoing medical supervision for optimal cardiovascular well-being.

Diet and Lifestyle for Blood Pressure Management

Maintaining healthy blood pressure levels is essential for overall cardiovascular health, especially for individuals with diabetes who are at increased risk of hypertension. A combination of dietary modifications and lifestyle changes can play a significant role in managing blood pressure effectively. In this section, we explore key dietary and lifestyle strategies to help control blood pressure and reduce the risk of heart disease.

Dietary Approaches
1. **DASH Diet (Dietary Approaches to Stop Hypertension)**:
   - **Principles**: The DASH diet emphasizes whole foods rich in nutrients such as fruits, vegetables, whole grains, lean proteins, and low-fat dairy products while limiting saturated fats, cholesterol, and sodium.
   - **Benefits**: Studies have shown that adopting a DASH-style eating pattern can significantly lower blood pressure and reduce the risk of heart disease.
   - **Implementation**: Focus on incorporating a variety of colorful fruits and vegetables, whole grains, lean proteins (such as poultry, fish, and legumes), and low-fat dairy products into your meals. Limit processed foods, high-fat meats, and added sugars.
2. **Reducing Sodium Intake**:

- **Importance**: High sodium intake is strongly associated with elevated blood pressure. Reducing sodium consumption can help lower blood pressure levels and reduce the risk of heart disease.
- **Strategies**: Read food labels carefully and choose low-sodium or sodium-free alternatives. Limit the use of table salt while cooking and avoid adding extra salt to meals. Use herbs, spices, and lemon juice to flavor foods instead of salt.

3. **Increasing Potassium-Rich Foods**:
   - **Benefits**: Potassium helps counteract the effects of sodium on blood pressure and promotes healthy blood vessel function. Consuming potassium-rich foods can help lower blood pressure levels.
   - **Sources**: Include potassium-rich foods such as bananas, sweet potatoes, spinach, avocados, and beans in your daily diet.

4. **Moderate Alcohol Consumption**:
   - **Guidelines**: Excessive alcohol consumption can raise blood pressure and increase the risk of heart disease. Limit alcohol intake to moderate levels, defined as up to one drink per day for women and up to two drinks per day for men.

Lifestyle Modifications

1. **Regular Physical Activity**:
   - **Benefits**: Engaging in regular physical activity helps lower blood pressure, improve cardiovascular fitness, and reduce the risk of heart disease. Aim for at least 150 minutes of moderate-intensity aerobic exercise or 75 minutes of vigorous-intensity aerobic exercise per week, along with muscle-strengthening activities on two or more days per week.
   - **Types of Exercise**: Include a variety of aerobic activities such as walking, jogging, cycling, swimming, or dancing. Incorporate strength training exercises using resistance bands, free weights, or bodyweight exercises.

2. **Maintaining a Healthy Weight**:
   - **Connection to Blood Pressure**: Being overweight or obese is a significant risk factor for hypertension. Losing excess weight can help lower blood pressure levels and improve overall cardiovascular health.
   - **Strategies**: Focus on achieving and maintaining a healthy weight through a combination of balanced eating, regular physical activity, and lifestyle changes.

3. **Stress Management**:
   - **Impact on Blood Pressure**: Chronic stress can contribute to elevated blood pressure levels. Implement stress management techniques to promote relaxation and reduce stress-related hypertension.
   - **Techniques**: Practice stress-reducing activities such as deep breathing exercises, meditation, yoga, tai chi, or mindfulness-based stress reduction. Engage in hobbies, spend time outdoors, and prioritize self-care activities to reduce stress levels.

4. **Quit Smoking**:
   - **Effects on Blood Pressure**: Smoking increases blood pressure and damages blood vessels, leading to an increased risk of heart disease and stroke. Quitting smoking can significantly improve blood pressure control and overall cardiovascular health.

Conclusion

Effective management of blood pressure requires a comprehensive approach that combines dietary modifications, regular physical activity, stress management techniques, and lifestyle changes. By adopting a heart-healthy diet, engaging in regular exercise, maintaining a healthy weight, managing stress effectively, and avoiding tobacco use, individuals with diabetes can take proactive steps to control blood pressure levels and reduce the risk of cardiovascular complications. It's essential to work closely with healthcare providers to develop personalized strategies for blood pressure management and monitor progress over time.

Chapter 4: Natural Solutions for Respiratory Conditions

Respiratory conditions such as asthma, allergies, and chronic obstructive pulmonary disease (COPD) can significantly impact an individual's quality of life, leading to symptoms such as wheezing, shortness of breath, coughing, and chest tightness. In this chapter, we explore natural solutions for managing respiratory conditions, including herbal remedies, lifestyle modifications, and techniques to improve respiratory health.

Herbal Remedies for Asthma and Allergies

Asthma and allergies are respiratory conditions characterized by inflammation and narrowing of the airways, leading to symptoms such as wheezing, shortness of breath, coughing, and chest tightness. While conventional treatments focus on symptom management through medications such as bronchodilators and corticosteroids, herbal remedies offer complementary approaches to support respiratory health. Below, we explore some of the best herbs for asthma and allergies, along with their benefits, preparation methods, optimal times for consumption, recommended quantities, and duration of use.

1. Boswellia (Boswellia serrata)
   - **Benefits**: Boswellia possesses anti-inflammatory properties that may help reduce airway inflammation and improve respiratory symptoms associated with asthma and allergies.
   - **Preparation**: Boswellia resin can be taken in supplement form, typically in capsules or tablets. Follow the manufacturer's instructions for dosage.
   - **When to Take**: Take Boswellia supplements as directed, preferably with meals to enhance absorption.
   - **Quantity and Duration**: Dosage recommendations may vary depending on the concentration of Boswellia extract. Follow the recommended dosage on the product label, and consult with a healthcare provider for personalized guidance on duration of use.
2. Ginger (Zingiber officinale)
   - **Benefits**: Ginger exhibits anti-inflammatory and bronchodilator properties, making it potentially beneficial for easing asthma symptoms and reducing airway inflammation.
   - **Preparation**: Ginger can be consumed fresh, as a tea, or in supplement form (e.g., capsules or extracts).
   - **When to Take**: Drink ginger tea or consume ginger supplements as needed to alleviate symptoms. For ongoing support, consider incorporating ginger into your daily routine.
   - **Quantity and Duration**: There is no standardized dosage for ginger, but a typical recommendation is 1 gram of ginger powder per day. Consult with a healthcare provider for personalized guidance on dosage and duration of use.
3. Turmeric (Curcuma longa)
   - **Benefits**: Curcumin, the active compound in turmeric, exhibits anti-inflammatory and antioxidant properties that may help alleviate airway inflammation and improve asthma symptoms.
   - **Preparation**: Turmeric can be consumed fresh, as a spice in cooking, or in supplement form (e.g., capsules or extracts).
   - **When to Take**: Incorporate turmeric into meals or take turmeric supplements with meals to enhance absorption.
   - **Quantity and Duration**: Dosage recommendations for turmeric supplements vary, but typical doses range from 500 mg to 2 grams per day. Consult with a healthcare provider for personalized guidance on dosage and duration of use.

4. Licorice Root (Glycyrrhiza glabra)
- **Benefits**: Licorice root possesses anti-inflammatory and expectorant properties, which may help soothe airway inflammation and reduce coughing associated with asthma and allergies.
- **Preparation**: Licorice root can be consumed as a tea, in liquid extracts, or in supplement form (e.g., capsules or tablets).
- **When to Take**: Drink licorice root tea or take licorice supplements as needed to relieve symptoms. Avoid long-term use of licorice supplements due to the risk of side effects.
- **Quantity and Duration**: Dosage recommendations for licorice supplements vary, but typical doses range from 200 mg to 600 mg per day. Consult with a healthcare provider for personalized guidance on dosage and duration of use.

5. Butterbur (Petasites hybridus)
- **Benefits**: Butterbur has been traditionally used for its anti-inflammatory and antihistamine properties, which may help alleviate allergy symptoms such as nasal congestion and sneezing.
- **Preparation**: Butterbur supplements are available in capsule or tablet form. Look for products that are labeled "PA-free" to avoid potentially harmful compounds.
- **When to Take**: Take butterbur supplements as directed, preferably with meals to minimize gastrointestinal side effects.
- **Quantity and Duration**: Dosage recommendations for butterbur supplements vary, but typical doses range from 50 mg to 150 mg twice daily. Consult with a healthcare provider for personalized guidance on dosage and duration of use.

Conclusion

Incorporating herbal remedies into your asthma and allergy management plan can offer additional support for respiratory health. However, it's essential to use caution and consult with a healthcare provider before starting any new herbal regimen, especially if you have underlying health conditions or are taking medications. Additionally, while herbs can provide symptom relief, they should not replace conventional treatments prescribed by a healthcare professional. With careful consideration and personalized guidance, herbal remedies can complement existing therapies and contribute to improved respiratory well-being.

Improving Respiratory Health Through Lifestyle

Respiratory health is influenced not only by medical treatments and herbal remedies but also by lifestyle choices and environmental factors. Adopting certain lifestyle practices can help support lung function, reduce the severity of respiratory symptoms, and enhance overall respiratory health. In this section, we explore various lifestyle modifications that individuals with respiratory conditions such as asthma, allergies, and chronic obstructive pulmonary disease (COPD) can incorporate into their daily routine to improve respiratory well-being.

1. Avoiding Environmental Triggers
- **Allergens**: Identify and minimize exposure to common allergens such as pollen, dust mites, pet dander, and mold. Use allergen-proof covers on pillows and mattresses, vacuum regularly, and keep indoor humidity levels low to reduce allergen exposure.
- **Air Pollution**: Limit exposure to outdoor air pollution by avoiding high-traffic areas and staying indoors during days with poor air quality. Use air purifiers at home to filter out pollutants and improve indoor air quality.
- **Tobacco Smoke**: Avoid smoking and exposure to secondhand smoke, as cigarette smoke can exacerbate respiratory symptoms and increase the risk of respiratory infections and lung diseases.

2. Maintaining a Healthy Weight
- **Impact on Lung Function**: Being overweight or obese can restrict lung expansion and reduce lung capacity, leading to breathing difficulties and exacerbating respiratory symptoms.

- **Healthy Eating**: Adopt a balanced diet rich in fruits, vegetables, whole grains, and lean proteins to support overall health and maintain a healthy weight. Avoid excessive consumption of processed foods, sugary beverages, and high-fat foods, which can contribute to weight gain and inflammation.

3. Regular Exercise
- **Benefits for Lung Health**: Engaging in regular physical activity strengthens respiratory muscles, improves lung function, and enhances overall cardiovascular fitness.
- **Types of Exercise**: Incorporate aerobic exercises such as walking, swimming, cycling, or jogging into your routine, aiming for at least 150 minutes of moderate-intensity exercise per week. Include strength training exercises to build muscle strength and endurance.

4. Proper Breathing Techniques
- **Diaphragmatic Breathing**: Practice deep breathing exercises to strengthen the diaphragm and improve lung capacity. Inhale deeply through your nose, allowing your abdomen to expand, then exhale slowly through your mouth, allowing your abdomen to contract.
- **Pursed Lip Breathing**: Use pursed lip breathing during activities that require increased exertion, such as climbing stairs or lifting heavy objects. Inhale through your nose for a count of two, then purse your lips as if blowing out a candle and exhale slowly for a count of four.

5. Managing Stress
- **Impact on Respiratory Symptoms**: Chronic stress can exacerbate respiratory symptoms and trigger asthma attacks or allergy flare-ups. Implement stress management techniques such as mindfulness meditation, yoga, tai chi, or deep breathing exercises to promote relaxation and reduce stress levels.
- **Quality Sleep**: Prioritize quality sleep to support overall health and reduce stress. Create a relaxing bedtime routine, maintain a consistent sleep schedule, and create a comfortable sleep environment conducive to restorative sleep.

6. Medication Adherence and Regular Check-ups
- **Follow Treatment Plans**: Adhere to prescribed medications and treatment plans recommended by healthcare providers to manage respiratory conditions effectively.
- **Regular Check-ups**: Schedule regular follow-up appointments with healthcare providers to monitor respiratory symptoms, assess lung function, and adjust treatment plans as needed.

Conclusion

By incorporating these lifestyle modifications into their daily routine, individuals with respiratory conditions can take proactive steps to support lung health, reduce the severity of respiratory symptoms, and enhance overall well-being. While lifestyle changes alone may not cure respiratory conditions, they can complement medical treatments and herbal remedies, contributing to improved respiratory health and a better quality of life. It's essential to consult with healthcare providers for personalized guidance and to address any concerns or questions about implementing lifestyle modifications. With dedication and perseverance, individuals can empower themselves to achieve optimal respiratory wellness.

Techniques to Enhance Air Quality at Home

Maintaining good indoor air quality is essential for respiratory health, especially for individuals with asthma, allergies, or other respiratory conditions. Indoor air pollutants such as dust, pet dander, mold spores, and volatile organic compounds (VOCs) can exacerbate symptoms and contribute to respiratory issues. Fortunately, there are several techniques you can implement to enhance air quality and create a healthier living environment for you and your family. Below are some effective strategies:

1. Proper Ventilation
- **Use Exhaust Fans**: Install and use exhaust fans in kitchens and bathrooms to remove moisture and pollutants generated during cooking or showering.
- **Open Windows**: Whenever weather permits, open windows to allow fresh outdoor air to circulate indoors and flush out indoor pollutants.

2. Air Purifiers
- **HEPA Filters**: Invest in high-efficiency particulate air (HEPA) purifiers equipped with HEPA filters to capture airborne particles, including dust, pollen, pet dander, and mold spores.
- **Activated Carbon Filters**: Consider air purifiers with activated carbon filters to absorb odors, VOCs, and other chemical pollutants from indoor air.

3. Houseplants
- **Natural Air Purifiers**: Incorporate indoor plants known for their air-purifying properties, such as spider plants, peace lilies, snake plants, and pothos. These plants can help remove harmful chemicals and improve indoor air quality.
- **Careful Maintenance**: Keep houseplants healthy by watering them appropriately and periodically wiping their leaves to remove dust and dirt.

4. Reduce Indoor Pollutants
- **Limit Smoking Indoors**: Avoid smoking indoors, as cigarette smoke contains numerous harmful chemicals that can pollute indoor air and exacerbate respiratory symptoms.
- **Control Humidity**: Use dehumidifiers to maintain indoor humidity levels between 30% and 50% to prevent mold growth and reduce the proliferation of dust mites.

5. Regular Cleaning
- **Dust and Vacuum**: Clean and dust surfaces regularly to remove accumulated dust, pet dander, and other allergens. Use a vacuum cleaner with a HEPA filter to trap fine particles and prevent them from recirculating into the air.
- **Wash Bedding**: Wash bedding, including sheets, pillowcases, and mattress covers, in hot water weekly to eliminate dust mites and allergens.

6. Avoid Harsh Chemicals
- **Choose Non-Toxic Cleaning Products**: Opt for environmentally friendly and non-toxic cleaning products to minimize exposure to harmful chemicals and VOCs.
- **Ventilate When Using Chemicals**: When using household cleaners or paints, ensure proper ventilation by opening windows or using exhaust fans to remove fumes and prevent indoor air pollution.

7. Maintain HVAC Systems
- **Change Air Filters**: Regularly replace air filters in heating, ventilation, and air conditioning (HVAC) systems to ensure optimal air flow and remove airborne particles effectively.
- **Professional Maintenance**: Schedule annual maintenance inspections for HVAC systems to identify and address any issues that could affect indoor air quality.

Conclusion

Implementing these techniques to enhance air quality at home can significantly improve respiratory health and overall well-being for everyone in the household. By reducing indoor pollutants, promoting proper ventilation, and maintaining a clean and healthy living environment, individuals can create a safer and more comfortable indoor environment conducive to respiratory wellness. Remember to prioritize regular cleaning, proper ventilation, and the use of air purifiers and houseplants to create a healthier home for you and your family.

Chapter 5: Addressing Skin Conditions with Herbs

Skin conditions, ranging from the occasional breakout to more chronic issues like eczema, psoriasis, and acne, can significantly impact an individual's quality of life. While conventional treatments offer relief, they sometimes come with side effects that can further irritate sensitive skin. This has led many to seek alternative, natural solutions. Among these, herbal remedies stand out for their potential to soothe, heal, and rejuvenate the skin with fewer side effects. This chapter delves into the world of herbs known for their skin-healing properties, offering insights into their benefits, preparation, application, and considerations for use.

Herbal Treatments for Acne, Eczema, and Psoriasis

Acne, eczema, and psoriasis are common skin conditions that can cause significant discomfort and affect an individual's self-esteem. Herbal treatments offer a natural way to manage these conditions by leveraging the anti-inflammatory, antimicrobial, and soothing properties of plants. Below, we explore some of the most effective herbs for treating acne, eczema, and psoriasis, including their benefits, how to prepare them, and guidelines for use.

1. Herbs for Acne
- **Tea Tree Oil (Melaleuca alternifolia)**
    - **Benefits**: Its antimicrobial properties make it effective against acne-causing bacteria, while its anti-inflammatory effects help reduce redness and swelling.
    - **Preparation**: Dilute tea tree oil with a carrier oil (such as jojoba or sweet almond oil) at a concentration of 5-10% tea tree oil to 90-95% carrier oil.
    - **Application**: Apply to the affected area using a cotton swab once or twice daily.
    - **Duration**: Results can vary, but many see improvement within a few weeks. Continuous use over several months can help maintain clear skin.
- **Green Tea (Camellia sinensis)**
    - **Benefits**: Rich in antioxidants and anti-inflammatory compounds, green tea can reduce sebum production and inflammation in acne-prone skin.
    - **Preparation**: Brew a strong cup of green tea and let it cool. Alternatively, use green tea extract.
    - **Application**: Use a cotton ball to apply cooled tea to the skin, or mix green tea extract into a carrier oil or cream and apply it to the skin.
    - **Duration**: Use daily for several weeks to months for best results.
2. Herbs for Eczema
- **Chamomile (Matricaria recutita)**
    - **Benefits**: Chamomile's anti-inflammatory properties can soothe eczema flare-ups and reduce skin irritation.
    - **Preparation**: Brew a strong chamomile tea and let it cool. Alternatively, chamomile essential oil can be diluted with a carrier oil.
    - **Application**: Apply the cooled tea with a clean cloth as a compress or add a few drops of diluted essential oil to the affected areas.
    - **Duration**: Use as needed during flare-ups to soothe the skin. Long-term use is generally safe.
- **Licorice Root (Glycyrrhiza glabra)**

- **Benefits:** Licorice root has anti-inflammatory and soothing effects beneficial for eczema-prone skin.
- **Preparation:** Prepare a licorice root decoction or use a cream containing licorice extract.
- **Application:** Apply licorice root decoction or cream to the affected areas twice daily.
- **Duration:** Improvement is often seen within a few weeks. It can be used as part of an ongoing skincare routine.

3. Herbs for Psoriasis

- **Aloe Vera (Aloe barbadensis miller)**
  - **Benefits:** Aloe vera can moisturize the skin, reduce redness and scaling associated with psoriasis.
  - **Preparation:** Use fresh aloe vera gel directly from the plant or purchase pure aloe vera gel.
  - **Application:** Apply aloe vera gel to the affected areas up to three times a day.
  - **Duration:** Continuous use is necessary to maintain symptom relief.
- **Turmeric (Curcuma longa)**
  - **Benefits:** The curcumin in turmeric has potent anti-inflammatory and antioxidant properties that can help reduce psoriasis flare-ups.
  - **Preparation:** Mix turmeric powder with water or a carrier oil to form a paste, or use turmeric capsules as a dietary supplement.
  - **Application:** Apply the paste to the affected areas or take capsules as directed on the package.
  - **Duration:** For topical applications, use daily for several weeks. When taking supplements, follow the package instructions or consult a healthcare provider.

General Guidelines for Using Herbs

- **Patch Test:** Always perform a patch test to ensure you don't have an allergic reaction to a new herb or oil.
- **Quality Matters:** Use high-quality, organic herbs and oils whenever possible to avoid contaminants.
- **Consultation:** Consult with a healthcare professional before starting any new herbal treatment, especially if you are pregnant, nursing, or taking other medications.
- **Patience and Consistency:** Natural remedies often require time to show effects. Consistency in application and patience is key to seeing results.

Herbal treatments offer a promising complement to conventional therapies for skin conditions. By understanding the specific benefits and proper use of each herb, individuals can harness these natural remedies to support skin health and alleviate the symptoms of acne, eczema, and psoriasis.

Diet's Impact on Skin Health

The connection between diet and skin health has long been recognized, underscoring the adage "you are what you eat." Nutritional science reveals that the quality of our diet directly impacts our skin's condition, affecting everything from its appearance to its aging process and susceptibility to various skin conditions. In this exploration, we delve into how diet influences skin health, highlighting specific nutrients that promote skin vitality and foods that might exacerbate skin issues.

Nutritional Foundations for Healthy Skin

1. **Antioxidants:**
   - **Role:** Combat oxidative stress, which can damage skin cells and contribute to aging and diseases.
   - **Sources:** Fruits and vegetables, particularly berries, tomatoes, carrots, spinach, and nuts, are rich in antioxidants such as vitamins C and E, selenium, and carotenoids.
   - **Impact:** Antioxidants help protect the skin from damage by free radicals and UV exposure, promoting a youthful appearance and reducing the risk of skin cancer.

2. **Healthy Fats**:
    *   **Role**: Support cell membrane health, reduce inflammation, and moisturize the skin from within.
    *   **Sources**: Avocados, olive oil, flaxseeds, and fatty fish like salmon and mackerel provide omega-3 fatty acids, which are essential for maintaining the skin's oil barrier.
    *   **Impact**: Omega-3 fatty acids can reduce the severity of skin conditions like acne and psoriasis by combating inflammation and dryness.
3. **Protein**:
    *   **Role**: Essential for the repair and regeneration of skin cells, collagen, and elastin production.
    *   **Sources**: Lean meats, poultry, fish, legumes, and tofu offer high-quality protein.
    *   **Impact**: Adequate protein intake ensures the skin has the necessary building blocks for repair and maintenance, supporting elasticity and firmness.
4. **Water**:
    *   **Role**: Hydrates the skin, maintains elasticity, and supports detoxification processes.
    *   **Impact**: Proper hydration can improve the skin's resilience, reduce the appearance of fine lines and wrinkles, and help clear acne and other skin conditions by flushing out toxins.

Foods That May Exacerbate Skin Conditions
1. **High Glycemic Index Foods**:
    *   Foods with a high glycemic index, such as white bread, pastries, and sugary drinks, can cause insulin levels to spike, leading to increased sebum production and exacerbation of acne.
2. **Dairy Products**:
    *   Some studies suggest a correlation between dairy consumption and acne severity, possibly due to hormones present in milk that can affect sebum production.
3. **Processed and Fried Foods**:
    *   These foods can promote inflammation throughout the body and skin, potentially worsening conditions like acne, eczema, and psoriasis.

Incorporating Skin-Healthy Foods into Your Diet
*   **Balance and Variety**: Aim for a balanced diet rich in colorful fruits and vegetables, lean proteins, healthy fats, and whole grains to cover the spectrum of essential nutrients for skin health.
*   **Hydration**: Drink plenty of water throughout the day, and consider foods with high water content like cucumbers, tomatoes, and watermelon.
*   **Moderation**: Limit the intake of processed foods, high glycemic index carbohydrates, and dairy, especially if you notice a link between these foods and skin flare-ups.

Conclusion

Diet plays a pivotal role in skin health, offering a powerful means to influence how our skin looks, feels, and ages. By prioritizing nutrient-rich foods and being mindful of those that may exacerbate skin issues, individuals can significantly impact their skin's health from the inside out. Adopting a holistic approach to nutrition not only benefits the skin but promotes overall health and well-being, underscoring the integral connection between diet and dermatological health.

External Applications and Skincare Routines

A comprehensive skincare routine is crucial for maintaining healthy, vibrant skin. External applications, including cleansers, moisturizers, exfoliants, and protective formulas, play a vital role in skin health. By understanding and implementing a tailored skincare regimen, individuals can address specific skin concerns, mitigate environmental damage, and promote long-term skin vitality. This section explores the components of an effective skincare routine, emphasizing the importance of natural and nourishing ingredients.

1. Cleansing
- **Purpose**: To remove dirt, oil, pollutants, and makeup that can clog pores and cause dullness and acne.
- **Recommendations**: Opt for gentle, sulfate-free cleansers that respect the skin's natural barrier. Ingredients like aloe vera, chamomile, and green tea offer soothing and antioxidant benefits. For acne-prone skin, cleansers with tea tree oil or salicylic acid can help reduce breakouts.
- **Routine**: Cleanse twice daily, in the morning and evening, to maintain clear pores and support skin health.

2. Exfoliation
- **Purpose**: To remove dead skin cells that accumulate on the surface, leading to a brighter complexion and improved absorption of skincare products.
- **Recommendations**: Natural exfoliants such as jojoba beads or ground walnut shells provide a gentle alternative to harsher synthetic abrasives. For chemical exfoliation, products containing alpha-hydroxy acids (AHAs) like glycolic acid or beta-hydroxy acids (BHAs) like salicylic acid can effectively renew skin texture.
- **Routine**: Exfoliate 1-2 times a week, adjusting frequency based on your skin's sensitivity and reaction.

3. Moisturizing
- **Purpose**: To hydrate and lock in moisture, maintaining the skin's elasticity and barrier function.
- **Recommendations**: Look for moisturizers with hyaluronic acid, glycerin, or squalane for deep hydration. Ingredients like ceramides, niacinamide, and natural oils (e.g., jojoba, almond, or rosehip oil) can nourish the skin and protect against environmental stressors.
- **Routine**: Apply moisturizer daily after cleansing and exfoliating to damp skin to maximize absorption.

4. Sun Protection
- **Purpose**: To protect the skin from harmful UV radiation, which can cause premature aging and increase the risk of skin cancer.
- **Recommendations**: Use broad-spectrum sunscreens with an SPF of 30 or higher. Mineral sunscreens containing zinc oxide or titanium dioxide offer physical protection and are less likely to irritate sensitive skin.
- **Routine**: Apply sunscreen every morning, reapplying every two hours when exposed to direct sunlight. Consider SPF-infused moisturizers for streamlined application.

5. Treatment Products
- **Purpose**: To address specific skin concerns such as acne, dark spots, wrinkles, or dehydration.
- **Recommendations**:
    - For acne, serums or spot treatments with salicylic acid, benzoyl peroxide, or tea tree oil can target breakouts.
    - To combat signs of aging, look for products with retinol, peptides, or antioxidants like vitamin C.
    - For hyperpigmentation, ingredients such as licorice extract, kojic acid, or vitamin C can help even out skin tone.
- **Routine**: Apply treatment products after cleansing and before moisturizing, focusing on areas of concern. Start with lower concentrations to assess skin tolerance.

6. Natural and DIY Skincare
- **Purpose**: To provide personalized and cost-effective skincare solutions using natural ingredients.
- **Recommendations**: Homemade masks, scrubs, and moisturizers can be crafted from kitchen ingredients. Honey, oatmeal, yogurt, and turmeric are popular for their soothing and anti-inflammatory properties.
- **Routine**: Incorporate DIY skincare treatments into your weekly regimen as a supplement to daily care, customizing ingredients to your skin's needs.

Conclusion

A thoughtful skincare routine is fundamental to maintaining skin health and addressing specific dermatological concerns. By selecting the right products and ingredients for each step of your regimen, you can nurture your skin's natural beauty and resilience. Remember, skincare is deeply personal; what works for one person may not work for another. Listen to your skin, adjust your routine as needed, and consult a dermatologist for persistent issues or tailored advice. Through consistent care and attention, you can achieve and maintain radiant, healthy skin.

Chapter 6: Mental Health and Stress Relief

Mental health, an integral component of overall well-being, encompasses our emotional, psychological, and social well-being. It influences how we think, feel, and act, especially under stress. Stress, a common response to challenges or pressures, can be beneficial in short bursts but detrimental to our health when it becomes chronic. This chapter delves into the interplay between mental health and stress, offering natural strategies and lifestyle adjustments for stress relief and improved mental well-being.

Herbs for Mood Improvement and Anxiety Reduction

The pursuit of mental wellness often leads individuals to explore natural remedies as complements or alternatives to conventional treatments. Among these, certain herbs have been recognized for their potential to enhance mood and alleviate anxiety. Below, we delve into some of the best herbs for these purposes, discussing their benefits, how to prepare them, optimal times for consumption, recommended quantities, and the duration of their use.

1. St. John's Wort (Hypericum perforatum)
   - **Benefits**: St. John's Wort is widely used for its antidepressant properties. It's believed to increase the levels of serotonin, a neurotransmitter associated with mood regulation.
   - **Preparation**: Available in capsules, tinctures, and teas. Ensure the product is standardized to contain 0.3% hypericin.
   - **When to Take**: Follow the manufacturer's instructions; typically, it's taken in divided doses (morning and evening).
   - **Quantity**: Commonly, 300 mg of standardized extract is taken three times daily.
   - **Duration**: Effects may take 2-4 weeks to appear. Consult with a healthcare provider for guidance on duration, as long-term use may be necessary for sustained benefits.
2. Lavender (Lavandula angustifolia)
   - **Benefits**: Lavender is renowned for its calming and sedative properties, helping reduce anxiety and improve sleep quality.
   - **Preparation**: Lavender oil can be used in aromatherapy, added to baths, or applied topically when diluted with a carrier oil. Lavender tea is also beneficial.
   - **When to Take**: For anxiety relief, use lavender oil in aromatherapy throughout the day or in the evening to promote relaxation before sleep.
   - **Quantity**: For teas, use 1-2 teaspoons of dried lavender per cup of boiling water. For essential oil, a few drops can be used in a diffuser or diluted in a bath.
   - **Duration**: Can be used as needed to alleviate anxiety or promote relaxation.
3. Chamomile (Matricaria recutita)
   - **Benefits**: Chamomile is known for its soothing effects, which can reduce anxiety and facilitate sleep.
   - **Preparation**: Chamomile tea is the most common form. It can also be taken as a supplement or used as an extract.
   - **When to Take**: Drink chamomile tea in the evening to help unwind before bedtime, or throughout the day to manage stress.
   - **Quantity**: For tea, steep 1-2 teaspoons of dried chamomile flowers in hot water for 10 minutes. Supplements should be taken according to the package instructions.
   - **Duration**: Safe for daily use; however, consult with a healthcare provider for long-term use.
4. Ashwagandha (Withania somnifera)

- **Benefits**: An adaptogen, ashwagandha helps the body manage stress and has been shown to reduce cortisol levels, enhance mood, and alleviate anxiety.
- **Preparation**: Available in capsules, powders, or tinctures.
- **When to Take**: Morning or evening, depending on personal response (some find it energizing, others find it sedating).
- **Quantity**: Dosages can vary widely; 300-500 mg of root extract per day is common.
- **Duration**: Effects may be noticed after 6-12 weeks of regular use. Consult a healthcare provider for advice on long-term use.

5. Lemon Balm (Melissa officinalis)
- **Benefits**: Lemon balm can improve mood and cognitive performance while reducing anxiety and promoting calmness.
- **Preparation**: Lemon balm tea is popular, but it can also be taken as a supplement or extract.
- **When to Take**: Consumed during the day for anxiety relief or in the evening to aid sleep.
- **Quantity**: For tea, steep 1-2 teaspoons of dried lemon balm in hot water for up to 10 minutes. Follow supplement instructions for extracts and capsules.
- **Duration**: Lemon balm can be used as needed, though regular use over weeks may provide cumulative benefits.

General Guidelines for Using Herbs for Mental Wellness
- **Consultation**: Always consult with a healthcare provider before starting any herbal regimen, especially if you are taking medications, as there can be interactions.
- **Quality**: Choose high-quality, reputable sources for herbs to ensure purity and potency.
- **Observation**: Monitor your body's response to herbal treatments, as individual reactions can vary.
- **Patience**: Natural remedies often take time to show their full effects, so patience and consistency in use are key.

Integrating these herbs into your wellness routine can offer natural support for managing mood and anxiety. However, they should complement a holistic approach to mental health that includes proper nutrition, exercise, stress management techniques, and professional support when necessary.

Daily Habits for Mental Wellness

Mental wellness encompasses our emotional, psychological, and social well-being. It affects how we think, feel, and act as we cope with life's stresses. Cultivating daily habits that promote mental wellness is crucial for maintaining balance and enhancing our ability to enjoy life. These habits can help mitigate the impacts of stress, anxiety, and depression, contributing to a more fulfilled and resilient existence. Here, we explore comprehensive strategies that form the cornerstone of daily mental wellness routines.

1. Mindful Morning Start
- **Practice**: Begin each day with a mindfulness practice, such as meditation or deep breathing exercises, to center yourself and set a positive tone for the day ahead.
- **Benefits**: This habit can reduce morning anxiety and stress, improving focus and mood throughout the day.

2. Nutritious Eating
- **Practice**: Incorporate a balanced diet rich in fruits, vegetables, whole grains, lean proteins, and healthy fats. Prioritize foods known to support brain health, such as those high in omega-3 fatty acids, antioxidants, and vitamins.
- **Benefits**: A nutritious diet can significantly impact mental health, enhancing mood, cognitive function, and energy levels.

3. Regular Physical Activity
- **Practice**: Engage in at least 30 minutes of moderate physical activity most days of the week. This could include walking, cycling, yoga, or any other exercise that you enjoy and can sustain long-term.

- **Benefits**: Exercise releases endorphins, often dubbed 'feel-good' hormones, which act as natural mood lifters. Regular activity also promotes better sleep, reduces anxiety, and boosts self-esteem.

4. Quality Sleep
- **Practice**: Establish a consistent sleep schedule by going to bed and waking up at the same times each day. Create a bedtime routine that promotes relaxation, such as reading or taking a warm bath.
- **Benefits**: Adequate sleep is essential for emotional regulation, cognitive function, and overall mental health. Consistent sleep patterns can help prevent mood swings and reduce the risk of depression.

5. Social Connections
- **Practice**: Make time for meaningful social interactions with friends, family, or community members. Even small interactions can make a difference.
- **Benefits**: Strong social connections are vital for emotional support, reducing feelings of loneliness and isolation. Engaging in social activities can also provide a sense of belonging and purpose.

6. Stress Management
- **Practice**: Incorporate stress-reduction techniques into your daily routine. This could include hobbies, creative arts, nature walks, or journaling—anything that helps you unwind and process your day.
- **Benefits**: Managing stress effectively can prevent chronic stress from impairing your mental health. It helps maintain a calm and clear mind, improving problem-solving and decision-making skills.

7. Digital Detox
- **Practice**: Set boundaries around your use of digital devices, especially social media. Consider dedicated times during the day when you disconnect from screens.
- **Benefits**: A digital detox can reduce the overwhelm from constant connectivity, lower anxiety levels, and improve face-to-face relationships. It also helps prevent information overload and improves sleep quality.

8. Practicing Gratitude
- **Practice**: End your day by reflecting on and writing down three things you are grateful for. This can be done in a journal or shared with a loved one.
- **Benefits**: Cultivating gratitude can shift your focus from what's lacking to what's abundant in your life, enhancing overall happiness and satisfaction. It promotes a positive mindset and resilience against adversity.

Conclusion

Integrating these daily habits for mental wellness creates a strong foundation for emotional and psychological health. By consistently practicing these habits, individuals can build resilience against life's stresses, enjoy improved relationships, and foster a positive outlook on life. Remember, mental wellness is a journey, not a destination. Be patient and kind to yourself as you incorporate these practices into your life, and seek professional help when needed to navigate more challenging mental health issues.

Stress Management and Relaxation Practices

In our fast-paced world, stress has become a pervasive issue, affecting both physical and mental health. Effective stress management is crucial for maintaining well-being and enhancing life quality. This segment explores various strategies and practices designed to manage stress and promote relaxation, offering a guide to developing a personalized stress-reduction routine.

Understanding Stress

Before delving into stress management techniques, it's essential to understand that stress is the body's response to any demand or challenge. While short-term stress can be beneficial, chronic stress can lead to numerous health problems, including anxiety, depression, heart disease, and weakened immune function. Recognizing the signs of stress is the first step toward managing it effectively.

Stress Management Techniques
1. **Mindfulness Meditation**
   - **Description**: Mindfulness involves paying attention to the present moment without judgment. Mindfulness meditation encourages awareness of thoughts, feelings, and bodily sensations.
   - **Practice**: Dedicate a few minutes each day to sit quietly, focus on your breath, and observe your thoughts and feelings without attachment.
   - **Benefits**: Reduces anxiety, improves mood, and enhances focus and clarity.
2. **Deep Breathing Exercises**
   - **Description**: Deep breathing techniques involve conscious, deliberate breathing designed to invoke the body's relaxation response.
   - **Practice**: Try the 4-7-8 technique—inhale deeply through the nose for 4 seconds, hold the breath for 7 seconds, and exhale slowly through the mouth for 8 seconds.
   - **Benefits**: Lowers stress levels, reduces blood pressure, and promotes calmness.
3. **Progressive Muscle Relaxation (PMR)**
   - **Description**: PMR is a technique for reducing stress and anxiety by tensing and then relaxing each muscle group in the body.
   - **Practice**: Starting with the toes and working your way up to the face, tense each muscle group for 5 seconds, then relax for 30 seconds, noticing the contrast between tension and relaxation.
   - **Benefits**: Helps identify areas of tension, reduces physical and psychological stress, and improves sleep quality.
4. **Yoga and Tai Chi**
   - **Description**: These ancient practices combine physical postures, breathing exercises, and meditation to balance the body and mind.
   - **Practice**: Join a class or follow online tutorials tailored to your experience level. Focus on the fluid movements and breath control inherent to each practice.
   - **Benefits**: Increases body awareness, reduces stress, improves mental clarity, and enhances flexibility and strength.
5. **Regular Physical Activity**
   - **Description**: Exercise is a powerful stress reliever that can improve your mood and decrease feelings of anxiety and depression.
   - **Practice**: Engage in at least 30 minutes of moderate-intensity exercise most days of the week, such as walking, cycling, swimming, or dancing.
   - **Benefits**: Releases endorphins (natural mood lifters), improves sleep, and boosts self-confidence.
6. **Nature Exposure**
   - **Description**: Spending time in natural environments can significantly reduce stress and improve overall well-being.
   - **Practice**: Make time for regular walks in parks, forest bathing, or simply sitting in a garden.
   - **Benefits**: Lowers stress hormone levels, enhances mood, and increases feelings of relaxation and calm.
7. **Art and Music Therapy**
   - **Description**: Engaging in creative activities such as drawing, painting, or listening to soothing music can serve as effective stress-relief tools.
   - **Practice**: Set aside time for artistic endeavors without focusing on the outcome, or create a playlist of calming music to listen to during stressful times.
   - **Benefits**: Facilitates emotional expression, reduces anxiety, and promotes relaxation.

Developing a Stress Management Plan

Creating a personalized stress management plan involves selecting techniques that resonate with you and integrating them into your daily routine. Consistency is key—regular practice yields the most significant benefits. Additionally, being proactive about stress management involves recognizing stressors and either altering your response to them or changing the situation when possible.

Conclusion

Effective stress management and relaxation practices are vital components of a healthy lifestyle. By incorporating a variety of techniques, individuals can not only mitigate the adverse effects of stress but also enhance their capacity for enjoyment, productivity, and emotional resilience. Remember, the journey to managing stress is personal and evolving; what works for one person may not work for another, so be open to exploring and adapting different practices to suit your needs and preferences.

Chapter 7: Enhancing Immune Function

In the pursuit of overall well-being, optimal immune function plays a pivotal role. Our immune system is our body's defense mechanism against infections, diseases, and various external and internal threats. Enhancing immune function involves adopting a holistic approach that includes dietary adjustments, lifestyle modifications, and the integration of natural remedies. This chapter delves into comprehensive strategies for bolstering the immune system, ensuring it operates efficiently and effectively.

Boosting Immunity with Specific Herbs and Foods

A strong immune system is fundamental to maintaining health and warding off illnesses. While no single food or herb can prevent illness entirely, incorporating certain immune-boosting herbs and foods into your diet can enhance your body's defense mechanisms. Here, we explore some of the most potent herbs and foods known for their immune-boosting properties, including their benefits, preparation methods, optimal times for consumption, recommended quantities, and duration of use.

Herbs for Enhancing Immune Function

1. **Echinacea (Echinacea purpurea)**
   - **Benefits**: Echinacea is renowned for its ability to prevent and alleviate common colds by enhancing the immune response. It's thought to increase the production of white blood cells, which fight infections.
   - **Preparation**: Echinacea can be consumed as tea, tinctures, or capsules.
   - **When to Take**: At the onset of cold symptoms or during cold seasons for prevention.
   - **Quantity**: Follow the manufacturer's instructions for supplements. For tea, steep 1-2 teaspoons of dried echinacea in hot water for 10-15 minutes.
   - **Duration**: Echinacea is typically taken at the onset of symptoms and continued for 7-10 days. It's not recommended for prolonged use due to concerns about impacting the immune system negatively over time.

2. **Astragalus (Astragalus membranaceus)**
   - **Benefits**: Astragalus is an adaptogen that boosts immunity and combats fatigue. It's believed to stimulate and increase white blood cells, which are vital for immune defense.
   - **Preparation**: Commonly used in soups or as a supplement in capsules or tinctures.
   - **When to Take**: Regularly during cold and flu season for preventive measures.
   - **Quantity and Duration**: For capsules and tinctures, follow the manufacturer's guidelines. Astragalus can be safely incorporated into your diet over longer periods as part of a balanced approach to immune support.

3. **Ginger (Zingiber officinale)**
   - **Benefits**: With its anti-inflammatory and antioxidative properties, ginger helps support the immune system and can reduce inflammation.
   - **Preparation**: Fresh ginger can be used in cooking, brewed as tea, or taken as supplements.
   - **When to Take**: Daily, incorporated into meals or as a morning or evening tea.
   - **Quantity**: For tea, use about 1-2 inches of fresh ginger per cup of boiling water. Adjust according to taste preference and tolerance.
   - **Duration**: Ginger is safe for daily consumption in food and tea. For supplements, adhere to the recommended dosage on the product label.

Foods to Boost Immunity

1. **Citrus Fruits**
   - **Benefits**: Rich in vitamin C, a crucial antioxidant for immune function and skin health. Vitamin C helps stimulate the production of white blood cells, key to fighting infections.
   - **Examples**: Oranges, lemons, limes, grapefruits, and tangerines.

- **Recommended Intake**: Incorporate a variety of citrus fruits into your daily diet during meals or as snacks.
2. **Garlic**
   - **Benefits**: Contains compounds that help the immune system fight germs. Garlic has been shown to enhance immune cell function and may have a mild antibacterial effect.
   - **Preparation**: Best consumed raw or lightly cooked to preserve its health benefits. Can be added to a wide range of dishes for flavor and health benefits.
   - **Recommended Intake**: 1-2 cloves per day can be beneficial for health when included as part of a balanced diet.
3. **Spinach**
   - **Benefits**: Spinach is packed with antioxidants and beta carotene, which may increase the infection-fighting ability of the immune system.
   - **Preparation**: Lightly cooked to enhance vitamin A and allow other nutrients to be released from oxalic acid.
   - **Recommended Intake**: Incorporate spinach into your diet several times a week for the best results.

Conclusion

Enhancing your immune system through herbs and foods is a holistic approach to maintaining health and preventing illness. By incorporating immune-boosting herbs like echinacea, astragalus, and ginger, along with nutrient-rich foods such as citrus fruits, garlic, and spinach, you can support your body's natural defenses. Remember, the key to benefiting from these herbs and foods lies in consistent and balanced consumption, coupled with a healthy lifestyle that includes adequate sleep, stress management, and physical activity. Always consult with a healthcare professional before adding new supplements to your routine, especially if you have existing health conditions or are taking medication.

Daily Practices for Disease Prevention

Maintaining optimal health and preventing disease is a multifaceted endeavor that involves a comprehensive approach to lifestyle management. By integrating specific daily practices into one's routine, individuals can significantly reduce the risk of developing various chronic diseases and enhance their overall well-being. This segment outlines essential daily practices aimed at disease prevention, focusing on nutrition, physical activity, mental health, and preventive healthcare.

Nutritional Habits
1. **Balanced Diet:**
   - **Practice**: Consume a variety of foods from all food groups to ensure a balanced intake of essential nutrients. Prioritize fruits, vegetables, whole grains, lean proteins, and healthy fats.
   - **Benefits**: A balanced diet supports body functions, strengthens the immune system, and reduces the risk of chronic diseases such as heart disease, diabetes, and cancer.
2. **Limit Processed Foods and Sugar:**
   - **Practice**: Minimize the intake of processed foods, sugary drinks, and snacks, which are often high in unhealthy fats, sugars, and sodium.
   - **Benefits**: Reducing these foods can decrease the risk of obesity, diabetes, and cardiovascular diseases.
3. **Hydration:**
   - **Practice**: Drink adequate amounts of water throughout the day. The amount can vary based on individual needs, but a general guideline is 8-10 glasses daily.
   - **Benefits**: Proper hydration is crucial for digestion, absorption of nutrients, and elimination of toxins, contributing to overall health maintenance.

Physical Activity
1. **Regular Exercise:**

- **Practice**: Engage in at least 150 minutes of moderate aerobic exercise or 75 minutes of vigorous exercise weekly, along with muscle-strengthening activities on two or more days.
- **Benefits**: Regular physical activity reduces the risk of chronic diseases, including heart disease, stroke, diabetes, and some cancers. It also supports mental health and well-being.

2. **Incorporate Movement Throughout the Day**:
   - **Practice**: Adopt habits that increase physical activity, such as taking the stairs, walking or cycling for short trips, and standing or stretching at regular intervals during sedentary activities.
   - **Benefits**: Increasing daily movement can help counteract the negative effects of prolonged sitting, contributing to cardiovascular health and weight management.

Mental Health and Stress Management
1. **Mindfulness and Relaxation Techniques**:
   - **Practice**: Dedicate time each day for mindfulness practices, meditation, or deep-breathing exercises to manage stress effectively.
   - **Benefits**: These practices can lower stress levels, reduce the risk of stress-related health issues, and enhance emotional well-being.
2. **Adequate Sleep**:
   - **Practice**: Ensure 7-9 hours of quality sleep per night, establishing a consistent sleep schedule and creating a restful sleeping environment.
   - **Benefits**: Adequate sleep is essential for physical health, cognitive function, and emotional regulation, reducing the risk of various chronic conditions.

Preventive Healthcare
1. **Regular Health Screenings**:
   - **Practice**: Adhere to recommended schedules for health screenings and check-ups, including blood pressure monitoring, cholesterol checks, diabetes screening, and cancer screenings.
   - **Benefits**: Early detection of health issues can lead to more effective management and treatment, significantly reducing the risk of severe complications.
2. **Vaccinations**:
   - **Practice**: Keep vaccinations up to date according to guidelines for age and health conditions.
   - **Benefits**: Vaccinations can prevent a range of infectious diseases, protecting individual health and contributing to community health through herd immunity.

Conclusion

Adopting these daily practices for disease prevention can profoundly impact one's health trajectory, reducing the risk of chronic diseases and enhancing quality of life. While individual practices contribute significantly to disease prevention, their collective implementation as part of a holistic lifestyle approach offers the most substantial benefits. Regular self-assessment and adjustments, coupled with healthcare professional consultations, can ensure these practices are effectively integrated into daily life, paving the way for a healthier future.

Sleep's Role in Immune Health

Sleep, an essential physiological process, plays a critical role in the maintenance and regulation of various bodily functions, including the immune system. The relationship between sleep and immune health is complex and bidirectional; not only does adequate sleep bolster the immune system, but the immune system, in turn, can regulate sleep patterns. This segment explores the intricacies of how sleep influences immune health, highlighting the mechanisms at play, the consequences of sleep deprivation, and strategies to enhance sleep quality for optimal immune function.

The Mechanisms Linking Sleep and Immune Function

1. **Cytokine Production**: During sleep, the body produces cytokines, proteins that are crucial for fighting infection and inflammation. Sleep deprivation can decrease the production of these protective cytokines, as well as antibodies and cells that combat infections, making the body more susceptible to illnesses.
2. **T-cell Function**: Sleep enhances the efficiency of T-cells, a type of white blood cell pivotal to the body's immune response. T-cells are better able to adhere to and destroy cells infected by viruses and other pathogens when the body gets enough rest.
3. **Stress Hormone Regulation**: Sleep helps regulate the levels of stress hormones, such as cortisol. Elevated cortisol levels can suppress immune function if the body does not have adequate rest to balance these hormone levels.

Consequences of Sleep Deprivation on Immune Health
1. **Increased Vulnerability to Illness**: Studies have shown that individuals who get less than seven hours of sleep per night are more likely to develop a cold when exposed to the virus compared to those who sleep more.
2. **Longer Recovery Times**: Lack of sleep can prolong recovery from illness due to the impaired production of cytokines and other immune cells.
3. **Chronic Inflammation**: Chronic sleep loss can lead to a state of low-grade, systemic inflammation, increasing the risk of developing chronic diseases, including cardiovascular disease, diabetes, and obesity.

Strategies for Enhancing Sleep Quality
1. **Establish a Consistent Sleep Schedule**: Going to bed and waking up at the same time every day, even on weekends, helps regulate your body's internal clock and can improve the quality of your sleep.
2. **Create a Restful Environment**: Make sure your bedroom is quiet, dark, and at a comfortable temperature. Consider using earplugs, eye shades, or white noise machines to create an environment conducive to sleep.
3. **Limit Exposure to Screens Before Bedtime**: The blue light emitted by phones, tablets, and computers can interfere with the production of melatonin, a hormone that regulates sleep-wake cycles. Avoid screens at least an hour before bedtime.
4. **Incorporate Relaxation Techniques**: Practices such as reading, taking a warm bath, or meditation can promote relaxation and make it easier to fall asleep.
5. **Be Mindful of Diet and Exercise**: Avoid heavy meals, caffeine, and alcohol close to bedtime, as they can disrupt sleep. Regular physical activity can help you fall asleep faster and enjoy deeper sleep, but try not to exercise too close to bedtime.
6. **Manage Stress**: Engaging in stress-reducing activities during the day can prevent stress from affecting your sleep. Techniques like deep breathing, yoga, and mindfulness meditation can be particularly effective.

Conclusion

Sleep is a fundamental pillar of immune health, with profound implications for the body's ability to fight infections and inflammation. By understanding the critical role of sleep in supporting the immune system, individuals can prioritize and adopt practices that enhance sleep quality, thereby bolstering their defense against illnesses and contributing to overall well-being. As research continues to unravel the complexities of sleep's impact on immune function, the adage "sleep is the best medicine" remains ever relevant, highlighting sleep's indispensable role in maintaining health and preventing disease.

Chapter 8: Women's Health: Natural Approaches

Women's health encompasses a broad spectrum of physical, mental, and emotional aspects, ranging from menstrual health and fertility to menopause and beyond. The unique physiological processes women experience throughout their lives can benefit greatly from natural approaches that support balance, wellness, and vitality. This chapter delves into natural strategies and remedies tailored specifically for women's health, emphasizing holistic care and preventive measures.

Natural Management of Menstrual and Menopausal Symptoms

Women's reproductive health encompasses various phases, each accompanied by its unique set of challenges. Menstrual and menopausal symptoms can significantly impact daily life, prompting many to seek natural methods for relief and management. This section explores holistic approaches to mitigating the symptoms associated with menstruation and menopause, emphasizing dietary, lifestyle, and herbal remedies.

Managing Menstrual Symptoms Naturally

Menstrual symptoms, including cramps, bloating, mood swings, and fatigue, can vary widely in intensity and duration. Natural management strategies focus on hormonal balance, pain relief, and overall wellness.

1. **Dietary Adjustments**:
    - **Anti-inflammatory Foods**: Incorporating foods rich in omega-3 fatty acids, such as salmon, flaxseeds, and walnuts, can help reduce menstrual pain. Fruits and vegetables high in antioxidants also combat inflammation.
    - **Magnesium-Rich Foods**: Dark leafy greens, nuts, seeds, and whole grains are excellent sources of magnesium, which can alleviate cramps and reduce bloating.
2. **Herbal Remedies**:
    - **Ginger**: Known for its anti-inflammatory properties, ginger can decrease the intensity and duration of pain. Consuming ginger tea or supplements starting a few days before menstruation may offer relief.
    - **Chamomile Tea**: Chamomile has calming effects, helping to soothe cramps and reduce menstrual discomfort. Its mild sedative effect can also improve sleep quality.
3. **Physical Activity and Yoga**:
    - Regular exercise, including yoga, can relieve menstrual cramps and improve mood. Specific yoga poses, like child's pose and cat-cow, can be particularly beneficial in easing menstrual discomfort.

Natural Approaches to Menopausal Symptoms

Menopause marks the end of a woman's reproductive years and is characterized by symptoms like hot flashes, night sweats, mood fluctuations, and sleep disturbances. Natural management focuses on hormonal balance and symptom relief.

1. **Phytoestrogens**:
    - Foods containing phytoestrogens, such as soy products, flaxseeds, and sesame seeds, may mimic estrogen in the body, helping to balance hormones naturally and alleviate menopausal symptoms.
2. **Herbal Supplements**:

- **Black Cohosh**: This herb is widely used for relieving menopausal symptoms, particularly hot flashes and mood swings. However, it should be used under the guidance of a healthcare professional due to potential interactions and side effects.
- **Dong Quai**: Often used in traditional Chinese medicine, Dong Quai is believed to offer relief from menopausal symptoms by affecting estrogen activity. It's commonly taken as a supplement or tea.

3. **Lifestyle Modifications**:
   - **Stress Management**: Techniques such as deep breathing, meditation, and mindfulness can reduce stress levels and mitigate mood swings associated with menopause.
   - **Sleep Hygiene**: Establishing a regular sleep schedule, creating a comfortable sleep environment, and practicing relaxation techniques before bed can improve sleep quality.

Additional Recommendations for Both Phases
- **Hydration**: Drinking plenty of water is essential during menstruation to replace lost fluids and during menopause to alleviate dryness symptoms.
- **Avoid Triggers**: Limiting caffeine, alcohol, and spicy foods can reduce menstrual pain and menopausal hot flashes.

Conclusion

Natural management of menstrual and menopausal symptoms offers a holistic approach to women's reproductive health. By combining dietary adjustments, herbal remedies, and lifestyle changes, women can navigate these phases with greater ease and comfort. However, it's important to consult with healthcare providers before trying new supplements or making significant lifestyle changes, especially for those with preexisting health conditions or who are taking medications. These natural strategies, tailored to individual needs and preferences, can significantly enhance quality of life during menstruation and menopause.

Herbs for Hormonal Balance and Reproductive Health

Hormonal balance is crucial for optimal reproductive health and overall well-being. Several herbs have been traditionally used and are supported by contemporary research for their ability to support hormonal regulation and enhance reproductive health in both men and women. This section explores the most effective herbs for these purposes, detailing their benefits, preparation methods, and guidelines for use.

1. Chaste Tree Berry (Vitex agnus-castus)
   - **Benefits**: Vitex is renowned for its ability to regulate menstrual cycles, relieve symptoms of PMS, and improve fertility by balancing female hormones. It specifically influences the pituitary gland, which controls hormone production.
   - **Preparation and Use**: Vitex is available in capsule, tincture, and tea forms. Capsules are commonly used for consistent dosing.
   - **When to Take**: Morning is ideal, as it can align with the body's natural rhythm. It should be taken daily for best results.
   - **Quantity and Duration**: Follow manufacturer's guidelines; a common dosage is 160-240 mg of extract daily. Vitex needs to be taken consistently for several months to experience benefits, often 3-6 months.

2. Maca (Lepidium meyenii)
   - **Benefits**: Maca root is an adaptogen that supports the endocrine system, enhancing fertility and libido in both men and women. It's known for improving energy levels and stamina.
   - **Preparation and Use**: Maca is available in powder, capsule, and liquid extract form. The powder can be added to smoothies, juices, or foods.
   - **When to Take**: Any time of day, preferably with food to aid digestion.
   - **Quantity and Duration**: Dosages of powder range from 1.5 to 5 grams daily. As an adaptogen, maca is best used for periods of several months, followed by a break.

3. Ashwagandha (Withania somnifera)

- **Benefits**: Ashwagandha is another adaptogen that helps the body manage stress, which can, in turn, support hormone balance. It's particularly beneficial for thyroid health and can enhance libido and fertility by regulating hormone levels.
- **Preparation and Use**: Available in capsules, powders, and tinctures. The powder can be mixed into beverages or foods.
- **When to Take**: It can be taken at any time, though some prefer it in the evening due to its calming effects.
- **Quantity and Duration**: Typical dosages range from 300-500 mg of extract twice daily. Continuous use for at least 6 weeks is recommended to observe benefits, with ongoing usage as needed.

4. Dong Quai (Angelica sinensis)
- **Benefits**: Often called "female ginseng," Dong Quai is a traditional Chinese herb used to regulate the menstrual cycle and alleviate menopausal symptoms. It's thought to act by affecting estrogen levels and improving blood health.
- **Preparation and Use**: Dong Quai can be taken as a tincture, in capsules, or as tea. It's often combined with other herbs for synergistic effects.
- **When to Take**: Daily, with consideration to menstrual cycle for those regulating menstruation.
- **Quantity and Duration**: Follow specific product dosing instructions due to varying concentrations. Use is often cyclic, discontinuing during menstruation.

5. Evening Primrose Oil (Oenothera biennis)
- **Benefits**: Rich in gamma-linolenic acid (GLA), evening primrose oil is beneficial for reducing PMS symptoms and supporting overall hormonal balance. It's also used for skin conditions like eczema, which can have hormonal components.
- **Preparation and Use**: Primarily taken in capsule form.
- **When to Take**: With meals to improve absorption of the oil.
- **Quantity and Duration**: Dosages typically range from 500-1300 mg daily. Benefits may be observed after several weeks of consistent use, with ongoing consumption as needed.

General Guidelines for Using Herbs for Hormonal Balance
- **Consultation**: Always consult a healthcare provider before starting any herbal supplement, especially for individuals with existing health conditions, those pregnant or breastfeeding, or persons taking medications, as interactions can occur.
- **Quality**: Opt for high-quality, reputable brands to ensure purity and potency of herbal supplements.
- **Patience**: Hormonal balance and reproductive health improvements often require consistent, long-term use of herbs. Patience and consistency are key.
- **Holistic Approach**: Combine herbal remedies with a balanced diet, regular exercise, and stress management practices for comprehensive benefits.

Herbs offer a natural avenue for supporting hormonal balance and enhancing reproductive health. By understanding and respecting the potency of these natural remedies, individuals can harness their benefits while minimizing risks.

Fertility Enhancement Through Natural Means

Fertility challenges are increasingly common among couples worldwide. While medical interventions offer solutions, many individuals and couples seek natural ways to enhance fertility due to their holistic benefits and lower side effects. This comprehensive approach combines dietary adjustments, lifestyle modifications, and the use of specific herbs to create an optimal environment for conception. Here, we delve into natural strategies for enhancing fertility, underlining the importance of a balanced approach to reproductive health.

Nutritional Support for Fertility
1. **Antioxidant-Rich Foods**:
    - **Role**: Antioxidants like vitamins C and E, selenium, and zinc help protect sperm and egg cells from damage by neutralizing harmful free radicals.

- **Sources**: Incorporate a diet rich in fruits (berries, citrus), vegetables (spinach, broccoli), nuts (almonds, walnuts), and seeds (flaxseeds, pumpkin seeds).
2. **Balanced Diet:**
    - **Importance**: A diet balanced in macronutrients (carbohydrates, proteins, and fats) and rich in micronutrients supports overall hormonal balance and reproductive health.
    - **Recommendations**: Focus on whole foods, lean proteins, healthy fats (avocado, olive oil), and whole grains to support fertility.

3. **Folic Acid:**
    - **Benefits**: Crucial for DNA synthesis, folic acid is essential before conception and during early pregnancy to prevent neural tube defects.
    - **Sources**: Leafy greens, beans, avocados, and fortified grains. Supplements are often recommended for women planning to conceive.

Lifestyle Modifications
1. **Maintain a Healthy Weight:**
    - **Impact**: Being significantly over or underweight can affect hormone levels and ovulation. Achieving and maintaining a healthy weight can improve fertility.
    - **Strategies**: Combine balanced nutrition with regular physical activity. Consider consulting a healthcare provider for personalized advice.
2. **Manage Stress:**
    - **Effects**: High stress levels can disrupt hormone balance and affect fertility. Stress management techniques can help create a more conducive environment for conception.
    - **Techniques**: Practice mindfulness, meditation, yoga, or deep-breathing exercises to reduce stress.
3. **Limit Toxins:**
    - **Advice**: Reduce exposure to environmental toxins and chemicals, including pesticides, plastics (BPA), and certain household cleaners, which can negatively impact fertility.
    - **Action Steps**: Opt for organic produce where possible, use glass or BPA-free containers, and choose natural cleaning products.
4. **Moderate Exercise:**
    - **Benefits**: Regular, moderate exercise supports overall health, including reproductive health, but excessive exercise may hinder fertility.
    - **Recommendations**: Aim for balanced activities like walking, swimming, and gentle yoga. Avoid overly strenuous routines if trying to conceive.

Herbal Remedies for Fertility Enhancement
1. **Chaste Tree Berry (Vitex agnus-castus):**
    - **Benefits**: Vitex supports hormonal balance, particularly in women with irregular menstrual cycles, enhancing ovulation and fertility.
    - **Use**: Take as directed by a healthcare professional, usually once daily in the morning.
2. **Maca (Lepidium meyenii):**
    - **Benefits**: Known to improve libido in both men and women, maca also supports sperm health and quantity.
    - **Use**: Incorporate maca powder into smoothies or take as capsules. Start with a low dose and adjust based on response.
3. **Ashwagandha (Withania somnifera):**
    - **Benefits**: This adaptogen can improve stress response, support hormone balance, and enhance male fertility by improving sperm quality.
    - **Use**: Available in powder or capsule form, follow the recommended dosages on the product label.

Holistic Approach to Fertility Enhancement

Enhancing fertility naturally is a holistic process that involves nurturing the body and mind. It's important for couples to adopt these practices together, supporting each other's health and well-being. Consistency and patience are key, as natural approaches can take time to manifest results. Always consult with healthcare professionals before starting any new supplements or making significant lifestyle changes, especially when related to fertility and conception.

Natural fertility enhancement emphasizes the body's inherent ability to heal and maintain balance, offering a nurturing path toward achieving pregnancy. Through mindful nutrition, lifestyle adjustments, and the judicious use of herbal remedies, couples can optimize their health and increase their chances of conception.

Chapter 9: Combating Chronic Inflammation

Chronic inflammation is an underlying factor in many serious diseases, including heart disease, diabetes, cancer, and autoimmune disorders. Unlike acute inflammation—a natural and beneficial process for healing—the chronic form can silently damage the body over years, often without noticeable symptoms. This chapter explores natural approaches to combating chronic inflammation through dietary choices, lifestyle modifications, and the integration of specific herbs known for their anti-inflammatory properties.

Anti-inflammatory Diet and Lifestyle Adjustments

An anti-inflammatory diet and lifestyle adjustments serve as foundational strategies in combating chronic inflammation. This approach emphasizes foods rich in antioxidants and phytonutrients that help reduce inflammatory responses in the body, alongside lifestyle practices that mitigate stress and promote overall well-being.

Anti-inflammatory Diet
1. **Whole Foods Over Processed Foods**:
    *   **Principle**: Prioritize whole, nutrient-dense foods while minimizing processed and refined foods high in sugar, unhealthy fats, and additives known to trigger inflammation.
    *   **Action Steps**: Incorporate a variety of fruits and vegetables, whole grains, lean protein sources, and healthy fats into your diet. Avoid or limit processed meats, white bread, pastries, and sugary beverages.
2. **Fatty Fish**:
    *   **Benefits**: Rich in omega-3 fatty acids (EPA and DHA), fatty fish like salmon, mackerel, sardines, and anchovies can reduce the levels of pro-inflammatory markers in the body.
    *   **Recommendation**: Aim for at least two servings of fatty fish per week.
3. **Antioxidant-Rich Foods**:
    *   **Benefits**: Foods high in antioxidants help neutralize free radicals, reducing oxidative stress and inflammation.
    *   **Sources**: Berries, leafy greens, nuts, seeds, and dark chocolate are excellent sources of various antioxidants, including vitamins C and E, flavonoids, and polyphenols.
4. **Spices and Herbs**:
    *   **Role**: Many herbs and spices have potent anti-inflammatory properties.
    *   **Examples**: Turmeric (containing curcumin), ginger, garlic, cinnamon, and rosemary not only enhance the flavor of foods but also offer health benefits. Incorporating these into daily meals can contribute to reducing inflammation.

Lifestyle Adjustments
1. **Regular Physical Activity**:
    *   **Impact**: Exercise stimulates the production of anti-inflammatory compounds in the body and helps manage weight, a key factor in controlling inflammation.
    *   **Recommendation**: Engage in at least 150 minutes of moderate aerobic activity or 75 minutes of vigorous activity weekly, plus muscle-strengthening exercises on two or more days a week.
2. **Stress Management**:
    *   **Importance**: Chronic stress triggers the release of pro-inflammatory cytokines. Managing stress effectively can help reduce inflammation.

- **Strategies**: Mindfulness, meditation, yoga, deep breathing exercises, and spending time in nature are effective ways to reduce stress levels.
3. **Adequate Sleep**:
   - **Benefits**: Quality sleep is crucial for regulating inflammatory responses and healing the body.
   - **Recommendation**: Aim for 7-9 hours of quality sleep per night. Establish a regular sleep schedule and create a restful environment free of electronic devices before bedtime.
4. **Hydration**:
   - **Role**: Proper hydration supports all body functions, including the efficient removal of toxins, which can contribute to inflammation when accumulated.
   - **Guideline**: Drink at least 8 cups (about 2 liters) of water daily, adjusting based on activity level and environmental conditions.
5. **Avoiding Smoking and Limiting Alcohol**:
   - **Reason**: Smoking and excessive alcohol consumption can exacerbate inflammation and disrupt the body's natural mechanisms for managing it.
   - **Action Steps**: Quit smoking and limit alcohol intake to moderate levels (up to one drink per day for women and up to two drinks per day for men).

Conclusion

An anti-inflammatory diet and lifestyle are key components in preventing and managing chronic inflammation, a silent contributor to many chronic diseases. By making conscious food choices and adopting lifestyle habits that promote well-being, individuals can significantly reduce inflammation and enhance their overall health. These adjustments require commitment and consistency, but the benefits for long-term health and quality of life are substantial. It's also important to consult with healthcare professionals when making significant changes to your diet and lifestyle, especially for individuals with existing health conditions.

Herbal Anti-inflammatories and Their Usage

The use of herbal remedies as anti-inflammatory agents has deep roots in traditional medicine, providing a natural approach to reducing inflammation and managing associated health conditions. Several herbs have been identified for their potent anti-inflammatory properties, supported by both traditional use and modern research. This section explores effective herbal anti-inflammatories, outlining their benefits, methods of preparation, guidelines on when and how much to take, and the duration of use for optimal benefits.

1. Turmeric (Curcuma longa)
   - **Benefits**: The active compound in turmeric, curcumin, has powerful anti-inflammatory and antioxidant properties. It's been shown to be effective in managing conditions like arthritis, gastrointestinal issues, and cardiovascular diseases.
   - **Preparation**: Turmeric can be used fresh or powdered in cooking, or taken as a supplement in capsule form. For enhanced absorption, combine turmeric with black pepper, which contains piperine.
   - **When to Take**: If using for general health, incorporate turmeric into daily meals. As a supplement, follow the manufacturer's instructions, typically with meals to improve absorption.
   - **Quantity**: For general health, incorporating turmeric into meals is sufficient. As a supplement, dosages of 500-2000 mg of curcumin per day are commonly used.
   - **Duration**: Long-term use is generally considered safe for dietary amounts. For supplements, consult a healthcare provider for advice on duration.
2. Ginger (Zingiber officinale)
   - **Benefits**: Ginger is renowned for its anti-inflammatory, antioxidant, and analgesic properties, making it beneficial for pain relief, gastrointestinal health, and reducing inflammation.

- **Preparation**: Fresh ginger can be used in cooking or brewed into tea. Ginger supplements are available as capsules, powders, or extracts.
- **When to Take**: Ginger can be consumed throughout the day in food or tea. For supplements, follow the recommended dosage on the product label, usually with meals.
- **Quantity**: A daily dose of 1-2 grams of powdered ginger is typically recommended for anti-inflammatory effects.
- **Duration**: Ginger can be consumed daily as part of a regular diet. For specific health conditions and higher doses (supplements), consult a healthcare provider.

3. Boswellia (Boswellia serrata)
- **Benefits**: Also known as Indian frankincense, Boswellia has been shown to reduce inflammation, particularly in conditions like osteoarthritis, rheumatoid arthritis, and inflammatory bowel disease.
- **Preparation**: Boswellia is available in capsules, tablets, and as a resin extract.
- **When to Take**: Follow the manufacturer's guidelines, typically with meals to enhance absorption.
- **Quantity**: Dosages can vary widely; common supplements contain 300-500 mg to be taken two to three times daily.
- **Duration**: Boswellia can be used for several months, but it's advisable to consult with a healthcare provider for personalized guidance, especially for long-term use.

4. Omega-3 Fatty Acids (Fish Oil)
- **Benefits**: While not an herb, omega-3 supplements derived from fish oil have significant anti-inflammatory effects, beneficial for heart health, cognitive function, and autoimmune conditions.
- **Preparation**: Omega-3 supplements are available in capsules or liquid form.
- **When to Take**: With meals to improve absorption and minimize any digestive discomfort.
- **Quantity**: Commonly, doses range from 500-1000 mg of EPA and DHA combined, per day.
- **Duration**: Long-term use is considered safe for most individuals, but it's important to consult with a healthcare provider, especially when used for specific health conditions.

General Guidelines for Using Herbal Anti-inflammatories
- **Consultation**: Always consult a healthcare professional before incorporating new herbal supplements into your regimen, particularly if you have existing health conditions or are taking other medications.
- **Quality and Purity**: Opt for high-quality, reputable brands to ensure the supplements are pure, potent, and free from contaminants.
- **Adverse Effects and Interactions**: Be aware of potential adverse effects and interactions with medications. Even natural remedies can have significant interactions with prescription drugs.

Herbal anti-inflammatories offer a natural path to managing inflammation and improving health. By understanding how to effectively incorporate these herbs into your wellness routine, alongside the necessary precautions and consultations with healthcare providers, individuals can harness the benefits of nature's pharmacy in supporting their health and well-being.

Understanding Inflammation's Role in Chronic Diseases

Inflammation is a natural process by which the body's immune system responds to injury, infection, or irritation. However, when inflammation becomes chronic, it can play a significant role in the development and progression of various chronic diseases. This detailed exploration sheds light on the mechanisms of inflammation, its connection to chronic diseases, and strategies for managing inflammation to mitigate disease risk.

The Dual Nature of Inflammation

1. **Acute Inflammation**: This is the body's immediate and temporary response to an injury or infection, characterized by redness, heat, swelling, and pain. It is a protective mechanism that eliminates the initial cause of cell injury, clears out damaged cells and tissues, and initiates tissue repair.
2. **Chronic Inflammation**: Unlike acute inflammation, chronic inflammation persists over time, often without a clear injury or infection to fight. This prolonged state of inflammation can lead to the damage of healthy cells and tissues, contributing to the development and exacerbation of chronic diseases.

Inflammation's Connection to Chronic Diseases

Chronic inflammation is increasingly recognized as a critical underlying mechanism in many chronic diseases, including:
1. **Cardiovascular Diseases**: Inflammation contributes to the development of atherosclerosis, where arteries become narrowed and hardened due to the buildup of plaque. This condition can lead to heart attacks and strokes.
2. **Diabetes**: Chronic low-grade inflammation affects insulin resistance, a hallmark of type 2 diabetes. Inflammatory markers are often elevated in individuals with this condition.
3. **Cancer**: Chronic inflammation has been linked to several steps in tumorigenesis, including initiation, promotion, malignant conversion, invasion, and metastasis. Inflammatory conditions can provide a microenvironment that supports tumor growth.
4. **Autoimmune Diseases**: Conditions like rheumatoid arthritis, lupus, and inflammatory bowel disease (IBD) are characterized by the immune system attacking the body's own tissues, driven in part by chronic inflammation.
5. **Neurodegenerative Diseases**: Chronic inflammation is also implicated in neurodegenerative diseases such as Alzheimer's disease and Parkinson's disease, where inflammation within the brain contributes to neuronal damage.

Strategies for Managing Chronic Inflammation

Managing chronic inflammation involves a holistic approach that includes dietary adjustments, lifestyle modifications, and, in some cases, medical interventions:
1. **Anti-inflammatory Diet**: Adopting a diet rich in antioxidants and omega-3 fatty acids can help counteract inflammation. Foods known for their anti-inflammatory properties include fatty fish, leafy greens, berries, nuts, and seeds.
2. **Regular Physical Activity**: Moderate exercise has been shown to reduce inflammatory markers in the body. It's recommended to engage in at least 150 minutes of moderate-intensity aerobic activity weekly.
3. **Stress Reduction**: Chronic stress can elevate levels of cortisol, a stress hormone that, when persistently high, can contribute to inflammation. Techniques such as mindfulness, meditation, and yoga can help manage stress.
4. **Adequate Sleep**: Ensuring sufficient, quality sleep is crucial, as sleep deprivation has been linked to increased inflammation. Aim for 7-9 hours of sleep per night.
5. **Avoiding Inflammatory Triggers**: Tobacco smoke, excessive alcohol consumption, and exposure to environmental toxins can all contribute to chronic inflammation. Minimizing exposure to these triggers is important for inflammation management.
6. **Monitoring and Medical Management**: For individuals with existing chronic diseases, regular monitoring and adherence to prescribed medical treatments are essential for managing inflammation. This may include the use of anti-inflammatory medications as directed by a healthcare provider.

Conclusion

Understanding the role of inflammation in chronic diseases highlights the importance of a proactive approach to health and wellness. By incorporating anti-inflammatory practices into daily life, individuals can significantly reduce their risk of chronic diseases and improve their overall health. Always consult with healthcare professionals when making significant changes to your diet, lifestyle, or medical regimen, especially if you have preexisting health conditions.

Chapter 10: Cancer Prevention and Support

Cancer remains one of the leading causes of death worldwide, prompting an ever-increasing focus on prevention strategies and supportive care. While not all cancers can be prevented, research suggests that lifestyle choices and environmental factors play a significant role in the risk of developing cancer. This chapter explores comprehensive strategies for cancer prevention and provides guidance on supportive care for individuals diagnosed with cancer, emphasizing the role of diet, lifestyle modifications, and natural approaches.

Introduction: A Holistic Approach to Cancer Prevention

Cancer prevention is a multifaceted endeavor that extends beyond the boundaries of medical interventions and genetic predispositions. It encompasses a holistic approach that integrates diet, lifestyle, mental health, and environmental factors to minimize the risk and support overall well-being. This introductory section lays the foundation for understanding how a comprehensive, proactive strategy can play a crucial role in reducing cancer risk and enhancing the quality of life.

The Pillars of Holistic Cancer Prevention

1. **Dietary Choices**: What we eat can significantly influence our cancer risk. A diet abundant in fruits, vegetables, whole grains, and lean proteins provides essential nutrients that support cellular health and reduce inflammation, a key contributor to cancer development. Conversely, diets high in processed foods, red meat, and sugars are linked to higher cancer risks. Thus, adopting a diet rich in antioxidants, phytochemicals, and anti-inflammatory foods becomes a cornerstone of cancer prevention.
2. **Physical Activity**: Regular exercise is not just about weight management; it's a powerful tool for cancer prevention. Physical activity helps regulate hormone levels, reduces inflammation, and improves immune function, all of which play roles in reducing cancer risk. The World Health Organization recommends at least 150 minutes of moderate-intensity or 75 minutes of high-intensity physical activity per week to derive these benefits.
3. **Mental and Emotional Well-being**: Stress, depression, and isolation can impact hormonal balance and immune function, potentially affecting cancer risk. Practices that promote mental and emotional well-being, such as mindfulness meditation, yoga, and social engagement, are vital components of a holistic cancer prevention strategy.
4. **Environmental and Lifestyle Factors**: Exposure to carcinogens in the environment—such as tobacco smoke, ultraviolet radiation, and certain chemicals—can significantly increase cancer risk. Minimizing exposure to these elements and adopting protective behaviors (e.g., using sunscreen, avoiding tobacco, limiting alcohol consumption) are essential preventive measures.
5. **Regular Screenings and Self-exams**: Early detection of cancer through regular screenings and being attuned to changes in one's body can drastically improve treatment outcomes. Adhering to recommended screening guidelines for breast, cervical, colorectal, and other cancers is a critical aspect of holistic cancer prevention.

Integrating Natural Approaches

Incorporating natural approaches, including the use of specific herbs and supplements known for their anti-cancer properties, can complement traditional preventive measures. For example, turmeric (containing curcumin), green tea, and cruciferous vegetables have been studied for their potential to inhibit cancer cell growth and protect against different types of cancer. However, it's essential to approach these remedies with caution, ensuring they do not interfere with conventional care or pre-existing conditions.

The Role of Personalized Care

Recognizing that each individual's risk factors, genetic predispositions, and lifestyle choices are unique is paramount in formulating a personalized holistic cancer prevention plan. Collaborating with healthcare providers to assess personal risk and develop a tailored prevention strategy that incorporates dietary, lifestyle, and natural approaches is essential for optimal outcomes.

Conclusion

A holistic approach to cancer prevention recognizes the complexity of cancer and the multifactorial influences on its development. By embracing a comprehensive strategy that integrates healthy dietary and lifestyle choices, mental and emotional health support, and mindful attention to environmental exposures, individuals can significantly contribute to their overall health and reduce their cancer risk. This proactive and inclusive perspective empowers individuals to take control of their health and supports a journey toward wellness and longevity.

Nutritional Guidelines for Cancer Prevention

The adage "Let food be thy medicine" underscores the critical role nutrition plays in preventing disease, including cancer. A growing body of evidence suggests that dietary patterns significantly influence cancer risk. These nutritional guidelines focus on optimizing intake of foods and nutrients known to support the body's natural defenses against cancer development.

Emphasize Plant-Based Foods
1. **Fruits and Vegetables**:
    - Rich in antioxidants, vitamins, minerals, and phytochemicals, fruits and vegetables combat oxidative stress and inflammation, both of which are linked to cancer. Aim for a variety of colors to ensure a broad spectrum of nutrients.
    - **Recommendation**: Incorporate at least 5 servings of fruits and vegetables daily, with an emphasis on leafy greens, berries, cruciferous vegetables (broccoli, cauliflower, Brussels sprouts), and bright-colored fruits and vegetables (carrots, tomatoes, bell peppers).
2. **Whole Grains**:
    - Whole grains contain fiber, which aids in digestive health and helps maintain a healthy weight, reducing cancer risk. They are also rich in antioxidants and phytochemicals.
    - **Recommendation**: Choose whole grains over refined grains. Include options like quinoa, barley, oats, brown rice, and whole-wheat products in your meals.

Limit Intake of Processed and Red Meats
- Processed meats (bacon, sausage, deli meats) and high amounts of red meat are associated with an increased risk of certain cancers, such as colorectal cancer.
- **Recommendation**: Limit red meat to no more than 18 ounces (cooked weight) per week and minimize processed meats. Opt for plant-based protein sources, poultry, or fish.

Incorporate Healthy Fats
1. **Omega-3 Fatty Acids**:
    - Found in fatty fish (salmon, mackerel, sardines), flaxseeds, chia seeds, and walnuts, omega-3s have anti-inflammatory properties that may help reduce cancer risk.
    - **Recommendation**: Include omega-3-rich foods in your diet 2-3 times per week or consider an omega-3 supplement after consulting with a healthcare provider.
2. **Limit Saturated and Trans Fats**:
    - Saturated fats (found in red meat and dairy products) and trans fats (found in some processed foods) can promote inflammation.
    - **Recommendation**: Choose lean protein sources and use cooking oils with healthy fats, such as olive oil, while limiting consumption of high-fat dairy and red meats.

Focus on Antioxidant-Rich Foods
- Antioxidants neutralize free radicals, reducing oxidative stress and cellular damage, which can lead to cancer.

- **Recommendation**: Beyond fruits and vegetables, include green tea, nuts, seeds, and spices like turmeric and ginger in your diet for their antioxidant properties.

Alcohol Consumption
- Alcohol is a known risk factor for various cancers, including breast, liver, colorectal, and esophageal cancer.
- **Recommendation**: If you choose to drink, do so in moderation. The American Cancer Society recommends no more than one drink per day for women and two drinks per day for men.

Dietary Supplements
- While getting nutrients from food sources is ideal, supplements may be necessary in some cases to address deficiencies.
- **Caution**: High-dose supplements can sometimes increase cancer risk. Consult with a healthcare professional before starting any new supplement, especially antioxidants during cancer treatment.

Maintaining a Healthy Weight
- Obesity and being overweight are linked to an increased risk of several cancers. A diet rich in plant-based foods and low in processed foods can help manage weight effectively.

Conclusion

Adopting a diet focused on plant-based foods, whole grains, healthy fats, and limited intake of processed and red meats can significantly contribute to cancer prevention. This approach, combined with regular physical activity and avoiding tobacco and excessive alcohol consumption, lays a solid foundation for reducing cancer risk and promoting overall health. Always consult healthcare professionals when making significant dietary changes, especially if you have existing health conditions or concerns.

Supportive Herbs for Cancer Prevention and Support

The integration of herbal medicine into cancer prevention and support strategies has gained attention for its potential to complement conventional treatments and improve quality of life. Certain herbs have shown promise in reducing cancer risk and aiding the body's response to cancer treatment through various mechanisms, including antioxidant activity, immune system modulation, and anti-inflammatory effects. Here, we explore some of the most researched herbs for cancer prevention and support, highlighting their benefits, evidence of effectiveness, and guidelines for use.

1. Turmeric (Curcuma longa)
- **Benefits**: The active compound in turmeric, curcumin, has potent anti-inflammatory and antioxidant properties. It has been studied for its potential to prevent cancer cell growth and enhance the effectiveness of chemotherapy.
- **Evidence**: Research indicates that curcumin can inhibit the proliferation of tumor cells in vitro and reduce inflammation, which is a significant contributor to cancer development.
- **Preparation and Use**: Turmeric can be incorporated into the diet as a spice or taken as a supplement in capsule form. Combining turmeric with black pepper enhances curcumin absorption.
- **When to Take**: If using supplements, follow the manufacturer's instructions, typically with meals to improve absorption.
- **Quantity and Duration**: Doses of curcumin supplements can range from 500 to 2,000 mg per day. Consult a healthcare provider for personalized advice, especially when used in conjunction with cancer treatment.
- **Safety Considerations**: High doses of curcumin may cause digestive upset in some individuals. Discuss with a healthcare professional before starting supplementation, especially during cancer treatment.

2. Green Tea (Camellia sinensis)
- **Benefits**: Green tea contains polyphenols like epigallocatechin-3-gallate (EGCG), which have been researched for their anti-cancer properties. EGCG may help prevent cancer cell proliferation and induce apoptosis (programmed cell death) in cancerous cells.

- **Evidence**: Epidemiological studies suggest a link between green tea consumption and a reduced risk of certain cancers, including breast, prostate, and colorectal cancers.
- **Preparation and Use**: Green tea can be consumed as a brewed tea or taken as an extract in capsule form.
- **When to Take**: If drinking green tea, spreading consumption throughout the day can maximize its benefits. For supplements, follow the product's dosing instructions.
- **Quantity and Duration**: For preventive purposes, 3-5 cups of green tea per day are often recommended. Supplements should be used according to the label's instructions.
- **Safety Considerations**: Excessive consumption of green tea (especially in supplement form) can interact with certain medications and affect liver health.

3. Milk Thistle (Silybum marianum)
- **Benefits**: Milk thistle is known for its liver-protective effects and contains silymarin, a compound studied for its potential to inhibit cancer cell growth and support liver health during chemotherapy.
- **Evidence**: Some studies suggest that silymarin has antioxidant, anti-inflammatory, and antiproliferative effects on various cancer cell lines.
- **Preparation and Use**: Milk thistle is available in capsules, liquid extracts, and teas.
- **When to Take**: Follow the manufacturer's instructions, typically with meals to enhance absorption.
- **Quantity and Duration**: Dosing can vary widely depending on the form; consult with a healthcare provider for guidance tailored to your needs.
- **Safety Considerations**: Milk thistle is generally considered safe, but it can interact with certain medications. Always consult a healthcare provider before starting new supplements.

4. Garlic (Allium sativum)
- **Benefits**: Garlic has been studied for its potential anticancer properties, attributed to its sulfur-containing compounds, which may help in detoxifying carcinogens and halting cancer cell growth.
- **Evidence**: Population studies have shown an association between increased garlic intake and reduced risk of certain cancers, including stomach and colorectal cancers.
- **Preparation and Use**: Garlic can be consumed raw or cooked as part of the diet or taken in supplement form.
- **When to Take**: If using supplements, follow the product's dosing instructions.
- **Quantity and Duration**: Incorporating garlic into daily meals is beneficial; for supplements, dosages typically range from 600 to 1,200 mg per day in divided doses.
- **Safety Considerations**: Garlic, especially in high doses or supplement form, can thin the blood and interact with blood-thinning medications.

Conclusion

Incorporating supportive herbs into cancer prevention and care strategies offers a natural complement to conventional treatments. However, it's essential to approach herbal supplementation with caution, considering potential interactions with treatments and individual health conditions. Consulting with healthcare professionals experienced in both oncology and herbal medicine is crucial to developing a safe and effective approach tailored to individual needs. These herbs, alongside a healthy diet and lifestyle, can contribute to a holistic cancer care plan aimed at enhancing quality of life and supporting overall health.

Integrating Natural Care with Conventional Treatments

Integrating natural care approaches with conventional cancer treatments represents a holistic strategy aimed at enhancing treatment efficacy, minimizing side effects, and improving patients' overall quality of life. This approach, often referred to as integrative oncology, combines the best of both worlds—utilizing surgery, chemotherapy, radiation, and other conventional methods alongside dietary, lifestyle, and complementary therapies. Developing a coherent and safe integrative plan requires careful consideration, open communication with healthcare providers, and a personalized approach based on the individual's unique medical history and treatment goals.

Foundations of Integrative Oncology
1. **Patient-Centered Care**:

- Emphasizes treating the patient as a whole, considering all aspects of their physical, mental, emotional, and spiritual health.
- Involves personalized care plans that address the patient's specific needs, preferences, and values.

2. **Evidence-Based Approach**:
   - Integrates therapies supported by scientific evidence into cancer care.
   - Requires ongoing research and clinical trials to evaluate the efficacy and safety of natural and complementary therapies in conjunction with conventional treatments.

Strategies for Integration

1. **Dietary Modifications**:
   - Enhances the nutritional status of patients, supporting their body's natural defenses and potentially improving outcomes of conventional treatments.
   - Includes anti-inflammatory diets rich in fruits, vegetables, whole grains, lean proteins, and healthy fats, aiming to reduce treatment side effects and promote recovery.

2. **Physical Activity**:
   - Regular, moderate exercise tailored to the patient's capabilities can help mitigate some side effects of cancer treatment, such as fatigue, and improve overall well-being.
   - Exercise programs should be designed with input from healthcare providers to suit the patient's current health status and treatment phase.

3. **Stress Reduction Techniques**:
   - Practices such as mindfulness meditation, yoga, and deep breathing exercises can help manage the emotional and psychological stress associated with cancer diagnosis and treatment.
   - Stress reduction is key to enhancing the quality of life and may positively affect treatment outcomes.

4. **Herbal and Supplemental Support**:
   - Certain herbs and supplements may complement conventional treatments, helping to manage side effects, enhance immune function, and potentially improve treatment efficacy.
   - It's critical to consult with healthcare providers before starting any new supplements to avoid interactions with conventional cancer treatments.

5. **Acupuncture and Other Complementary Therapies**:
   - Acupuncture, massage therapy, and reflexology can help alleviate some treatment side effects, such as nausea, pain, and stress.
   - These therapies should be provided by licensed practitioners with experience in working with cancer patients.

Navigating Integration Safely

1. **Open Communication**:
   - Patients should discuss all aspects of their care, including the use of natural and complementary therapies, with their oncology team.
   - This open dialogue ensures that all providers are aware 255ft he patient's treatment plan, reducing the risk of adverse interactions and enhancing care coordination.

2. **Professional Guidance**:
   - Seek guidance from professionals trained in integrative oncology who can provide evidence-based recommendations tailored to the individual's treatment plan.
   - This includes consulting dietitians, physical therapists, and complementary therapy practitioners who specialize in oncology.

3. **Monitoring and Adjustment**:
   - Integrative care plans should be regularly reviewed and adjusted based on treatment progress, changes in the patient's condition, and emerging scientific evidence.

- Continuous monitoring helps maximize benefits, minimize risks, and adapt to the patient's evolving needs.

Conclusion

Integrating natural care with conventional cancer treatments offers a comprehensive approach that addresses the multifaceted challenges of cancer care. By combining the strengths of both domains, patients can access a broader spectrum of supportive measures designed to enhance treatment efficacy, manage side effects, and improve quality of life. Achieving successful integration requires careful planning, evidence-based decision-making, and collaborative care teams committed to the holistic well-being of each patient.

Chapter 11: Easing Migraines and Headaches

Migraines and headaches, ranging from mild tension headaches to severe migraines, affect a significant portion of the population. These conditions can be debilitating, impacting daily life, productivity, and overall well-being. While conventional medicine offers various treatments, many individuals seek additional relief through natural and complementary approaches. This chapter explores strategies for easing migraines and headaches, focusing on prevention, natural remedies, lifestyle modifications, and the integration of holistic practices.

Identifying Triggers and Natural Preventative Measures for Migraines and Headaches

Migraines and headaches can have a wide range of triggers, from environmental factors to dietary habits and stress. Identifying these triggers is a crucial step in managing and preventing attacks. Natural preventative measures, alongside awareness of personal triggers, can significantly reduce the frequency and severity of migraines and headaches. This section delves into common triggers and outlines natural strategies for prevention.

Common Triggers for Migraines and Headaches
1. **Dietary Factors**:
   - Certain foods and additives are known to trigger migraines in some individuals. Common culprits include aged cheeses, processed foods, red wine, chocolate, caffeine, and food additives like monosodium glutamate (MSG) and nitrates.
2. **Stress**:
   - High stress levels are a well-documented trigger for both migraines and tension headaches. Stress can also exacerbate the intensity and duration of an attack.
3. **Hormonal Changes**:
   - For some women, fluctuations in estrogen levels, particularly around menstrual cycles, can trigger migraines.
4. **Environmental Factors**:
   - Changes in weather or barometric pressure, bright lights, loud noises, and strong smells can provoke migraines in susceptible individuals.
5. **Sleep Patterns**:
   - Both too much and too little sleep, along with disturbances in sleep patterns, can trigger migraines and headaches.

Natural Preventative Measures
1. **Dietary Modifications**:
   - **Keep a Food Diary**: Track what you eat and note any headache occurrences to identify potential food-related triggers.
   - **Maintain a Balanced Diet**: Emphasize whole foods, fruits, vegetables, whole grains, and lean proteins. Hydration is also key; drink plenty of water throughout the day.
2. **Stress Management Techniques**:
   - **Mindfulness and Meditation**: Practices like mindfulness meditation, deep-breathing exercises, and yoga can reduce stress levels and potentially decrease the frequency of migraine attacks.
   - **Regular Physical Activity**: Exercise is a powerful stress reducer. Even moderate activities like walking or cycling can help manage stress effectively.
3. **Regulating Sleep**:

- **Establish a Regular Sleep Schedule**: Go to bed and wake up at the same time every day, even on weekends.
- **Create a Restful Environment**: Ensure your sleeping environment is conducive to good quality sleep. Consider factors like mattress comfort, room temperature, and light exposure.

4. **Avoiding Environmental Triggers**:
   - **Adapt Your Surroundings**: Use earplugs in noisy environments and sunglasses in bright light. Air purifiers can help if specific odors trigger your migraines.

5. **Supplements and Herbal Remedies**:
   - **Magnesium**: Some studies suggest that magnesium deficiency may be linked to headaches and migraines. Magnesium supplements or magnesium-rich foods might help prevent attacks.
   - **Riboflavin (Vitamin B2) and Coenzyme Q10 (CoQ10)**: These supplements have shown potential in reducing migraine frequency for some individuals.
   - **Feverfew and Butterbur**: Herbal supplements like feverfew and butterbur have been traditionally used for migraine prevention, though butterbur should be used with caution due to potential liver toxicity.

6. **Acupuncture and Biofeedback**:
   - These therapies have shown promise in reducing headache frequency and severity. Acupuncture involves the insertion of thin needles into specific body points, while biofeedback teaches control over certain bodily processes that reduce pain.

Implementing Preventative Strategies

Preventing migraines and headaches often requires a multi-faceted approach tailored to the individual's specific triggers and lifestyle. Implementing dietary changes, managing stress, regulating sleep, and considering supplements or alternative therapies can collectively contribute to significant improvements. Importantly, these strategies should complement, not replace, medical treatments prescribed by healthcare professionals. Regular consultations and open discussions with healthcare providers will ensure that your prevention plan is both effective and safe.

Effective Herbal Remedies and Dosages for Migraines and Headaches

Migraines and headaches can be challenging to manage, but several herbal remedies have shown promise in providing relief. These natural treatments work by addressing various underlying causes of headaches, including inflammation, muscle tension, and nerve pain. Here's an in-depth look at some of the most effective herbs for migraines and headaches, their benefits, how to prepare and take them, recommended dosages, and duration of use.

1. Feverfew (Tanacetum parthenium)
   - **Benefits**: Feverfew has been widely studied for its effectiveness in preventing migraines. It works by reducing inflammation and the release of substances that can trigger migraines.
   - **Preparation and Use**: Feverfew is available in capsules, tablets, and teas. Some people choose to eat fresh feverfew leaves.
   - **When to Take**: For prevention, feverfew should be taken daily.
   - **Quantity**: The recommended dose varies, but studies have used doses ranging from 50-150 mg of feverfew extract daily.
   - **Duration**: Feverfew is meant for long-term use to prevent migraines. Benefits may take several weeks to become evident.

2. Butterbur (Petasites hybridus)
   - **Benefits**: Butterbur is another herb with strong evidence supporting its use in migraine prevention. It's believed to reduce spasms in cerebral blood vessels and has anti-inflammatory properties.
   - **Preparation and Use**: Butterbur is available in capsules and extracts. Ensure you're using a product labeled PA-free (pyrrolizidine alkaloids-free), as PAs can be harmful to the liver.

- **When to Take**: Daily for migraine prevention.
- **Quantity**: A typical dose is 75 mg twice daily of a PA-free butterbur extract.
- **Duration**: Like feverfew, butterbur is used for long-term management. It may take 2-3 months to see a reduction in migraine frequency.

3. Peppermint (Mentha piperita)
- **Benefits**: Peppermint oil can alleviate the pain and discomfort of headaches, particularly tension headaches, through its cooling, muscle-relaxing, and pain-relieving effects.
- **Preparation and Use**: Peppermint oil is applied topically. It should be diluted with a carrier oil (like coconut or jojoba oil) before being massaged into the temples and forehead.
- **When to Take**: Use at the onset of headache symptoms.
- **Quantity**: A few drops of peppermint oil diluted in one tablespoon of carrier oil.
- **Duration**: Use as needed to relieve headache symptoms.

4. Ginger (Zingiber officinale)
- **Benefits**: Ginger can help reduce headache severity and duration due to its anti-inflammatory and anti-nausea properties, making it particularly useful for migraines.
- **Preparation and Use**: Ginger can be consumed as tea, in capsules, or fresh. For tea, steep 1-2 teaspoons of freshly grated ginger in boiling water for 10-15 minutes.
- **When to Take**: At the onset of migraine or headache symptoms.
- **Quantity**: For fresh ginger or tea, 1-2 teaspoons per cup of tea. For supplements, follow the manufacturer's recommendations.
- **Duration**: Use as needed for symptom relief.

General Guidelines for Using Herbal Remedies
- **Consultation**: Always consult a healthcare provider before starting any new herbal treatment, especially if you are pregnant, breastfeeding, or on medication, as herbs can interact with medications.
- **Quality**: Choose high-quality, reputable sources for herbs and supplements to ensure safety and efficacy.
- **Monitoring**: Keep track of your headache or migraine frequency, severity, and any potential side effects from herbal remedies to assess effectiveness and make necessary adjustments.

Incorporating these herbal remedies into your migraine and headache management plan can offer natural, effective relief and prevention. However, individual responses to herbs can vary, and what works for one person may not work for another. Therefore, it's essential to approach treatment with patience and openness to finding the right combination of remedies and lifestyle changes that work for you.

Lifestyle Adjustments for Migraine Sufferers

Living with migraines can be challenging, but making specific lifestyle adjustments can significantly reduce the frequency and severity of attacks. These changes involve modifying daily habits to avoid known triggers, incorporating practices that promote overall well-being, and managing stress effectively. Here's a comprehensive guide to lifestyle adjustments specifically designed for individuals who suffer from migraines.

Regular Sleep Patterns
1. **Consistency is Key**: Establish a regular sleep schedule by going to bed and waking up at the same time every day, including weekends. Irregular sleep patterns can trigger migraines in many individuals.
2. **Optimize Your Sleep Environment**: Ensure your bedroom is conducive to sleep. This means a comfortable mattress and pillows, a cool room temperature, and minimal noise and light.

Stress Management
1. **Identify Stressors**: Keep a diary to identify stress triggers and your responses to them. Understanding the relationship between stress and your migraines is the first step in managing them.

2. **Relaxation Techniques**: Incorporate relaxation practices into your daily routine, such as deep breathing exercises, progressive muscle relaxation, mindfulness meditation, or gentle yoga.

Diet and Nutrition

1. **Maintain a Balanced Diet**: Eat regular meals to avoid low blood sugar levels, which can trigger migraines. Include a variety of fruits, vegetables, whole grains, and lean proteins in your diet.
2. **Hydration**: Dehydration is a common trigger for migraines. Aim to drink at least 8 glasses of water a day, more if you're active or it's hot.
3. **Identify and Avoid Food Triggers**: Common culprits include aged cheeses, processed foods, chocolate, caffeine, and alcohol, especially red wine. Keep a food diary to track what you eat and how it relates to your migraine patterns.

Physical Activity

1. **Regular Exercise**: Engage in regular, moderate exercise like walking, swimming, or cycling. Exercise promotes overall well-being and can reduce the frequency and severity of migraines by relieving stress and improving sleep.
2. **Start Slowly**: If you're new to exercise or find that intense activity triggers your migraines, start with light exercise and gradually increase intensity.

Environmental Adjustments

1. **Lighting**: Bright or flickering lights can trigger migraines for some people. Use natural lighting when possible, and consider anti-glare screens for computers and devices.
2. **Noise**: Loud or constant noise can also be a trigger. Use earplugs in noisy environments if necessary.

Ergonomics and Posture

1. **Workstation Setup**: If you spend long hours at a desk, ensure your workstation is ergonomically set up to reduce strain on your neck and shoulders, which can contribute to migraines.
2. **Take Regular Breaks**: Practice the 20-20-20 rule: every 20 minutes, look at something 20 feet away for 20 seconds. Get up and move around regularly.

Medication Management

1. **Use Medication Wisely**: Overuse of headache medication can lead to rebound headaches. Work with your healthcare provider to find the most effective medication for your situation and adhere to their prescribed regimen.

Holistic Therapies

1. **Complementary Treatments**: Consider acupuncture, massage therapy, or biofeedback, which some people find helpful for managing migraines. Always consult with a healthcare provider before starting new treatments.

Conclusion

Adopting these lifestyle adjustments requires time and may involve trial and error to discover what works best for you. The key is consistency and a proactive approach to managing your migraines. Partner with healthcare professionals who understand migraines to develop a comprehensive management plan. By making these changes, many individuals find they can reduce the impact of migraines on their lives, leading to improved health and quality of life.

Chapter 12: Natural Remedies for the Common Cold and Flu

The common cold and flu are viral infections that affect millions of people annually, leading to a range of uncomfortable symptoms like congestion, sore throat, cough, and fever. While there is no cure for these illnesses, natural remedies can offer relief from symptoms, shorten the duration of illness, and boost the immune system to fend off future infections. This chapter explores a comprehensive approach to managing cold and flu symptoms through natural means, including herbal remedies, dietary adjustments, and supportive practices.

Introduction: Winning Over Colds and Flu Naturally

Navigating through the cold and flu season, or even sporadic bouts of these illnesses, calls for more than just reactive measures. The key lies in a holistic approach that not only focuses on alleviating symptoms after they've appeared but also on bolstering the body's natural defenses to prevent the onset of illness. This introduction sets the stage for understanding how natural remedies, lifestyle adjustments, and proactive wellness practices can empower individuals to effectively combat and triumph over colds and flu.

The Prevalence and Impact of Colds and Flu

Colds and flu are among the most common infectious diseases, with millions of cases reported annually worldwide. Characterized by symptoms such as coughing, sneezing, sore throat, congestion, and fatigue, these viral infections can range from mildly inconvenient to severely debilitating. Beyond individual discomfort, they contribute to significant absenteeism from work and school, underscoring the need for effective prevention and treatment strategies.

The Natural Approach to Prevention and Healing

A natural approach to colds and flu encompasses a broad spectrum of strategies designed to support the body's immune system, alleviate symptoms, and hasten recovery. This approach is rooted in the understanding that the body possesses an innate ability to heal itself, provided it has the right support. Key components of this strategy include:

1. **Strengthening Immune Function**: Enhancing the body's natural defenses through diet, supplementation, and lifestyle practices is foundational to preventing colds and flu.
2. **Symptom Relief Through Natural Remedies**: A variety of herbs and natural substances have been traditionally used and are supported by contemporary research for their potential to relieve the symptoms of colds and flu, reduce the duration of illness, and improve overall well-being.
3. **Holistic Wellness Practices**: Incorporating practices that promote overall health, such as adequate sleep, stress management, and physical activity, plays a crucial role in maintaining immune health and resilience against infections.
4. **Nutritional Support**: A nutrient-rich diet that includes plenty of antioxidants, vitamins, and minerals supports immune function and helps the body resist and recover from infections.

Embracing a Proactive Wellness Mindset

Adopting a proactive wellness mindset involves making conscious choices daily that contribute to health and well-being. It means prioritizing activities and habits that bolster immunity, being mindful of early signs of illness and addressing them promptly with natural remedies, and understanding the importance of rest and recovery.

Conclusion

Winning over colds and flu naturally is a multifaceted endeavor that emphasizes prevention, natural symptom relief, and the promotion of holistic health. By understanding and applying the principles of natural care and immune support, individuals can enhance their ability to prevent and recover from these common illnesses. The subsequent sections will delve into specific natural remedies, dietary recommendations, and lifestyle adjustments that constitute an effective natural arsenal against colds and flu, empowering readers to take charge of their health in a holistic and proactive manner.

Immune-Boosting Herbs and Their Preparations for Cold and Flu

The use of herbs for bolstering the immune system and combating the symptoms of colds and flu is a time-honored tradition. Several herbs stand out for their efficacy, backed by both historical use and modern research. Below, we explore these immune-boosting herbs, detailing their specific benefits, how to prepare them, and guidelines for their use.

1. Echinacea (Echinacea spp.)
   - **Benefits**: Echinacea is renowned for its ability to enhance the immune response, potentially reducing the duration and severity of cold and flu symptoms. It is thought to stimulate the activity of immune cells that fight infections.
   - **Preparation and Use**: Echinacea can be consumed as a tea, tincture, or in capsule form. To make tea, steep 1-2 teaspoons of dried echinacea in hot water for 10-15 minutes.
   - **When to Take**: At the first sign of cold or flu symptoms. It's most effective when used at the onset of symptoms.
   - **Quantity and Duration**: For teas, 1-2 cups three times a day. Tinctures and capsules should be taken according to the product's instructions, typically for 7-10 days.
2. Elderberry (Sambucus nigra)
   - **Benefits**: Elderberry is well-regarded for its antiviral properties, particularly against flu viruses. It can reduce symptom severity and duration.
   - **Preparation and Use**: Elderberry is available in syrups, gummies, lozenges, and teas. For homemade elderberry syrup, simmer dried elderberries with water and honey to form a syrup.
   - **When to Take**: At the onset of symptoms or during cold and flu season for prevention.
   - **Quantity and Duration**: Follow the dosing instructions on commercial products. For homemade syrup, 1 tablespoon (15 ml) every 3-4 hours for adults during active symptoms.
3. Ginger (Zingiber officinale)
   - **Benefits**: Ginger has potent anti-inflammatory and antioxidative properties, offering relief from nausea and sore throat associated with flu and colds. It also has antiviral effects.
   - **Preparation and Use**: Fresh ginger can be used to make tea. Simmer a small piece of ginger root in water for 10-20 minutes, depending on the desired strength. Honey and lemon may be added for taste and extra benefits.
   - **When to Take**: As needed for symptom relief, especially for nausea or throat discomfort.
   - **Quantity and Duration**: Ginger tea can be consumed 2-3 times a day. Use about 1 inch of ginger root per cup of water for tea.
4. Garlic (Allium sativum)
   - **Benefits**: Garlic is known for its immune-boosting and antimicrobial properties. It can help prevent colds and accelerate recovery.
   - **Preparation and Use**: Garlic is most beneficial when consumed raw, as cooking can diminish some of its therapeutic properties. It can be minced and added to foods or taken as a supplement.
   - **When to Take**: At the onset of cold or flu symptoms or regularly during cold and flu season for prevention.
   - **Quantity and Duration**: For raw garlic, 1-2 cloves per day. If using supplements, follow the manufacturer's recommendations.
5. Astragalus (Astragalus membranaceus)

- **Benefits**: Astragalus root is used in Traditional Chinese Medicine to boost immunity and prevent colds and respiratory infections. It is considered an adaptogen, helping to protect the body against physical, mental, or emotional stress.
- **Preparation and Use**: Astragalus can be added to soups, brewed as tea, or taken as a supplement in capsule or tincture form.
- **When to Take:** For prevention during cold and flu season.
- **Quantity and Duration**: For tea, simmer 4-6 grams of dried astragalus root in water for about 30 minutes. Drink 1-2 cups daily. Follow dosing instructions for supplements.

General Guidelines for Using Herbal Remedies

- **Consultation**: Always consult with a healthcare provider before starting any new herbal remedy, especially if you have existing health conditions or are taking medications.
- **Quality Matters**: Choose high-quality, reputable brands for supplements, and ensure that herbs are sourced from reliable suppliers.
- **Listen to Your Body**: Pay attention to how your body responds to these remedies and adjust accordingly. Not all remedies are suitable for everyone, and some may experience allergic reactions or gastrointestinal upset.

Incorporating these immune-boosting herbs into your regimen can offer natural support against colds and flu, enhancing your body's ability to fight off these infections. Remember, while these remedies can be effective for symptom relief and immune support, they are most beneficial when used as part of a holistic approach to health that includes proper nutrition, hydration, rest, and stress management.

Supportive Dietary Practices During Illness

When battling a cold or flu, the body requires additional nutrition to support the immune system and accelerate recovery. Adopting supportive dietary practices during illness can make a significant difference in the duration and severity of symptoms. This comprehensive approach to nutrition focuses on hydrating fluids, nutrient-dense foods, and specific dietary adjustments that can aid in the body's healing process.

Hydration is Key

1. **Fluid Intake**: Increasing fluid intake is crucial during illness to prevent dehydration, especially if fever is present. Fluids help thin mucus, making it easier to expel, and ensure the body's cells are well-hydrated to function optimally.
2. **What to Drink**: Water is the best choice for staying hydrated. Herbal teas, broth, and electrolyte-replenishing drinks can also be beneficial. Warm beverages can provide soothing relief for sore throats and congestion.

Nutrient-Dense Foods

1. **Vitamins and Minerals**: Foods rich in vitamins C and D, zinc, and selenium support immune function. Citrus fruits, leafy greens, nuts, seeds, and lean proteins are excellent sources. Incorporating a variety of these foods can help cover the spectrum of essential nutrients needed for recovery.
2. **Antioxidant-Rich Foods**: Antioxidants combat oxidative stress and inflammation, which are heightened during illness. Berries, dark chocolate, and spices like turmeric and ginger are high in antioxidants.

Easy-to-Digest Foods

1. **Simple, Comforting Foods**: When appetite is reduced, and the body is weak, simple and comforting foods can be more appealing and easier to digest. Porridge, soup, and stew are gentle on the stomach and can provide the necessary nutrients without overwhelming the digestive system.
2. **Probiotic and Prebiotic Foods**: Supporting gut health is vital during and after illness, as a significant portion of the immune system is housed in the gut. Yogurt, kefir, and fermented foods

supply probiotics, while bananas, onions, and garlic offer prebiotics that nourish beneficial gut bacteria.

Foods to Avoid
1. **Processed and Sugary Foods**: These can exacerbate inflammation and provide little nutritional value. Limiting or avoiding sugary drinks, snacks, and processed foods can help the body direct its energy toward healing.
2. **Heavy, Fatty Foods**: High-fat foods can be harder to digest and may strain the digestive system when the body is already taxed from fighting an infection.

Specific Dietary Adjustments
1. **Small, Frequent Meals**: Consuming smaller, more frequent meals can be easier on the digestive system and ensure a steady intake of nutrients throughout the day.
2. **Listening to Your Body**: Appetite can vary widely during illness. It's important to listen to your body's cues and eat when hungry, but not to force-feed if the appetite is lacking. Hydration should remain a priority.

Incorporating Healing Herbs and Spices
1. **Ginger and Turmeric**: Both have anti-inflammatory properties and can be added to teas, soups, and other dishes to boost flavor and health benefits.
2. **Honey**: A natural cough suppressant and sore throat soother, honey can be added to tea or warm water. (Note: Honey should not be given to children under one year of age.)

Conclusion
Adopting supportive dietary practices during illness can significantly aid the body's healing process. Focusing on hydration, nutrient-dense foods, easy-to-digest meals, and avoiding certain foods can help manage symptoms and shorten the duration of colds and flu. As always, it's essential to listen to your body and consult with healthcare professionals regarding dietary changes, especially for individuals with pre-existing health conditions or dietary restrictions.

Hydration and Rest Strategies for Recovery

Recovering from illnesses like the common cold or flu involves more than just medication; it requires a holistic approach where hydration and rest play pivotal roles. These strategies not only alleviate symptoms but also expedite the healing process by supporting the body's natural defenses. This comprehensive overview delves into effective hydration and rest techniques tailored for recovery, emphasizing their significance in overcoming illness.

Hydration: The Cornerstone of Recovery
1. **The Importance of Staying Hydrated**:
   - Hydration is crucial during illness because it helps to thin mucus, making it easier to expel, supports the lymphatic system in transporting immune cells, and aids in detoxifying the body.
2. **Effective Hydration Strategies**:
   - **Water**: The simplest and most effective way to stay hydrated. Aim for at least 8-10 glasses a day, increasing intake if fever or increased sweating is present.
   - **Electrolyte-Rich Fluids**: Beverages like coconut water, electrolyte-replenishing drinks, or even a homemade solution of water, salt, and sugar can help maintain electrolyte balance, especially important if vomiting or diarrhea occurs.
   - **Broths and Soups**: Warm broths not only provide hydration but also offer comforting relief from respiratory symptoms. The steam can help open nasal passages, while the nutrients support overall health.

- **Herbal Teas**: Teas such as ginger, peppermint, or chamomile are soothing choices that can provide hydration and specific benefits like reducing nausea or promoting relaxation.
3. **Signs of Adequate Hydration**:
   - Monitoring the color of urine is an easy way to gauge hydration levels; pale yellow indicates good hydration, while dark urine suggests a need for more fluids.

Rest: Facilitating Healing Through Sleep
1. **The Healing Power of Sleep**:
   - Sleep plays a critical role in recovery by enhancing immune function and allowing the body to repair and rejuvenate. During sleep, the production of cytokines increases, aiding in fighting off infections.
2. **Strategies to Enhance Restful Sleep**:
   - **Establish a Comfortable Sleep Environment**: Ensure the room is dark, quiet, and cool. Consider using a humidifier to add moisture to the air, which can ease breathing.
   - **Maintain a Regular Sleep Schedule**: Going to bed and waking up at consistent times reinforce the body's natural sleep-wake cycle, promoting better quality sleep.
   - **Limit Screen Time Before Bed**: Exposure to blue light from screens can disrupt the production of melatonin, the hormone that regulates sleep. Limit screens an hour before bedtime to improve sleep quality.
   - **Relaxation Techniques**: Practices such as deep breathing, progressive muscle relaxation, or meditation can help calm the mind and prepare the body for sleep.
3. **Naps and Resting**:
   - While a good night's sleep is important, short naps or simply resting can be beneficial during the day, especially when the body is fighting an illness. Listen to your body and rest when needed without oversleeping during the day to maintain nighttime sleep quality.

Conclusion

Hydration and rest are fundamental components of the recovery process from colds, flu, and other illnesses. By implementing effective hydration strategies and fostering a conducive environment for rest and sleep, individuals can support their body's healing mechanisms, alleviate symptoms, and reduce the overall duration of illness. Remember, these practices should complement, not replace, medical treatment and professional advice when dealing with severe or prolonged illness. Prioritizing hydration and rest underscores the importance of a holistic approach to health and recovery.

Chapter 13: Men's Health: Prostate Support and Vitality

M en's health, particularly as it relates to the prostate, is a crucial aspect of overall well-being that often does not receive the attention it deserves. The prostate, a small gland found in men, plays a pivotal role in the reproductive system but can become a source of concern, especially with advancing age. Conditions like benign prostatic hyperplasia (BPH), prostatitis, and prostate cancer can significantly impact a man's quality of life. This chapter delves into strategies for prostate support and enhancing overall vitality, focusing on preventive measures, nutritional guidelines, and lifestyle modifications.

Introduction: Enhancing Men's Health and Vitality

In today's fast-paced world, men's health often takes a backseat until noticeable problems arise. However, a proactive approach focusing on enhancing overall health and vitality can significantly improve quality of life and reduce the risk of common male health issues, including those related to prostate health, cardiovascular disease, and mental well-being. This introduction lays the groundwork for understanding the holistic strategies that contribute to men's health, emphasizing the importance of prevention, awareness, and lifestyle choices in fostering longevity and vitality.

The Pillars of Men's Health

Men's health encompasses a broad spectrum, requiring attention to physical, mental, and emotional well-being. Key pillars include:

1. **Nutritional Wellness**: A balanced diet rich in nutrients supports cellular health, hormone balance, and weight management. It's the foundation for preventing chronic diseases and enhancing energy levels and physical performance.
2. **Physical Activity**: Regular exercise is crucial for maintaining cardiovascular health, muscle strength, flexibility, and mental health. It also plays a significant role in preventing obesity, type 2 diabetes, and maintaining a healthy prostate.
3. **Mental and Emotional Well-being**: Stress, depression, and anxiety can significantly impact men's health. Cultivating resilience through stress management techniques, social connections, and hobbies is vital for maintaining a balanced state of mind.
4. **Preventive Healthcare**: Regular health check-ups, screenings, and being informed about men's health risks are essential for early detection and management of potential health issues.
5. **Lifestyle Modifications**: Lifestyle choices, including smoking cessation, moderating alcohol consumption, and ensuring adequate sleep, directly influence men's health outcomes.

Enhancing Vitality Through Natural Means

Enhancing men's health and vitality involves more than addressing individual symptoms or conditions; it requires a holistic approach that integrates natural and lifestyle interventions:

1. **Herbal Support**: Certain herbs, such as saw palmetto, ashwagandha, and ginseng, have been traditionally used to support men's health, including prostate health, energy levels, and stress management.
2. **Dietary Focus**: Emphasizing heart-healthy fats, lean proteins, and antioxidant-rich fruits and vegetables can improve cardiovascular health and support prostate wellness. Nutrients such as omega-3 fatty acids, zinc, selenium, and vitamins D and E are particularly beneficial.

3. **Physical Fitness**: A combination of cardiovascular exercises, strength training, and flexibility practices like yoga can enhance physical vitality, improve mood, and reduce the risk of chronic conditions.
4. **Mind-Body Practices**: Techniques such as meditation, deep breathing, and mindfulness can help manage stress and its physical manifestations, contributing to overall vitality.
5. **Community and Relationships**: Building strong social connections and engaging in meaningful activities contribute to emotional well-being and resilience.

Conclusion

Men's health and vitality are influenced by a complex interplay of factors, including diet, exercise, mental health, and lifestyle choices. By adopting a comprehensive approach that addresses these areas proactively, men can significantly enhance their health, reduce the risk of common diseases, and maintain a high quality of life. The following sections will delve deeper into specific strategies for supporting prostate health, managing stress, and promoting cardiovascular wellness, providing practical tips for men to implement in their daily lives.

Herbs Specifically Beneficial for Men's Health: Prostate Support and Vitality

Men's health, particularly as it pertains to prostate support and overall vitality, can benefit significantly from the inclusion of specific herbs known for their therapeutic properties. These herbs not only offer support for prostate health but also contribute to hormonal balance, vitality, and wellness. Below, we explore some of the most effective herbs for men's health, their benefits, how to prepare and administer them, and guidelines regarding quantity and duration of use.

1. Saw Palmetto (Serenoa repens)
- **Benefits**: Saw palmetto is one of the most well-researched herbs for prostate health. It's commonly used to treat symptoms of benign prostatic hyperplasia (BPH) due to its ability to inhibit the conversion of testosterone to dihydrotestosterone (DHT), a hormone associated with prostate enlargement.
- **Preparation and Use**: Available in capsules, tablets, and liquid extracts. The extract form is most commonly used for prostate support.
- **When to Take**: Follow the manufacturer's instructions, usually with meals to enhance absorption.
- **Quantity and Duration**: Typical doses range from 160 to 320 mg of standardized extract daily. Long-term use (up to 6 months) has been studied and is generally considered safe.

2. Stinging Nettle (Urtica dioica)
- **Benefits**: Stinging nettle root is used for its benefits in reducing BPH symptoms and urinary issues. It works in part by inhibiting the binding of sex hormone-binding globulin to receptors, thereby potentially reducing the size of the prostate.
- **Preparation and Use**: Nettle can be taken as a tea, capsule, or tincture. For tea, steep 1-2 teaspoons of dried root in hot water for 10 minutes.
- **When to Take**: If using tea, 2-3 cups daily. Capsules and tinctures should be taken according to product guidelines.
- **Quantity and Duration**: For capsules, dosages of 300-600 mg daily are common. Continuous use for several weeks to months is often necessary to see benefits.

3. Pumpkin Seeds (Cucurbita pepo)
- **Benefits**: Pumpkin seeds are rich in zinc, a mineral essential for prostate health and overall male fertility. They also contain phytosterols that may help reduce the size of the prostate.
- **Preparation and Use**: Pumpkin seeds can be consumed raw or roasted as a snack. Pumpkin seed oil is also available in capsule form.
- **When to Take**: If eating seeds, a handful (about 30 grams) per day. If using oil capsules, follow the product's dosing instructions.

- **Quantity and Duration**: Continuous use is generally considered safe, with regular dietary inclusion recommended.

4. Pygeum (Pygeum africanum)
- **Benefits**: Pygeum is used for reducing symptoms of BPH and prostatitis. It contains compounds that help reduce inflammation and improve urinary symptoms associated with an enlarged prostate.
- **Preparation and Use**: Available in capsules or as an extract.
- **When to Take**: Follow the dosing instructions on the product label, typically with meals.
- **Quantity and Duration**: Doses of 100-200 mg of pygeum extract daily are commonly used. Benefits may take several weeks to manifest.

5. Ginseng (Panax ginseng)
- **Benefits**: While not specific to the prostate, ginseng is renowned for its overall vitality and energy-boosting properties. It can support stamina, mental performance, and sexual health in men.
- **Preparation and Use**: Ginseng can be consumed as tea, capsules, or liquid extracts.
- **When to Take**: Morning or early afternoon to avoid potential interference with sleep.
- **Quantity and Duration**: For general vitality, doses of 200-400 mg daily for capsules or 1-2 cups of tea. Use for up to three months before taking a break or as directed by a healthcare provider.

General Guidelines for Using Herbs
- **Consultation**: Always consult with a healthcare provider before starting any new herbal regimen, especially for individuals with existing medical conditions or those taking medications.
- **Quality**: Opt for high-quality, reputable brands and sources for herbs to ensure purity and potency.
- **Monitoring**: Pay attention to your body's response to these herbal remedies. Adjustments in dosage or discontinuation may be necessary based on individual reactions and outcomes.

Incorporating these herbs into a regimen for men's health, particularly for prostate support and vitality, can offer significant benefits. However, their effectiveness can be enhanced when combined with a healthy diet, regular physical activity, and proper stress management techniques, underscoring the importance of a holistic approach to wellness.

Exercise and Stress Reduction for Overall Vitality

The synergy of exercise and stress reduction plays a pivotal role in enhancing men's overall vitality, including mental, physical, and emotional well-being. Regular physical activity and effective stress management not only contribute to immediate health benefits but also set the foundation for long-term resilience against chronic diseases, including those affecting prostate health. This detailed exploration offers insights into how integrating exercise and stress reduction can significantly improve quality of life and overall vitality.

The Importance of Regular Exercise
1. **Cardiovascular Health**: Exercise strengthens the heart, improves circulation, and helps regulate cholesterol levels and blood pressure, reducing the risk of heart disease.
2. **Weight Management**: Maintaining a healthy weight through regular physical activity is crucial for reducing the risk of several chronic conditions, such as type 2 diabetes, certain cancers, and even BPH (Benign Prostatic Hyperplasia).
3. **Muscle Strength and Flexibility**: Strength training and flexibility exercises maintain muscle mass, support joint health, and prevent injuries, contributing to physical resilience and independence as men age.
4. **Mental Health**: Exercise is a powerful mood booster, thanks to the release of endorphins. It's effective in reducing symptoms of depression, anxiety, and stress, promoting a sense of well-being.

Incorporating Exercise into Daily Life
1. **Find Activities You Enjoy**: The key to consistent exercise is engagement. Whether it's cycling, swimming, team sports, or resistance training, choosing activities that you look forward to makes regular practice more sustainable.

2. **Set Realistic Goals**: Begin with attainable goals and gradually increase intensity and duration. Aiming for at least 150 minutes of moderate aerobic activity or 75 minutes of vigorous activity per week is recommended.
3. **Integrate Physical Activity**: Incorporate movement into daily routines—take stairs instead of elevators, walk or cycle for short trips, and stand or stretch regularly if your job involves prolonged sitting.

Effective Stress Reduction Techniques

1. **Mindfulness and Meditation**: Practices like mindfulness meditation have been shown to lower stress levels, enhance focus, and improve emotional regulation. Even a few minutes daily can yield significant benefits.
2. **Deep Breathing Exercises**: Techniques such as diaphragmatic breathing or the 4-7-8 method can quickly alleviate acute stress, promoting relaxation and reducing anxiety.
3. **Yoga and Tai Chi**: These ancient practices combine physical postures, breathing exercises, and meditation to reduce stress, improve flexibility, and support overall health.
4. **Quality Sleep**: Adequate rest is essential for stress recovery. Establish a regular sleep schedule, create a restful environment, and avoid screens before bedtime to improve sleep quality.

Lifestyle Modifications to Enhance Vitality

1. **Balanced Diet**: Nutrition plays a critical role in managing stress and maintaining energy levels. A diet rich in vegetables, fruits, lean proteins, and whole grains, while low in processed foods and sugars, supports both physical and mental health.
2. **Social Connections**: Maintaining strong relationships and social activities can provide emotional support, reduce feelings of isolation, and contribute to a more fulfilled life.
3. **Hobbies and Interests**: Engaging in activities that bring joy and satisfaction can act as a counterbalance to stress, enhancing life's quality and vitality.

Conclusion

The integration of regular exercise and effective stress reduction practices is essential for men seeking to improve their overall vitality and health. By adopting a holistic approach that includes physical activity, mindful practices, and supportive lifestyle choices, men can significantly enhance their well-being, reducing the risk of chronic conditions and improving quality of life. Remember, the journey to health is personal and evolving; start small, be consistent, and adjust as needed to meet your body's changing needs.

Chapter 14: Allergy Relief and Management

Allergies, a common yet often debilitating condition, affect millions of individuals worldwide. They occur when the immune system reacts to a foreign substance—such as pollen, bee venom, pet dander, or certain foods—that doesn't cause a reaction in most people. This overreaction can lead to various symptoms, ranging from mild irritations, like sneezing and itching, to more severe conditions, including anaphylaxis. Effective allergy management and relief entail a combination of avoiding known allergens, using medications to relieve symptoms, and adopting natural and lifestyle strategies to reduce exposure and improve overall immune health.

Introduction: Breathing Easier with Natural Remedies

In the quest for relief from respiratory ailments such as allergies, asthma, and recurrent respiratory infections, many individuals are turning towards natural remedies as complementary or alternative solutions. The appeal of these remedies lies in their potential to offer relief with fewer side effects, work in harmony with the body's natural healing processes, and sometimes even address underlying causes rather than merely suppressing symptoms. This introduction delves into the world of natural remedies aimed at improving respiratory health, highlighting the importance of a holistic approach that encompasses lifestyle changes, dietary adjustments, and the use of specific herbs and supplements known for their respiratory benefits.

The Holistic View on Respiratory Health

Respiratory health issues can significantly impact quality of life, making breathing—a process most take for granted—a constant struggle. Traditional medicine often offers effective treatments for immediate relief, but incorporating natural remedies into one's healthcare regimen can provide additional support by:

1. **Strengthening the Respiratory System**: Enhancing the overall health of the lungs and respiratory tract to resist and recover from infections more effectively.
2. **Reducing Inflammation**: Many respiratory issues involve inflammation. Natural remedies can help manage this inflammation, reducing symptoms and discomfort.
3. **Supporting Immune Function**: A robust immune system is crucial in fighting off the pathogens that cause respiratory illnesses. Certain natural supplements can bolster immune defenses.
4. **Detoxifying and Cleansing**: Some natural therapies aim to detoxify the body, potentially reducing the burden of toxins that can exacerbate respiratory conditions.
5.

Embracing Natural Remedies

Natural remedies encompass a wide array of practices and products, including but not limited to:

1. **Herbal Treatments**: Numerous herbs have been traditionally used to support respiratory health. These range from anti-inflammatory options like turmeric and ginger, to herbs that act as expectorants or antihistamines, such as licorice root and butterbur.
2. **Supplements**: Vitamins and minerals that support immune health, like Vitamin C, Vitamin D, and Zinc, can also contribute to better respiratory function.
3. **Aromatherapy and Essential Oils**: The use of essential oils, through methods like diffusion or topical application, can offer symptomatic relief for various respiratory conditions. Peppermint, eucalyptus, and tea tree oil are popular choices for their decongestant and antimicrobial properties.
4. **Dietary Adjustments**: Incorporating anti-inflammatory foods and those rich in antioxidants can support lung health. Simultaneously, reducing intake of foods that trigger allergic reactions or increase mucus production can alleviate symptoms.

5. **Lifestyle Changes**: Practices such as nasal irrigation, steam inhalation, and breathing exercises can improve respiratory health. Regular exercise and avoiding exposure to pollutants and allergens are also critical.

Navigating the Path to Better Breathing

While natural remedies can offer significant benefits, they should be approached with care. Not all remedies are suitable for everyone, and interactions with prescribed medications can occur. It's essential to:

1. **Research**: Understand the potential benefits and risks associated with any remedy.
2. **Consult**: Speak with healthcare professionals before starting any new treatment, especially if you have ongoing health issues or are taking other medications.
3. **Personalize**: Tailor your approach to suit your specific needs, conditions, and lifestyle.

Conclusion

Breathing easier with natural remedies is about more than just symptom management; it's about adopting a holistic approach to respiratory health that strengthens the body's defenses, reduces exposure to irritants, and addresses underlying issues. By carefully selecting and integrating natural remedies into their care regimen, individuals can achieve greater control over their respiratory health, improving their quality of life and wellbeing.

Identifying Allergens and Reducing Exposure

For individuals suffering from allergies, identifying specific allergens and minimizing exposure to these triggers is crucial for managing symptoms and improving quality of life. Allergens can vary widely, from environmental factors like pollen and pet dander to food items such as nuts and dairy. This detailed exploration provides strategies for identifying common allergens, assessing personal triggers, and implementing measures to reduce exposure effectively.

Identifying Common Allergens

1. **Environmental Allergens**: These include pollen from trees, grasses, and weeds; dust mites; mold spores; pet dander; and cockroach droppings. They are predominant causes of respiratory allergies, leading to symptoms like sneezing, runny nose, itchy eyes, and asthma.
2. **Food Allergens**: Common food allergens include peanuts, tree nuts, milk, eggs, wheat, soy, fish, and shellfish. Food allergies can cause a range of symptoms from mild (rashes, gastrointestinal discomfort) to severe (anaphylaxis).
3. **Chemical Allergens**: Chemicals found in cleaning products, perfumes, cosmetics, and certain types of industrial materials can trigger allergic reactions for some people. Symptoms may include skin rashes, headaches, and respiratory issues.

Assessing Personal Triggers

1. **Keep a Symptom Diary**: Track daily activities, environments, foods consumed, and any symptoms experienced to identify patterns and potential triggers.
2. **Allergy Testing**: Consult with an allergist for professional allergy testing, which can include skin prick tests, blood tests, and elimination diets for food allergies. These tests can help pinpoint specific allergens responsible for reactions.

Reducing Exposure to Allergens

1. **Environmental Allergens**:
   - **Pollen**: Stay indoors on high pollen count days, keep windows closed, and use air conditioning with HEPA filters. Shower and change clothes after being outside.
   - **Dust Mites**: Use allergen-proof mattress and pillow covers, wash bedding in hot water weekly, and maintain low humidity levels in the home.
   - **Mold**: Fix leaks and damp areas promptly, use dehumidifiers in moist areas like basements, and clean bathrooms and kitchens regularly with mold-killing products.
   - **Pet Dander**: Bathe pets regularly, keep them out of bedrooms and off upholstered furniture, and clean the home frequently, including floors and surfaces.

2. **Food Allergens**:
   - **Read Labels**: Always check food labels for potential allergens. Be aware of cross-contamination risks and food processing practices that may introduce allergens.
   - **Communicate**: Inform restaurant staff about any food allergies when dining out to ensure meals are prepared safely.
3. **Chemical Allergens**:
   - **Choose Products Wisely**: Opt for fragrance-free, hypoallergenic products for cleaning, personal care, and cosmetics.
   - **Ventilation**: Ensure good ventilation when using cleaning agents or chemicals and wear protective gear if necessary.

Lifestyle Adjustments
1. **Air Purification**: Use air purifiers with HEPA filters to reduce indoor allergen levels.
2. **Flooring**: Hard flooring, rather than carpet, can reduce the accumulation of dust mites, pet dander, and pollen indoors.
3. **Avoidance**: For food allergies, develop a plan for avoiding allergens, including safe snacking options and emergency meals.

Conclusion

Effectively managing allergies requires a multifaceted approach focused on identifying specific allergens, understanding personal triggers, and taking proactive steps to reduce exposure. By combining environmental adjustments, dietary caution, and lifestyle modifications with professional medical advice and allergy testing, individuals can achieve significant relief from allergy symptoms and enhance their overall well-being.

Herbal Remedies for Allergy Symptoms

Allergies can significantly impact the quality of life, leading many individuals to seek natural remedies for symptom relief. Several herbs have shown promise in managing allergy symptoms by supporting the immune system, reducing inflammation, and acting as natural antihistamines. Below are some of the most effective herbs for allergies, including their benefits, preparation methods, suggested dosages, and duration of use.

1. Butterbur (Petasites hybridus)
   - **Benefits**: Butterbur has been studied for its effectiveness in reducing nasal symptoms of hay fever without the drowsiness associated with some antihistamines. It works by blocking leukotrienes, substances that can trigger allergy symptoms.
   - **Preparation and Use**: Butterbur is available in capsules or extracts. Ensure the product is labeled PA-free (pyrrolizidine alkaloids-free) to avoid liver toxicity.
   - **When to Take**: Use as directed on the product label, typically before meals.
   - **Quantity and Duration**: Studies have used doses ranging from 50-100 mg twice daily. Due to concerns about long-term safety, it's recommended to use butterbur for seasonal allergy relief rather than year-round.

2. Quercetin
   - **Benefits**: Quercetin is a natural flavonoid that acts as an antioxidant and antihistamine. It can help stabilize mast cells to prevent them from releasing histamine and reduce inflammation, providing relief from allergy symptoms.
   - **Preparation and Use**: Quercetin supplements are widely available. It's also found naturally in foods like onions, apples, and berries.
   - **When to Take**: For best results, start taking quercetin 6-8 weeks before allergy season begins.
   - **Quantity and Duration**: Typical dosages range from 500-1000 mg taken twice daily. Consult a healthcare provider for personalized advice.

3. Stinging Nettle (Urtica dioica)

- **Benefits**: Stinging nettle has a long history of use for relieving allergy symptoms, particularly nasal congestion, sneezing, and itching. It is believed to have antihistamine and anti-inflammatory properties.
- **Preparation and Use**: Nettle can be consumed as a freeze-dried supplement, tea, or tincture. For tea, steep 1-2 teaspoons of dried nettle leaves in boiling water for 10-15 minutes.
- **When to Take**: Use at the onset of allergy symptoms or during peak allergy seasons.
- **Quantity and Duration**: For freeze-dried capsules, dosages of 300-500 mg daily are common. For tea, 2-3 cups daily during allergy season.

4. Spirulina
- **Benefits**: This blue-green algae has been shown to reduce symptoms of allergic rhinitis, including nasal discharge, sneezing, nasal congestion, and itching.
- **Preparation and Use**: Spirulina is available in powder, tablet, or capsule form.
- **When to Take**: With meals to improve absorption.
- **Quantity and Duration**: Studies have used doses ranging from 1-2 grams per day. Consult a healthcare provider to determine the appropriate dosage and duration for your needs.

5. Bromelain
- **Benefits**: Found in pineapple, bromelain is an enzyme that can help reduce nasal swelling and thin mucus, making it easier to breathe.
- **Preparation and Use**: Bromelain supplements are available in capsule or tablet form.
- **When to Take**: On an empty stomach unless directed otherwise on the product label.
- **Quantity and Duration**: Dosages can vary widely; 400-500 mg three times a day is a common recommendation for allergy-related sinus discomfort. It is typically used on a short-term basis.

General Guidelines for Using Herbal Remedies
- **Consultation**: Always consult with a healthcare professional before beginning any new herbal treatment, especially if you have existing health conditions or are taking other medications.
- **Quality**: Choose high-quality, reputable brands to ensure the purity and potency of herbal supplements.
- **Allergies to Herbs**: Be aware that some individuals may have allergic reactions to certain herbs. Start with a lower dose to assess tolerance.

Herbal remedies offer a natural adjunct to conventional allergy treatments, potentially easing symptoms through various mechanisms. Incorporating these herbs, along with dietary and lifestyle modifications, can provide holistic support for individuals seeking relief from allergies.

Dietary Changes to Alleviate Allergies

Diet plays a crucial role in managing and alleviating allergy symptoms. Certain foods can exacerbate allergic reactions, while others might help reduce inflammation, bolster the immune system, and act as natural antihistamines. By making strategic dietary changes, individuals suffering from allergies can potentially see a significant reduction in symptoms. This exploration delves into the dietary adjustments beneficial for those with allergies, focusing on what to incorporate, reduce, or eliminate for better allergy management.

Incorporating Anti-inflammatory Foods
1. **Omega-3 Fatty Acids**: Foods rich in omega-3 fatty acids, like salmon, flaxseeds, chia seeds, and walnuts, can help reduce the body's inflammatory response to allergens.
2. **Fruits and Vegetables**: A diet high in fruits and vegetables provides antioxidants and phytonutrients, such as quercetin found in apples, onions, and berries, which may help stabilize mast cells and reduce histamine release.
3. **Probiotics**: Fermented foods like yogurt, kefir, sauerkraut, and kombucha contain probiotics, which support gut health. A healthy gut microbiome is linked to improved immune function and may help manage allergic reactions.

Reducing Histamine Levels in the Diet

Some individuals are sensitive to histamine, a compound found in various foods that can exacerbate allergy symptoms.

1. **Foods to Avoid**: Aged cheeses, smoked meats, fermented products, and alcohol, especially red wine and beer, are high in histamine and might worsen symptoms for some people.
2. **Fresh Foods**: Opting for fresh rather than processed or aged foods can help manage dietary histamine intake.

Eliminating Allergenic Foods

For food-specific allergies, identifying and eliminating the offending food(s) is essential.

1. **Common Allergens**: The most common food allergens include dairy, eggs, peanuts, tree nuts, soy, wheat, fish, and shellfish. An elimination diet, guided by a healthcare professional, can help identify sensitivities.
2. **Reading Labels**: Always read food labels carefully to avoid hidden allergens and be aware of cross-contamination risks.

Supporting the Liver

The liver plays a vital role in processing and eliminating toxins, including allergens.

1. **Liver-supportive Foods**: Incorporate foods that support liver health, such as beets, carrots, leafy greens, green tea, and herbs like milk thistle and dandelion root.

Hydration

Staying well-hydrated helps maintain mucosal lining health, which can act as a barrier against allergens.

1. **Water Intake**: Aim to drink at least 8 glasses of water daily. Herbal teas can also contribute to hydration needs.

Lifestyle and Dietary Habits

1. **Meal Timing and Composition**: Eating smaller, more frequent meals can help maintain steady blood sugar levels, supporting overall immune function.
2. **Cooking at Home**: Preparing meals at home allows for better control over ingredients and can help avoid accidental exposure to allergens.

Conclusion

Dietary changes offer a viable strategy for managing and alleviating allergy symptoms. By focusing on anti-inflammatory foods, reducing histamine intake, eliminating specific allergens, and supporting overall health through nutrition, individuals can potentially experience fewer allergy symptoms. It's important to approach dietary changes with mindfulness and, when possible, the guidance of a healthcare professional, especially when dealing with severe food allergies. This holistic approach to allergy management can complement medical treatments, leading to an overall improvement in quality of life.

Chapter 15: A 30-Day Disease Prevention Routine

I n the pursuit of long-term health and disease prevention, consistency in daily habits is key. A 30-day routine focused on disease prevention can set the foundation for a lifestyle that naturally supports the body's defenses against illnesses. This comprehensive plan includes dietary recommendations, physical activity, mental wellness practices, and sleep hygiene—all pivotal for bolstering the immune system and minimizing the risk of chronic diseases. Here's a detailed guide to embarking on a 30-day journey toward improved health and disease prevention.

Week 1: Establishing the Basics

Day 1-7 Focus: Hydration, Nutrition, and Gentle Movement

1. **Hydration**: Start each day with a glass of water upon waking. Aim for at least 8 glasses of water throughout the day. Incorporate herbal teas like green tea, which offers antioxidant benefits.

2. **Nutrition**: Introduce more whole foods into your diet. Focus on consuming a variety of fruits and vegetables, lean proteins, whole grains, and healthy fats. Begin to reduce intake of processed foods, sugars, and saturated fats.

3. **Physical Activity**: Incorporate gentle movement. Aim for at least 30 minutes of moderate activity daily, such as walking, yoga, or cycling.

4. **Mental Wellness**: Dedicate 10 minutes each morning or evening to mindfulness or meditation to reduce stress and promote mental clarity.

Week 2: Enhancing Nutritional Intake

Day 8-14 Focus: Antioxidant-rich Foods, Probiotics, and Omega-3s

1. **Antioxidants**: Increase intake of antioxidant-rich foods. Add berries, nuts, dark leafy greens, and colorful vegetables to your meals.

2. **Probiotics**: Introduce probiotic-rich foods like yogurt, kefir, kombucha, or sauerkraut to support gut health.

3. **Omega-3 Fatty Acids**: Include omega-3 sources in your diet, such as salmon, chia seeds, or walnuts, to reduce inflammation and support brain health.

4. **Sleep Hygiene**: Establish a bedtime routine that allows for 7-9 hours of sleep. Limit screen time an hour before bed to improve sleep quality.

Week 3: Building Physical and Mental Resilience

Day 15-21 Focus: Increasing Exercise Intensity and Stress Management

1. **Exercise**: Gradually increase the intensity or duration of your physical activity. Consider strength training exercises to build muscle and support metabolism.

2. **Stress Management**: Incorporate stress-reducing activities into your routine, such as journaling, spending time in nature, or engaging in a hobby.

3. **Sleep**: If not already consistent, prioritize going to bed and waking up at the same time each day to regulate your body's clock.

4. **Hydration**: Continue to focus on hydration, especially around workouts, to aid in recovery and overall health.

Week 4: Solidifying Habits and Mindful Living

Day 22-30 Focus: Mindful Eating, Advanced Physical Activity, and Reflection

1. **Mindful Eating**: Practice being present during meals. Focus on chewing thoroughly and appreciating the flavors and textures of your food to improve digestion and satisfaction.

2. **Advanced Physical Activity**: Introduce new forms of exercise or increase challenge levels, such as interval training, to enhance cardiovascular health and endurance.

3. **Reflection**: Spend time reflecting on the changes you've made and the effects they've had on your mental and physical well-being. Note any improvements in energy, mood, or physical health.

4. **Planning Ahead**: Begin to plan how you will incorporate these habits into a long-term routine. Consider setting new health goals for the coming months.

Conclusion

Embarking on a 30-day disease prevention routine is an excellent way to reset and focus on habits that contribute to long-term health. This period is not just about making temporary changes but about establishing sustainable habits that can significantly reduce the risk of chronic diseases and enhance overall vitality. By focusing on nutrition, physical activity, mental wellness, and sleep, individuals can lay a strong foundation for a healthier lifestyle that supports disease prevention well beyond the initial 30 days.

Daily Checklist for Holistic Health Practices

Adopting a holistic approach to health encompasses nurturing the body, mind, and spirit through balanced daily practices. A comprehensive daily checklist can serve as a guide to integrating holistic health practices into your routine, ensuring a well-rounded approach to wellness. This checklist includes essential activities and habits that support physical health, mental well-being, and emotional balance.

Morning

1. **Hydration**: Start your day with a glass of water to rehydrate your body after sleep. Consider adding lemon for detoxification and a vitamin C boost.

2. **Mindfulness Practice**: Dedicate 5-10 minutes to meditation or deep breathing exercises to center your thoughts and set a positive tone for the day.

3. **Movement**: Engage in at least 30 minutes of physical activity. Morning is an ideal time for yoga, a brisk walk, or any exercise that energizes you for the day ahead.

4. **Nutritious Breakfast**: Consume a balanced breakfast that includes proteins, healthy fats, and whole grains to fuel your body and mind. Incorporate fruits or vegetables for added nutrients.

5. **Intention Setting**: Take a moment to set intentions for the day. Reflect on your goals, what you wish to accomplish, and how you want to feel.

Midday

1. **Healthy Snacking**: Choose snacks that are high in nutrients and low in processed sugars, such as nuts, seeds, or fresh fruit.

2. **Hydration**: Continue to drink water throughout the day. Aim for at least 8 glasses in total to ensure proper hydration.

3. **Mindful Eating**: Practice mindful eating during lunch. Focus on your meal, chew thoroughly, and enjoy the flavors and textures.

4. **Short Walk**: If possible, take a brief walk after lunch. A short stroll can aid digestion and invigorate you for the rest of the day.

5. **Breathing Break**: Take a few minutes for deep breathing or a quick relaxation exercise to reduce stress and recharge.

Evening

1. **Digital Detox**: Allocate time away from screens at least an hour before bedtime to reduce blue light exposure and prepare your mind for sleep.

2. **Reflective Journaling**: Spend a few minutes reflecting on your day, noting successes, areas for improvement, and feelings in a journal.

3. **Gratitude Practice**: Write down three things you are grateful for each day. This practice fosters positivity and contentment.

4. **Nutritious Dinner**: Have a balanced dinner with a variety of nutrients. Include lean proteins, whole grains, and a large portion of vegetables.

5. **Preparation for Sleep**: Engage in a relaxing activity before bed, such as reading, gentle stretching, or taking a warm bath, to signal to your body that it's time to wind down.

6. **Sleep Hygiene**: Ensure your sleeping environment is conducive to rest. Keep the room cool, dark, and quiet. Aim for 7-9 hours of quality sleep.

Weekly Additions

- **Nature Time**: Spend time in nature at least once a week to connect with the outdoors and ground yourself.

- **Social Connection**: Cultivate meaningful relationships by connecting with friends or family.

- **Self-Care Ritual**: Incorporate a self-care activity that you enjoy, such as a hobby, spa day at home, or creative project.

This daily checklist for holistic health practices emphasizes the importance of consistency in nurturing all aspects of well-being. By integrating these practices into your daily and weekly routines, you can build a strong foundation for holistic health, promoting balance, vitality, and happiness in your life.

Herbal Supplements and Dietary Plan for Holistic Health

Integrating herbal supplements into a balanced dietary plan can significantly enhance holistic health by providing essential nutrients, supporting bodily functions, and potentially preventing various health issues. This comprehensive guide outlines a strategic approach to selecting herbal supplements and structuring a dietary plan that aligns with the principles of holistic well-being.

Selecting Herbal Supplements

When considering herbal supplements, focus on those known for their health-promoting properties, safety, and effectiveness. It's crucial to choose high-quality products from reputable sources and consult with a healthcare provider, especially if you have existing health conditions or are taking medications. Below are some commonly recommended herbal supplements for holistic health:

1. **Turmeric (Curcuma longa)**: Contains curcumin, a compound with potent anti-inflammatory and antioxidant properties. Beneficial for joint health, cognitive function, and cardiovascular health.

2. **Ginger (Zingiber officinale)**: Offers digestive support, relieves nausea, and has anti-inflammatory effects that can benefit overall wellness.

3. **Ashwagandha (Withania somnifera)**: An adaptogen that helps the body manage stress, supports adrenal function, and enhances mood and energy levels.

4. **Omega-3 Supplements (Fish Oil or Flaxseed Oil)**: Essential fatty acids that support heart health, cognitive function, and reduce inflammation.

5. **Probiotics**: Support gut health by maintaining a healthy balance of intestinal flora, crucial for digestion, immune function, and mental health.

Daily Dietary Plan

A holistic dietary plan emphasizes whole foods, minimizes processed foods, and includes a wide variety of nutrients. Here's a sample daily plan incorporating herbal supplements:

Morning:

- **Breakfast**: Oatmeal with fresh berries, chia seeds, and a dollop of yogurt. Green tea or a turmeric latte.
- **Supplement**: Probiotic with a glass of water.

Mid-Morning Snack:

- **Snack**: A small handful of almonds and an apple.
- **Hydration**: Herbal tea, such as ginger or peppermint, or water.

Lunch:

- **Main**: Grilled chicken or chickpea salad with mixed greens, avocado, cherry tomatoes, cucumbers, and olive oil dressing.
- **Supplement**: Omega-3 supplement (fish oil or flaxseed oil).

Afternoon Snack:

- **Snack**: Carrot sticks with hummus.
- **Hydration**: Water or herbal infusion.

Dinner:

- **Main**: Baked salmon or lentil stew, quinoa, and steamed broccoli.
- **Side**: A small portion of sauerkraut for probiotic benefits.
- **Supplement**: Ashwagandha supplement (consult with a healthcare provider for the best time, as some individuals may find it energizing while others may find it sedating).

Evening:

- **Relaxation**: Herbal tea, such as chamomile, to support relaxation and sleep.

Weekly Additions

- **Incorporate Diverse Foods**: Each week, try to include different fruits, vegetables, whole grains, lean proteins, and healthy fats to ensure a broad intake of nutrients.

- **Plan for Meatless Days**: Incorporate one or two plant-based days into your weekly plan to diversify your diet with legumes, nuts, and seeds.

General Guidelines

- **Stay Hydrated**: Aim for 8-10 glasses of water daily, adjusting based on activity level and climate.

- **Mindful Eating**: Focus on the experience of eating; chew thoroughly and avoid distractions during meals to improve digestion and satisfaction.

- **Adjust Portions and Timing**: Listen to your body's hunger and fullness cues. Eating smaller, more frequent meals can support metabolism and energy levels.

Conclusion

A holistic approach to health that combines carefully selected herbal supplements with a balanced dietary plan can significantly enhance well-being. This strategy supports various body systems, promotes mental and emotional health, and contributes to long-term disease prevention. Remember, individual needs may vary, so it's important to tailor this plan to your specific health goals, preferences, and nutritional requirements. Consulting with healthcare professionals can provide personalized guidance and ensure that any supplements and dietary changes complement existing health regimens.

Exercise and Mindfulness Activities Schedule for Holistic Health

A well-rounded health routine incorporates both physical activity and mindfulness practices, enhancing not only physical fitness but also mental and emotional well-being. Creating a structured schedule that includes both elements can help establish consistency, build resilience, and foster a deeper connection between mind and body. Here is a detailed plan for integrating exercise and mindfulness into your daily routine, adaptable to varying fitness levels and lifestyles.

Week Overview

The goal is to balance various types of physical activities with daily mindfulness practices, ensuring a comprehensive approach to health. This plan can be adjusted based on individual needs, preferences, and time constraints.

Monday: Cardio Focus and Meditation

- **Morning**: Begin the day with 10 minutes of meditation upon waking. Focus on breath awareness to center your thoughts and set a positive tone for the day.

- **Evening Exercise**: 30 minutes of cardiovascular exercise. Options include brisk walking, jogging, cycling, or a cardio class. Cardiovascular workouts improve heart health and endurance.

Tuesday: Strength Training and Gratitude Journaling

- **Morning Gratitude Practice**: Spend 5 minutes writing in a gratitude journal. Listing things you're thankful for can enhance mood and perspective.

- **Evening Exercise**: 30 minutes of strength training focusing on major muscle groups. Use free weights, resistance bands, or bodyweight exercises like squats and push-ups.

Wednesday: Yoga and Mindful Walking

- **Morning**: Start with a 20-minute yoga session to stretch and strengthen the body while cultivating mindfulness through focused movement and breath.

- **Evening Mindfulness Activity**: Go for a 20-minute mindful walk. Engage all your senses, noticing the sights, sounds, and smells around you without judgment.

Thursday: High-Intensity Interval Training (HIIT) and Deep Breathing Exercises

- **Morning Deep Breathing**: Practice 5 minutes of deep breathing exercises to energize the body and clear the mind.

- **Evening Exercise**: Engage in 20 minutes of HIIT. Alternate between high-intensity exercises (like jumping jacks or burpees) and rest periods to boost metabolism.

Friday: Restorative Yoga and Visualization

- **Morning Visualization**: Spend 5-10 minutes visualizing your goals and the positive outcomes you desire. Visualization can enhance motivation and clarity.

- **Evening Activity**: 30 minutes of restorative yoga. Focus on relaxation and deep stretching to unwind and release tension from the week.

Saturday: Active Recreation and Digital Detox

- **Daytime Activity**: Choose an enjoyable active recreational activity that gets you moving and outdoors if possible. Consider hiking, swimming, or playing a sport with friends or family.

- **Evening Digital Detox**: Spend the evening free from screens. Read, engage in hobbies, or spend quality time with loved ones to enhance personal connections and relaxation.

Sunday: Leisurely Walk and Guided Meditation

- **Morning Leisure Walk**: Start the day with a leisurely 30-minute walk. Use this time to reflect on the past week and set intentions for the week ahead.

- **Evening Meditation**: End the week with a 15-minute guided meditation session. There are many apps and online resources available for guided meditations focusing on various themes, such as stress relief or gratitude.

Additional Tips for Success

- **Flexibility**: Listen to your body and adjust the intensity and type of exercise as needed. The goal is to enhance health, not to push through pain or discomfort.

- **Consistency Over Intensity**: Regular, moderate activity is more beneficial in the long term than sporadic, intense workouts.

- **Mindfulness in Daily Activities**: Try to incorporate mindfulness into everyday activities, not just during designated times. Be fully present whether you're eating, working, or spending time with others.

Creating a balanced schedule of exercise and mindfulness activities promotes a holistic approach to health, emphasizing the importance of nurturing the body, mind, and spirit in unison. By committing to this routine, individuals can enjoy improved physical fitness, mental clarity, and emotional resilience.

Conclusion: Empowering Your Health Journey

Embarking on a health journey is a deeply personal and transformative process that extends beyond the pursuit of disease prevention or physical fitness. It's about cultivating a lifestyle that harmonizes the body, mind, and spirit, leading to a state of holistic well-being. This journey is unique for each individual, shaped by personal goals, experiences, and challenges. As we conclude this guide on fostering holistic health, it's important to reflect on the key elements that empower your health journey, ensuring it is sustainable, fulfilling, and adaptive to your evolving needs.

Embracing a Holistic Perspective

Holistic health recognizes the interconnectedness of physical, mental, and emotional aspects of well-being. Empowerment comes from understanding that nurturing each aspect contributes to overall health. This approach encourages you to view health not merely as the absence of disease but as a dynamic state of balance and vitality. By integrating practices that support all facets of your well-being, you're more likely to achieve and maintain optimal health.

Personalization and Flexibility

Your health journey is yours alone, and what works for one person may not work for another. Personalization is key. Listen to your body and be mindful of how different foods, activities, and practices affect you. Flexibility allows you to adapt your health plan as you progress, accommodating changes in your lifestyle, preferences, and goals. Remember, the path to holistic health is not linear but a continuous process of learning and adapting.

Education and Self-Awareness

Empowerment is rooted in education and self-awareness. The more you understand about your body and the factors that influence your health, the better equipped you are to make informed decisions. Continue to seek knowledge about nutrition, exercise, mindfulness, and other areas relevant to your health. Self-awareness helps you recognize your progress, understand your limits, and identify when changes are needed.

Community and Support

While the journey is personal, support from others can be incredibly empowering. Sharing experiences, challenges, and successes with a community or support group provides motivation, accountability, and a sense of belonging. Whether it's family, friends, or online communities, surround yourself with people who encourage and uplift you.

Celebrating Milestones

Acknowledging and celebrating milestones, no matter how small, reinforce positive behaviors and motivate you to continue on your path. Set realistic, achievable goals, and take time to appreciate your progress. Celebrating these achievements helps maintain momentum and keeps you focused on your long-term vision for health.

Resilience and Compassion

Encountering setbacks is a natural part of any journey. What matters is how you respond to them. Cultivate resilience by viewing challenges as opportunities to learn and grow. Be compassionate with yourself, recognizing that perfection is not the goal—continued effort and commitment are. Self-compassion fosters a healthier relationship with yourself and supports enduring change.

Moving Forward

As you move forward on your health journey, remember that empowerment comes from within. It's about making choices that align with your values, goals, and well-being. By embracing a holistic approach, personalizing your path, and approaching challenges with resilience and compassion, you lay the foundation for a vibrant, healthy life. Your health journey is an ongoing process of growth and discovery, one that holds the potential for profound transformation and fulfillment.

Appendix: Preparing Herbal Remedies

Creating herbal remedies at home allows you to harness the natural benefits of herbs in forms that can be easily incorporated into your health routine. Here's a detailed guide on making tinctures, teas, and salves, which are among the most versatile and commonly used herbal preparations.

Making Herbal Tinctures

Tinctures are concentrated herbal extracts made using alcohol to extract the active compounds from herbs.

Materials Needed:

- Dried or fresh herbs
- High-proof alcohol (at least 40% alcohol by volume, such as vodka or brandy)
- Clean glass jar with a tight-fitting lid
- Cheesecloth or fine mesh strainer
- Amber or dark-colored glass bottles for storage

Steps:

1. **Prepare the Herbs**: If using fresh herbs, chop them finely to increase the surface area for extraction. Dried herbs should be lightly crushed.

2. **Jar Filling**: Fill the glass jar ⅓ to ½ with herbs. The amount can vary depending on the herb's potency and the desired strength of the tincture.

3. **Add Alcohol**: Pour the alcohol over the herbs until the jar is nearly full, ensuring the herbs are completely submerged to prevent mold growth.

4. **Seal and Label**: Close the jar tightly and label it with the herb's name, the type of alcohol used, and the date.

5. **Store and Shake**: Keep the jar in a cool, dark place. Shake it daily to help the extraction process.

6. **Strain**: After 4-6 weeks, strain the tincture through cheesecloth or a fine mesh strainer into another clean jar. Press or squeeze the herbs to extract as much liquid as possible.

7. **Bottle**: Transfer the strained tincture into amber or dark-colored glass bottles. Label the bottles with the herb's name and the date of completion.

Brewing Herbal Teas

Herbal teas (infusions) are a gentle way to enjoy the benefits of herbs.

Materials Needed:

- Dried or fresh herbs
- Boiling water
- Teapot or jar

- Strainer or tea infuser
- Mug or cup

Steps:

1. **Prepare Herbs**: Measure 1-2 teaspoons of dried herbs per cup of water. Adjust the amount to taste or depending on the herb's strength.

2. **Boil Water**: Heat water until it reaches a rolling boil.

3. **Steep**: Place the herbs in the teapot or jar, pour the boiling water over them, and cover. Steep for 5-15 minutes, depending on the desired strength and the herb used.

4. **Strain and Serve**: Strain the tea into a mug or cup using a strainer or remove the tea infuser. Enjoy as is or sweeten with honey if desired.

Crafting Herbal Salves

Salves are used topically to soothe skin, aid in healing, or relieve pain.

Materials Needed:

- Dried herbs
- Carrier oil (such as olive, coconut, or almond oil)
- Beeswax
- Double boiler or a heat-proof bowl and pot
- Cheesecloth or fine mesh strainer
- Clean containers for the salve

Steps:

1. **Infuse Oil**: Place the herbs and carrier oil in a double boiler or heat-proof bowl over a pot of simmering water. Use about 1 cup of oil for every ¼ cup of dried herbs. Gently heat for 2-3 hours, avoiding boiling, to infuse the oil.

2. **Strain**: Remove the mixture from heat and strain it through cheesecloth or a fine mesh strainer to remove the herbs, squeezing to extract as much oil as possible.

3. **Add Beeswax**: Return the infused oil to the double boiler and add beeswax. Use about 1 ounce (28 grams) of beeswax per cup of infused oil for a standard consistency. Adjust for a softer or harder salve.

4. **Melt and Mix**: Heat gently until the beeswax is completely melted into the oil, stirring to ensure an even mixture.

5. **Pour and Cool**: Carefully pour the hot mixture into clean containers. Let it cool and solidify at room temperature.

6. **Label**: Once cooled, label the containers with the herb(s) used, the date, and any specific instructions for use.

Creating tinctures, teas, and salves at home is a rewarding way to engage with herbal medicine and tailor remedies to your specific health needs. Always start with high-quality, organic herbs to ensure the purity and effectiveness of your homemade remedies.

Storage and Usage Instructions for Herbal Remedies

Proper storage and correct usage are crucial for maintaining the efficacy and safety of herbal remedies. Whether you've prepared tinctures, teas, or salves, adhering to guidelines ensures that these natural products provide the intended health benefits while minimizing any potential risks. This detailed guide covers the essentials of storing and using herbal remedies, from optimal conditions to shelf life and administration tips.

Storing Herbal Remedies

Tinctures:

- **Conditions**: Store in a cool, dark place, such as a cupboard or a pantry, away from direct sunlight, moisture, and heat sources. The ideal storage temperature is between 54°F (12°C) and 77°F (25°C).

- **Containers**: Use dark glass bottles (amber or cobalt) to protect the tincture from light, which can degrade active compounds over time. Ensure the cap is tight to prevent evaporation.

- **Shelf Life**: Properly stored, alcohol-based tinctures have a long shelf life, typically lasting 2-5 years. Vinegar or glycerin-based tinctures have a shorter shelf life, generally around 1-2 years.

Herbal Teas (Dried Herbs):

- **Conditions**: Keep dried herbs in a cool, dry place, away from sunlight, moisture, and strong odors that could affect their flavor and potency.

- **Containers**: Airtight containers are essential to prevent moisture from spoiling the herbs. Glass jars, metal tins, or mylar bags with oxygen absorbers are good options.

- **Shelf Life**: When stored properly, dried herbs used for teas can last up to 1-2 years. Signs of degradation include loss of aroma, discoloration, and diminished flavor.

Salves:

- **Conditions**: Store salves in a cool, dry place to prevent melting and preserve consistency. Avoid leaving them in hot environments, like a car on a sunny day.

- **Containers**: Use clean, airtight containers, preferably made of glass or metal, to protect the salve from contamination and oxidation.

- **Shelf Life**: Herbal salves generally have a shelf life of 1-2 years, depending on the carrier oil's stability. If the salve changes in smell, color, or texture, it should be discarded.

Usage Instructions

Tinctures:

- **Dosage**: Follow the recommended dosage on the product label or as advised by a healthcare professional. A common dosage is 1-2 droppers full (about 1-2 mL) taken 2-3 times daily, but this can vary.

- **Administration**: Tinctures can be taken directly under the tongue for fast absorption or diluted in a small amount of water or juice.

- **Precautions**: Alcohol-based tinctures may not be suitable for everyone, including children, pregnant women, and individuals with a history of alcohol dependence.

Herbal Teas:

- **Preparation**: Use 1-2 teaspoons of dried herbs per cup of boiling water. Steep covered for 5-15 minutes, depending on the desired strength.

- **Frequency**: Herbal teas can generally be enjoyed 2-3 times daily unless otherwise indicated. Pay attention to your body's response, as some herbs can have strong effects.

- **Precautions**: Ensure the herb is safe for consumption and be aware of potential interactions with medications or existing health conditions.

Salves:

- **Application**: Apply a small amount of salve to the affected area, gently massaging into the skin. Use as needed, typically 2-3 times daily.

- **Patch Test**: Before widespread use, conduct a patch test by applying a small amount to a discreet skin area to check for adverse reactions.

- **Precautions**: Salves are for external use only. Avoid applying to open wounds or broken skin unless the product is specifically designed for such use.

Conclusion

Proper storage extends the shelf life of herbal remedies, ensuring they remain potent and safe to use. By following these storage and usage instructions, you can maximize the benefits of your herbal remedies. Always start with quality ingredients, and don't hesitate to consult healthcare professionals for guidance on herbal supplement use, especially in relation to specific health conditions or treatments.

The Essential
BARBARA O'NEILL
COOKBOOK

Revitalize Your Health in 30 Days! Discover Natural, Wholesome Recipes and Smart Eating Habits Tailored for Optimal Well-being

Janet Moore

Introduction: The Philosophy Behind the Recipes

At the heart of this book lies a philosophy deeply rooted in the conviction that food is much more than sustenance—it is medicine, a source of healing, and a pathway to a richer, more vibrant life. This philosophy does not view nutrition through the narrow lens of dieting or restrictions. Instead, it embraces food as a celebration of nature's diversity, a testament to the interconnectedness of life, and a profound opportunity to influence our health and wellbeing positively.

Harmony with Nature

The recipes and teachings within these pages are born out of a deep respect for the natural world and its cycles. We believe that by aligning our eating habits with the rhythms of nature, we can foster a state of balance and health that resonates through every aspect of our being. This philosophy advocates for whole, unprocessed foods that carry the life force of the earth, foods that are grown and harvested with care, and that nourish not only our bodies but also our souls.

The Healing Power of Whole Foods

Central to our philosophy is the understanding that whole foods, particularly those that are plant-based, possess an inherent power to heal and rejuvenate our bodies. These foods are rich in essential nutrients, antioxidants, and phytochemicals that work synergistically to reduce inflammation, boost immunity, and enhance our overall health. The recipes you will find here are designed to showcase the beauty and nutritional bounty of these ingredients, combining them in ways that maximize their healing potential.

Culinary Alchemy

The art of cooking is, at its core, a form of alchemy—a transformative process that turns simple ingredients into nourishing meals that can heal the body and delight the senses. Our recipes are more than just instructions; they are invitations to engage in this alchemy, to experiment with flavors and textures, and to discover the joy of creating meals that do more than fill the stomach. They heal, energize, and inspire.

A Holistic Approach

We understand that true health encompasses the body, mind, and spirit, and our approach to nutrition reflects this holistic view. The recipes and guidance offered in this book are designed not just to feed the body but to nourish the mind and spirit as well. We emphasize the importance of mindfulness in eating—savoring each bite, being present in the moment, and appreciating the food that sustains us.

Empowerment through Knowledge

Knowledge is the foundation of empowerment, and through this book, we aim to equip you with the understanding and skills you need to take control of your health through nutrition. We delve into the science behind the healing power of foods, the significance of balancing macronutrients, and the importance of choosing ingredients that are organic, non-GMO, and sustainably sourced. This knowledge serves as the bedrock upon which you can build a lifestyle that supports your health and wellness goals.

A Journey of Transformation

Ultimately, the philosophy behind the recipes is about transformation—a journey from where you are now to where you want to be in terms of your health and wellbeing. It's a journey that doesn't promise quick fixes or miracle cures but offers something far more valuable: a sustainable path to a healthier, more vibrant life. By embracing the principles outlined in this book, you are taking the first step on this journey.

We invite you to join us in this culinary adventure, to explore the healing power of food, and to discover the joy and satisfaction that comes from nourishing yourself in a way that is aligned with the rhythms of the earth and the needs of your body. Welcome to a world where cooking is an act of love, eating is a celebration of life, and every meal is a step on the path to wellness.

How to Use This Book for Maximum Health Benefit

Embarking on a journey towards improved health and wellness through nutrition is a transformative process that requires guidance, practice, and patience. This book has been meticulously designed not only as a collection of recipes but as a comprehensive guide to nurturing your body and soul with every meal. To harness the full potential of this resource, consider the following strategies for integrating its teachings into your daily life.

1. Embrace the Philosophy

Before diving into the recipes, take the time to absorb the underlying philosophy detailed in the Introduction. Understanding the holistic approach to nutrition and health will enhance your appreciation of the recipes and advice provided, allowing you to fully engage with the process of nourishing yourself in a more mindful and informed manner.

2. Start with Self-Reflection

Assess your current eating habits, health status, and wellness goals. This self-reflection will serve as your personal roadmap, guiding you towards the sections and recipes that align most closely with your needs. Whether you're looking to combat specific ailments, improve your overall vitality, or simply explore a more plant-based diet, this book offers pathways tailored to diverse objectives.

3. Progress at Your Own Pace

Transformation doesn't happen overnight. Allow yourself the flexibility to progress through the book at a pace that feels comfortable and sustainable for you. Begin by integrating one or two recipes into your weekly meal plan, gradually incorporating more as you become accustomed to new ingredients and cooking techniques.

4. Engage with Each Section Holistically

Maximize your health benefits by engaging deeply with each section of the book. Beyond the recipes, explore the foundational principles of healing nutrition, the importance of whole foods, and the role of hydration and organic choices. Integrating these principles into your lifestyle will amplify the benefits of the individual recipes.

5. Utilize the Additional Resources

Make full use of the appendices and additional resources provided at the end of the book. From the comprehensive shopping lists to the glossary of ingredients and their health benefits, these tools are designed to support your journey, making the transition to a healthier lifestyle as seamless as possible.

6. Experiment and Personalize

View the recipes as a starting point for your culinary exploration. Feel encouraged to experiment with substitutions that cater to your personal taste preferences or dietary restrictions. Personalization is key to sustainable change; finding what works best for you will make the process more enjoyable and effective.

7. Reflect and Adapt

Regular reflection on your progress and how your body responds to changes in your diet is crucial. Use the insights gained from this reflection to adapt your approach, experimenting with different recipes or principles to find the perfect balance for your body's unique needs.

8. Share the Journey

Health and wellness are not solitary pursuits. Share your journey with friends and family, whether by preparing meals together, discussing the insights you've gained, or even tackling the 30-Day Meal Plan as a group. Community support can be incredibly motivating and enriching.

9. Be Mindful and Patient

Adopting a new approach to eating is an opportunity to cultivate mindfulness and patience. Be present with the process, from selecting ingredients to preparing meals and eating. Recognize that each step is a part of your journey towards better health.

10. Keep Learning and Growing

Consider this book not just as a resource but as a companion on your journey to wellness. As you evolve, revisit sections for deeper understanding or new inspiration. The path to health is ongoing, and continued learning and adaptation will keep you moving forward.

By following these strategies, you'll be well-equipped to utilize this book to its fullest potential, transforming your approach to nutrition and health. Welcome to a journey of discovery, healing, and vibrant living.

Part I: Foundations of Healing Nutrition

Embarking on the path of healing nutrition is akin to laying the groundwork for a temple of wellness. In this foundational part of your journey, we establish the core principles that will guide your way to profound health transformations. This section is designed to equip you with the knowledge, understanding, and appreciation of the nutritional philosophies that underpin the healing recipes and lifestyle changes recommended in this book. Let's delve into the crucial components that form the bedrock of healing nutrition.

Chapter 1: The Core Principles of Dr. O'Neill's Nutritional Teachings

At the heart of Dr. O'Neill's nutritional philosophy is the belief that the body possesses an inherent ability to heal itself, given the right conditions and nourishments. This chapter distills decades of research, practice, and insights into a set of core principles that underpin the transformative power of healing nutrition. Embracing these principles can guide you towards sustained health, vitality, and well-being.

Principle 1: The Primacy of Whole Foods

Nature's Design: Dr. O'Neill emphasizes that foods in their whole, unprocessed form are the most harmonious with our body's natural processes. Whole foods provide a complex blend of nutrients, fiber, and energy in forms precisely designed by nature. This principle encourages a diet centered around fruits, vegetables, whole grains, nuts, seeds, and legumes, with minimal processed or refined foods.

Principle 2: Plant-Based at the Core

Vitality Through Plants: A diet rooted in plant-based foods is rich in phytonutrients, antioxidants, vitamins, and minerals, contributing to reduced inflammation, improved gut health, and lower risk of chronic diseases. While not necessarily advocating for a strictly vegan or vegetarian lifestyle, Dr. O'Neill stresses the importance of making plant-based foods the cornerstone of your diet.

Principle 3: Nutritional Synergy

The Whole is Greater: The interaction between different nutrients in our diet can amplify their benefits. This concept of synergy suggests that the nutritional value of a whole food cannot be replicated by consuming its individual components in isolation. By eating a variety of whole foods, we provide our body with a symphony of nutrients that work together to promote optimal health.

Principle 4: The Importance of Hydration

Water as Life's Elixir: Water is fundamental to every cellular function in the body, yet it is often overlooked in discussions of nutrition. Dr. O'Neill advises not only drinking adequate amounts of water but also consuming foods high in water content. Proper hydration supports digestion, nutrient absorption, and detoxification processes.

Principle 5: Mindful Eating

Conscious Consumption: How we eat is as important as what we eat. Mindful eating involves being fully present during meals, savoring each bite, and listening to the body's hunger and satiety signals. This practice encourages a deeper connection with food, reduces overeating, and enhances digestion.

Principle 6: Individualized Nutrition

One Size Does Not Fit All: Recognizing that each person's body is unique, Dr. O'Neill advocates for personalized nutrition. Factors such as age, gender, health status, and lifestyle must be considered when determining the optimal diet for an individual. Experimentation and adjustment are key to finding what works best for you.

Principle 7: The Healing Power of Herbs and Spices

Nature's Pharmacy: Beyond their ability to enhance flavor, herbs and spices possess potent medicinal properties. Incorporating a diverse array of these natural wonders into your diet can boost immunity, reduce inflammation, and contribute to overall health. Dr. O'Neill encourages the exploration of global cuisines and traditions to diversify your intake of these powerful ingredients.

Principle 8: The Role of Gut Health

Foundation of Wellness: A healthy gut microbiome is essential for digestion, nutrient absorption, immune function, and even mental health. A diet rich in fiber, probiotics, and prebiotics nurtures a diverse and balanced gut flora, laying the groundwork for good health.

Principle 9: Sustainability and Ethical Eating

Harmony with the Earth: True health extends beyond the individual to the health of the planet. Choosing locally sourced, organic, and ethically produced foods minimizes our environmental footprint and supports sustainable agricultural practices.

Principle 10: Continuous Learning and Adaptation

Journey, Not Destination: The landscape of nutrition and health science is ever-evolving. Staying informed about the latest research, being open to new ideas, and being willing to adapt your dietary practices as new evidence emerges are essential aspects of a holistic approach to health.

By integrating these core principles into your daily life, you embrace a holistic approach to nutrition that nurtures not only your physical body but also your mental and emotional well-being. Dr. O'Neill's teachings invite you on a journey of discovery, where the ultimate goal is not just to live but to thrive.

Chapter 2: Understanding Foods: What to Embrace and What to Avoid

Navigating the vast landscape of food choices can often feel overwhelming. With an abundance of conflicting information and new diets emerging constantly, it's crucial to ground your nutritional choices in a clear understanding of what foods serve your health and which ones undermine it. This chapter demystifies these choices by outlining a comprehensive guide on what to embrace and what to avoid for optimal health.

Foods to Embrace

Whole, Plant-Based Foods: The cornerstone of a healing diet, these are foods in their most natural state. Fruits, vegetables, whole grains, nuts, seeds, and legumes are packed with essential nutrients, fiber, and antioxidants that support overall health. They are the foundation of a diet that promotes vitality and longevity.

- **Fruits and Vegetables:** A rainbow of colors on your plate ensures a broad range of vitamins, minerals, and phytochemicals. Aim for variety and seasonality to maximize nutritional intake and enjoy the best flavors.

- **Whole Grains:** Quinoa, brown rice, oats, and barley provide sustained energy and are rich in fiber, which is crucial for digestive health.

- **Legumes:** Beans, lentils, and chickpeas are excellent protein sources and rich in fiber, making them staples in a health-conscious diet.

- **Nuts and Seeds:** Almonds, walnuts, flaxseeds, and chia seeds are excellent sources of healthy fats, proteins, and various essential micronutrients.

Clean Proteins: Opt for sustainably sourced, clean proteins. This includes plant-based proteins and, for those who include animal products in their diets, options like wild-caught fish, organic poultry, and grass-fed meats. These choices minimize exposure to hormones, antibiotics, and harmful contaminants.

Healthy Fats: Embrace sources of monounsaturated and polyunsaturated fats, including avocados, olive oil, and fatty fish like salmon. These fats are crucial for brain health, inflammation reduction, and overall cellular function.

Herbs and Spices: Not only do they elevate the flavor of dishes, but they also offer significant health benefits, including anti-inflammatory and antioxidant properties.

Foods to Avoid

Processed and Refined Foods: These are often stripped of nutrients and filled with added sugars, unhealthy fats, and preservatives. Processed foods can disrupt metabolic health, contribute to weight gain, and increase the risk of chronic diseases.

- **Added Sugars:** Found in sodas, sweets, and many packaged foods, added sugars contribute to a host of health issues, including obesity, diabetes, and heart disease.

- **Refined Grains:** White bread, pasta, and other products made from refined grains lack the fiber and nutrients found in their whole counterparts.

- **Trans Fats and Hydrogenated Oils:** Often found in fried foods, baked goods, and processed snack foods, these fats can raise bad cholesterol levels and lower good cholesterol levels, increasing the risk of heart disease.

Excessive Sodium: A high intake of sodium, commonly found in processed and packaged foods, can lead to hypertension and cardiovascular diseases. Opting for fresh foods and seasoning with herbs and spices can help manage sodium intake.

Artificial Additives: Colorants, preservatives, artificial sweeteners, and flavor enhancers are ubiquitous in the modern food supply. These additives can have various adverse health effects and are best minimized in a healing diet.

Embracing Balance and Mindfulness

While this guide offers a framework for understanding what foods to embrace and what to avoid, it's also important to approach your diet with balance and mindfulness. Extreme restrictions can lead to a fraught relationship with food, while mindful indulgence can contribute to a balanced, joyful approach to eating. Listen to your body, enjoy food's pleasures, and make informed choices that align with your health goals and ethical values.

By incorporating these guidelines into your daily life, you can navigate the complex world of food choices with confidence. Embracing whole, nutrient-dense foods and avoiding those that undermine health can lead to lasting wellness and vitality.

Chapter 3: The Vital Role of Whole Foods and Plant-Based Ingredients in Your Diet

I n an era where processed foods dominate the culinary landscape, turning towards whole foods and plant-based ingredients represents a profound shift back to the basics of nutrition. This chapter delves into the transformative impact that whole, unprocessed foods, with an emphasis on plant-based ingredients, can have on our health, well-being, and the environment. By understanding and embracing the vitality offered by these foods, we can unlock the door to enhanced health and longevity.

The Essence of Whole Foods

Whole foods are those that have been minimally processed or are completely unaltered from their natural state. This includes a vast array of fruits, vegetables, grains, nuts, seeds, legumes, meats, fish, and dairy products. The key characteristic of whole foods is their complexity; they contain a full spectrum of nutrients (vitamins, minerals, fiber, and antioxidants) that work synergistically to nourish the body.

Nutritional Synergy: Whole foods provide nutrients that work together in harmony to promote optimal health. For instance, the vitamin C found in oranges enhances iron absorption from spinach when consumed together, showcasing the body's need for a varied, whole-food diet.

Fiber Richness: Whole foods, particularly plant-based varieties, are rich in dietary fiber, which is essential for digestive health, helps regulate blood sugar levels, and can aid in weight management by promoting a feeling of fullness.

The Power of Plant-Based Ingredients

Plant-based ingredients are derived from plants, including vegetables, fruits, grains, nuts, seeds, and legumes, and do not include animal products. While not everyone may choose a fully plant-based diet, incorporating more plant-based foods has been shown to offer significant health benefits.

Disease Prevention: Diets high in plant-based ingredients are linked to a lower risk of developing chronic diseases such as heart disease, diabetes, and certain cancers. The antioxidants and phytochemicals found in plants play a crucial role in reducing inflammation and protecting the body from oxidative stress.

Heart Health: The high fiber content and healthy fats in plant-based foods contribute to cardiovascular health by lowering cholesterol levels and improving blood pressure.

Environmental Sustainability: Beyond personal health benefits, shifting towards a diet that emphasizes plant-based ingredients significantly reduces one's environmental footprint. Plant-based diets require less water and land, and produce fewer greenhouse gas emissions compared to diets high in animal products.

Integrating Whole Foods and Plant-Based Ingredients into Your Diet

Start with Small Changes: Incorporate more fruits and vegetables into your meals, aiming for variety and color to ensure a broad spectrum of nutrients. Replace refined grains with whole grains like quinoa, brown rice, and whole wheat.

Explore Plant-Based Proteins: Experiment with plant-based protein sources such as lentils, chickpeas, tempeh, and black beans. These can be excellent replacements for meat in many recipes.

Snack Smart: Choose whole-food snacks like nuts, seeds, fruit, and vegetables instead of processed snack foods. These options are not only healthier but also more satisfying.

Learn New Recipes: Embrace the adventure of discovering new plant-based recipes. Cooking at home allows you to control the ingredients and explore the diversity of flavors that whole, plant-based foods offer.

Mindful Eating: Pay attention to the food you eat, savor each bite, and listen to your body's hunger and fullness cues. Mindful eating can enhance the enjoyment of whole foods and help you tune into your body's nutritional needs.

The shift towards whole foods and plant-based ingredients is more than a dietary change; it's a lifestyle transformation that promotes holistic health, sustainability, and a deeper connection to the natural world. By prioritizing these elements in your diet, you embark on a journey towards a more vibrant, healthful, and conscientious way of living.

Chapter 4: Hydration: Understanding Its Critical Role in Health

Water, the most basic yet essential element of life, plays a pivotal role in maintaining our health and well-being. Despite its crucial importance, hydration is often overlooked in discussions about nutrition and health. This chapter explores the multifaceted role of hydration in the body, underscoring its impact on physical functions, mental performance, and overall health. Understanding and prioritizing proper hydration can significantly enhance your quality of life and support your body's natural healing processes.

The Fundamental Role of Water in the Body

Water constitutes about 60% of the adult human body and is a key component of every cell, tissue, and organ. It serves numerous vital functions, including:

- **Nutrient Transport:** Water is essential for transporting nutrients and oxygen to cells, facilitating the absorption of vitamins, minerals, and other essential nutrients.

- **Temperature Regulation:** Through the process of perspiration and evaporation, water helps maintain the body's temperature within a narrow, healthy range.

- **Detoxification:** Water aids in the removal of waste products and toxins from the body through urination, perspiration, and bowel movements.

- **Lubrication and Cushioning:** Water acts as a lubricant for joints and helps protect sensitive tissues and organs in the body, including the brain, spinal cord, and fetus during pregnancy.

- **Digestive Health:** Adequate hydration is critical for proper digestion. It helps break down food, absorb nutrients, and prevent constipation.

Recognizing the Signs of Dehydration

Dehydration occurs when you use or lose more fluid than you take in, and your body doesn't have enough water to carry out its normal functions. Recognizing the early signs of dehydration is essential for preventing its adverse effects. Symptoms include:

- Thirst

- Dry mouth, lips, and eyes

- Reduced urine output, often with a darker color

- Fatigue and weakness

- Headache

- Dizziness or lightheadedness

Chronic dehydration can lead to more severe health issues, such as urinary tract infections, kidney stones, and even kidney failure. It can also impair cognitive functions, reducing concentration, alertness, and short-term memory.

How Much Water Do You Need?

Hydration needs can vary greatly depending on factors such as age, weight, climate, physical activity levels, and health status. While the "8x8 rule" — drinking eight 8-ounce glasses of water a day — is a good general guideline, your individual needs may vary. Listening to your body and drinking when you feel thirsty is generally an adequate measure for most healthy individuals. However, during intense exercise, in hot climates, or if you're pregnant or breastfeeding, your needs increase.

Enhancing Hydration Through Foods

While drinking water is the most direct way to hydrate, many foods, particularly fruits and vegetables, can also significantly contribute to your daily water intake. Foods like cucumbers, celery, watermelon, oranges, and strawberries are over 90% water by weight. Incorporating these foods into your diet can help maintain hydration and provide a rich source of vitamins, minerals, and antioxidants.

Strategies for Staying Hydrated

- **Start Your Day with Water:** Drinking a glass of water first thing in the morning is a great way to kickstart your hydration for the day.

- **Carry a Water Bottle:** Having water on hand at all times makes it easier to drink throughout the day.

- **Set Reminders:** In today's busy world, it's easy to forget to drink water. Setting reminders on your phone or computer can help maintain consistent hydration.

- **Flavor Your Water:** If you find plain water unappealing, adding a slice of lemon, lime, cucumber, or a few berries can enhance the taste, making it more enjoyable to drink.

Hydration is a foundational aspect of health that supports every cellular and systemic function in the body. By understanding its critical role and adopting strategies to ensure adequate fluid intake, you can significantly enhance your health, vitality, and well-being.

Chapter 5: The Significance of Organic and Non-GMO Foods

I n the quest for optimal health and nutrition, the quality and source of the foods we consume are of paramount importance. The growing awareness and concern over the impact of agricultural practices on food quality, environmental sustainability, and health have brought organic and non-GMO (Genetically Modified Organism) foods to the forefront of nutritional consciousness. This chapter explores the significance of these foods within the context of a healing diet, shedding light on their benefits and considerations for individuals aiming to nourish their bodies in the most healthful way possible.

Understanding Organic Foods

What Makes Food Organic?

Organic food refers to produce and other ingredients that are grown without the use of synthetic pesticides, fertilizers, genetically modified organisms, antibiotics, or growth hormones. The organic certification process, governed by strict national and international standards, ensures that farmers and producers adhere to practices that promote ecological balance, conserve biodiversity, and minimize pollution and waste.

Health Benefits of Organic Foods

- **Reduced Exposure to Pesticides:** Organic foods have significantly lower pesticide residues compared to conventionally grown produce. Pesticides have been linked to a range of health issues, including neurological effects, hormone disruption, and increased risk of certain cancers.

- **Higher Nutritional Content:** Some studies suggest that organic foods may have higher levels of certain nutrients, including antioxidants. Antioxidants play a critical role in protecting the body from oxidative stress and inflammation.

- **Antibiotic Resistance:** Organic animal products come from animals that are not given antibiotics or growth hormones. Consuming these products helps combat antibiotic resistance, a growing public health concern.

The Role of Non-GMO Foods

Genetic Modification Explained

GMOs are organisms whose genetic material has been artificially manipulated in a laboratory through genetic engineering. This technology creates combinations of plant, animal, bacteria, and virus genes that do not occur in nature or through traditional crossbreeding methods.

Why Choose Non-GMO?

- **Health and Safety Concerns:** While the long-term health impacts of GMOs are still under study, many consumers choose non-GMO foods to avoid potential risks. Concerns include allergies, antibiotic resistance, and the unknown effects of long-term consumption of genetically modified foods.

- **Environmental Impact:** GMO crops often require the use of specific pesticides and herbicides, some of which have been linked to environmental degradation, such as loss of biodiversity and the development of pesticide-resistant weeds.

Integrating Organic and Non-GMO Foods into Your Diet

Reading Labels: Learn to identify labels that indicate organic and non-GMO certifications. In many countries, organic foods carry a certification seal, and non-GMO products are often labeled as such.

Prioritizing Purchases: If budget constraints make it challenging to buy everything organic, prioritize according to your consumption patterns and the Environmental Working Group's (EWG) "Dirty Dozen" and "Clean Fifteen" lists, which identify produce with the highest and lowest pesticide residues.

Local and Seasonal Eating: Purchasing organic and non-GMO foods from local farmers' markets not only supports local agriculture but also ensures that you're getting fresh, nutrient-dense foods. Eating seasonally is also more sustainable and can be more cost-effective.

Growing Your Own: Starting a garden, even a small one, can be a rewarding way to ensure you have access to fresh, organic produce. Herbs, tomatoes, and leafy greens are among the easiest foods to grow, even in limited spaces.

The decision to incorporate organic and non-GMO foods into your diet is a personal yet impactful choice that can contribute to your health, the well-being of the planet, and the promotion of sustainable agricultural practices. By making informed choices about the foods we consume, we can support our health and the health of our environment.

Chapter 6: Combating Common Ailments with Specific Nutrients

The adage "Let food be thy medicine and medicine be thy food" underscores the intrinsic power of nutrition to combat various ailments. By understanding and leveraging the specific nutrients that target common health issues, we can significantly enhance our body's ability to heal and maintain optimal health. This chapter delves into how certain nutrients can play a pivotal role in preventing and managing common ailments, offering a natural pathway to bolster health and well-being.

Nutrients for Heart Health

Omega-3 Fatty Acids: Found abundantly in fatty fish (like salmon, mackerel, and sardines), flaxseeds, chia seeds, and walnuts, omega-3 fatty acids are crucial for heart health. They help reduce inflammation, lower blood pressure, decrease triglycerides, and reduce the risk of heart disease.

Fiber: Soluble fiber, found in oats, legumes, apples, and pears, can help lower cholesterol levels by binding to cholesterol in the digestive system and removing it from the body. This, in turn, helps reduce the risk of heart disease.

Nutrients for Bone Health

Calcium and Vitamin D: These nutrients work in tandem to promote bone health. Calcium supports bone structure, while vitamin D enhances calcium absorption. Dairy products, fortified plant milks, leafy green vegetables, and sunlight exposure are vital sources of these nutrients.

Magnesium and Vitamin K: Magnesium, found in nuts, seeds, whole grains, and green leafy vegetables, is crucial for bone health. Vitamin K, found in green leafy vegetables, fish, meat, and eggs, is essential for bone mineralization.

Nutrients for Immune Support

Vitamin C: A potent antioxidant found in citrus fruits, strawberries, bell peppers, and broccoli, vitamin C supports the immune system by stimulating the production of white blood cells, which help protect the body against infection.

Zinc: This mineral, found in meat, shellfish, legumes, seeds, and nuts, is crucial for immune function and wound healing. Zinc helps the immune system fight off invading bacteria and viruses.

Nutrients for Digestive Health

Probiotics: These beneficial bacteria, found in fermented foods like yogurt, kefir, sauerkraut, and kimchi, help maintain the health of the gut microbiome, which is vital for digestion, nutrient absorption, and immune function.

Prebiotics: Prebiotic fibers feed the beneficial bacteria in the gut. They are found in foods like bananas, onions, garlic, leeks, asparagus, and whole grains.

Nutrients for Mental Health

B Vitamins: Particularly B12 (found in animal products and fortified foods) and folate (found in green leafy vegetables, legumes, and fortified grains), these vitamins play critical roles in brain health and the production of neurotransmitters responsible for mood regulation.

Omega-3 Fatty Acids: Besides their benefits for heart health, omega-3 fatty acids are also crucial for brain health. They can improve mood, cognitive function, and protect against age-related mental decline.

Implementing Nutrient-Focused Strategies

- **Diverse Diet:** Incorporating a wide variety of foods into your diet ensures you receive a broad spectrum of nutrients to support overall health and combat specific ailments.

- **Supplementation:** In some cases, supplements may be necessary to meet specific nutrient needs, especially for nutrients like vitamin D and B12. However, it's best to consult with a healthcare provider before starting any supplementation.

- **Lifestyle Factors:** Alongside nutrition, other lifestyle factors such as physical activity, adequate sleep, stress management, and avoiding harmful substances play a crucial role in preventing and managing health issues.

By prioritizing these nutrients in your diet, you can create a powerful, natural toolkit for combating common ailments and enhancing your health. Remember, while food can significantly impact health, it's also essential to consult with healthcare professionals for personalized advice and treatment for specific health conditions.

Chapter 7: The Importance of a Balanced pH: Alkaline vs. Acidic Foods

The concept of balancing the body's pH through diet has gained attention in the realm of nutrition and holistic health. The pH scale, which runs from 0 to 14, measures how acidic or alkaline a substance is. Pure water is neutral, at a pH of 7; substances with a pH less than 7 are considered acidic, while those with a pH greater than 7 are alkaline. The human body meticulously maintains the pH of its blood at around 7.4, slightly alkaline, a critical factor for overall health. This chapter explores the significance of dietary choices in influencing the body's pH balance and the impact of acidic and alkaline foods on health and well-being.

Understanding Body pH and Health

The body's ability to maintain its blood pH within a tight range is vital for supporting essential functions. Enzymes that catalyze life-sustaining chemical reactions have optimal pH levels at which they function best. Deviations from the ideal pH can disrupt these processes, affecting health adversely.

While the body has robust mechanisms to maintain pH balance, including the respiratory system and kidneys, diet plays a role in influencing the body's overall pH balance. The modern diet, rich in processed foods, meat, and refined grains, tends to be more acidic, which can challenge the body's regulatory systems.

Alkaline vs. Acidic Foods

Acidic Foods: Foods considered to be acidic include meat, poultry, fish, dairy products, eggs, grains, and alcohol. While these foods can be part of a healthy diet, the concern arises when they dominate our food intake, potentially burdening the body's pH-regulating mechanisms.

Alkaline Foods: Alkaline-promoting foods include most fruits and vegetables, nuts, and legumes. These foods contribute to an alkaline load in the body, supporting its natural pH balance.

The Potential Benefits of an Alkaline Diet

Enhanced Bone Health: Some research suggests that an alkaline diet may benefit bone health by reducing the loss of calcium in urine and promoting the preservation of bone mass.

Improved Muscle Mass: Older adults eating more alkaline diets have been shown to have improved muscle mass. This is possibly due to the diet's impact on growth hormone levels and the reduction of muscle wasting.

Chronic Disease Prevention: There is ongoing research into the alkaline diet's potential to lower the risk of chronic diseases, including hypertension and stroke, through its effects on reducing inflammation and improving cardiovascular health.

Implementing a pH-Balanced Diet

Increase Intake of Fruits and Vegetables: Aim to fill half your plate with a variety of fruits and vegetables at each meal. These foods not only support alkalinity but also provide essential vitamins, minerals, and fiber.

Moderate Consumption of Acid-Producing Foods: While not needing to be eliminated, acidic foods such as meat and dairy should be consumed in moderation. Balance these with alkaline foods to maintain dietary equilibrium.

Choose Whole, Unprocessed Foods: Minimizing the intake of highly processed foods, which can contribute to acidity, supports not only pH balance but overall health.

Hydration: Drinking plenty of water can help flush the system and support the body's natural pH-regulating mechanisms.

Considerations and Balance

While the concept of balancing dietary pH holds potential health benefits, it's crucial to approach it with balance and flexibility. The human body is adept at managing pH balance, and drastic dietary changes are generally not required for healthy individuals. Instead, focusing on a diet rich in whole, nutrient-dense foods, predominantly plants, can naturally support the body's pH balance and overall health.

Embracing a diet that supports a healthy pH balance is about more than just alkalinity; it's about fostering a holistic approach to eating that emphasizes the quality and variety of foods. By making informed choices, we can support our body's natural mechanisms, promoting health, vitality, and well-being.

Chapter 8: Integrating Superfoods into Daily Meals

The term "superfoods" refers to nutrient-rich foods considered especially beneficial for health and well-being. While no official scientific definition of a superfood exists, these foods are typically loaded with antioxidants, vitamins, and minerals that can help ward off diseases, improve energy levels, and enhance overall health. This chapter explores practical ways to incorporate a variety of these powerful foods into your daily meals, making it easier to reap their health benefits without drastically altering your diet.

Understanding Superfoods

Superfoods span a diverse range of edible items, from leafy greens and berries to nuts, seeds, and ancient grains. Each comes with its unique profile of health-promoting properties. For instance, berries are known for their high antioxidant content, which can protect the body from oxidative stress and inflammation. Leafy greens, like spinach and kale, are rich in vitamins A, C, E, and K, as well as calcium and several phytochemicals.

Breakfast

Start Your Day with a Superfood Smoothie: A smoothie made with spinach or kale, mixed berries, a banana for sweetness, and a tablespoon of flaxseed or chia seeds can deliver a potent nutrient kick. Add a scoop of protein powder or a handful of nuts for extra protein.

Superfood Toppings on Oatmeal or Yogurt: Enhance your morning oatmeal or yogurt with a sprinkle of chia seeds, hemp seeds, or ground flaxseeds. Top with fresh berries, sliced bananas, and a drizzle of honey for additional superfood benefits and flavor.

Lunch

Super Salad: Create a base of mixed leafy greens (spinach, kale, arugula) and top with slices of avocado, a handful of nuts (walnuts, almonds), and some quinoa or chickpeas for protein. Dress with olive oil and lemon juice for an extra antioxidant boost.

Wrap It Up: Use whole grain or spinach wraps and fill them with a combination of grilled vegetables, hummus, a sprinkle of seeds (pumpkin, sunflower), and fresh greens for a nutrient-dense meal.

Dinner

Incorporate Ancient Grains: Swap out white rice or pasta with ancient grains like quinoa, farro, or barley. These grains offer higher protein content and a rich array of nutrients. Serve as a side dish or incorporate into salads, soups, and stews.

Add Superfoods to Soups and Stews: Lentil or bean-based soups and stews can be easily enhanced with superfoods. Add kale, spinach, or Swiss chard in the last few minutes of cooking to preserve their nutrients. Sprinkle some turmeric for its anti-inflammatory properties.

Snacks

Nuts and Seeds: A handful of almonds, walnuts, or pumpkin seeds makes for a nutritious snack that's easy to eat on the go. These are high in healthy fats, fiber, and protein, helping to keep you full and energized.

Berries and Fruits: Keep fresh or dried berries and other fruits like apples and oranges handy for a quick, nutrient-packed snack. Pair with a small serving of cottage cheese or Greek yogurt for added protein.

Beverages

Green Tea: Replace your afternoon coffee with a cup of green tea. It's rich in antioxidants, including catechins, which have been linked to various health benefits, including reduced inflammation and improved brain function.

Water with Lemon or Berries: Enhance your water by adding slices of lemon or a few berries. This not only improves taste but adds a nutritional punch.

Integrating Superfoods Seamlessly

- **Think Variety:** No single food holds the key to good health. A varied diet ensures a broad spectrum of nutrients and benefits.

- **Make It a Habit:** Incorporate superfoods into meals and snacks you already enjoy to make them a regular part of your diet.

- **Prep Ahead:** Prepare superfood snacks and meal components in advance to make healthy choices easy and convenient throughout the week.

By integrating superfoods into your daily meals, you can enjoy a diet that's not only rich in essential nutrients but also varied and delicious. The key is to start with small changes and gradually incorporate more superfoods into your diet, allowing you to experience their health benefits without feeling overwhelmed by major dietary overhauls.

Chapter 9: Simplifying Meal Planning for Busy Lives

In today's fast-paced world, maintaining a healthy diet can seem like a daunting task, especially for those with demanding schedules. However, with a bit of organization and some simple strategies, it's entirely possible to enjoy nutritious and delicious meals without spending hours in the kitchen. This chapter is dedicated to simplifying meal planning for busy lives, offering practical tips and tricks to streamline the process, reduce stress, and ensure you can enjoy healthy meals throughout the week.

Embrace the Power of Planning

Weekly Meal Planning: Dedicate a small amount of time each week to plan your meals. This doesn't have to be complicated. Start by listing meals for the week ahead, considering breakfast, lunch, dinner, and snacks. This plan will serve as your roadmap, saving you time on decision-making throughout the week and making grocery shopping more efficient.

Create a Master Grocery List: Based on your meal plan, create a comprehensive grocery list, categorizing items by department (produce, dairy, pantry staples) to make your shopping trip quicker and more organized.

Simplify with Theme Nights

To make meal planning even easier, consider setting theme nights each week, such as Meatless Monday, Taco Tuesday, or Stir-Fry Friday. Themes not only make planning more straightforward but also add variety to your meals, ensuring you and your family stay excited about dinner time.

Batch Cooking and Prep

Cook Once, Eat Multiple Times: Prepare larger batches of staples like grains, proteins, and vegetables at the start of the week. For instance, cooking a big batch of quinoa, roasting a tray of mixed vegetables, and grilling chicken breasts can provide versatile ingredients that can be mixed and matched to create different meals throughout the week.

Prep Ingredients in Advance: Washing and chopping vegetables, marinating proteins, and portioning out snacks on the weekend can save a significant amount of time during the week. Store these prepped ingredients in clear containers in the refrigerator for easy access.

Embrace Freezer-Friendly Meals

Prepare meals that freeze well, such as soups, stews, casseroles, and meatballs. Doubling a recipe and freezing half for a future date is an excellent way to ensure you have healthy meals on hand for busy nights, reducing the temptation to order takeout.

Quick and Healthy Meal Ideas

Stock your pantry, fridge, and freezer with quick-cooking and healthy staples, such as canned beans, frozen vegetables, eggs, whole grain pasta, and pre-cooked grains. These ingredients can be turned into meals in less than 30 minutes. Examples include stir-fries, omelets, pasta dishes, and hearty salads.

Utilize Technology

Meal Planning Apps and Tools: Numerous apps and online tools can streamline the meal planning process, from generating meal ideas based on what you have in your pantry to creating grocery lists and meal plans.

Online Grocery Shopping: If time is tight, consider using online grocery shopping services. Many offer the option to save your shopping list, making it quick and easy to reorder staples each week.

Learn to Love Leftovers

View leftovers as a bonus meal rather than a chore. Many meals can be repurposed in creative ways, turning last night's dinner into today's lunch. For example, roasted vegetables can become a filling for omelets or wraps, and grilled chicken can be sliced into salads or sandwiches.

Sharing the Responsibility

If possible, share the meal planning and preparation responsibilities with family members or roommates. Even young children can help with simple tasks, making mealtime a shared effort that reduces the burden on any one person.

Simplifying meal planning for busy lives is about finding strategies that work for your unique schedule and preferences. By incorporating these tips, you can ensure that eating healthily doesn't become another source of stress but rather a seamless and enjoyable part of your daily routine.

Chapter 10: Energizing Breakfasts Recipes

Almond Butter and Banana Oatmeal

- **Preparation Time:** 5 minutes
- **Cooking Time:** 10 minutes
- **Servings:** 2

Ingredients:

- 1 cup rolled oats
- 2 cups almond milk (or water)
- 1 ripe banana, sliced
- 2 tablespoons almond butter
- 1 teaspoon cinnamon
- 1 tablespoon chia seeds (optional for added texture and nutrients)
- A drizzle of honey or maple syrup (optional)

Procedure:

1. In a medium saucepan, bring the almond milk to a boil. Add the rolled oats and cinnamon, reduce the heat, and simmer for about 10 minutes, stirring occasionally until the oats are soft and the mixture has thickened.
2. Remove from heat. Stir in the almond butter and chia seeds until well combined.
3. Divide the oatmeal into bowls. Top each serving with sliced banana and a drizzle of honey or maple syrup, if desired.
4. Serve warm and enjoy the comforting and nutritious breakfast.

Macronutrients (per serving):

- **Calories:** 385 kcal
- **Carbohydrates:** 54 g
- **Protein:** 12 g
- **Fat:** 14 g

Vitamins:

- High in Vitamin E from almond butter
- Rich in Potassium and Vitamin C from bananas

Apple Cinnamon Quinoa Porridge

- **Preparation Time:** 5 minutes
- **Cooking Time:** 20 minutes
- **Servings:** 2

Ingredients:

- 1 cup quinoa, rinsed
- 2 cups almond milk
- 1 large apple, diced
- 2 teaspoons cinnamon
- 1 tablespoon maple syrup (optional)
- 1/4 cup walnuts, chopped (for topping)
- 1 tablespoon flaxseeds (for topping)

Procedure:

1. Combine quinoa, almond milk, diced apple, and cinnamon in a medium saucepan. Bring the mixture to a boil over medium heat.
2. Reduce the heat to low, cover, and simmer for 15-20 minutes, or until the quinoa is cooked through and has absorbed most of the liquid. Stir occasionally to prevent sticking.
3. Once the quinoa is cooked and creamy, remove from heat. Stir in maple syrup for added sweetness if desired.
4. Serve hot, garnished with chopped walnuts and flaxseeds for added texture and nutrients.

Macronutrients (per serving):

- **Calories:** 380 kcal
- **Carbohydrates:** 58 g
- **Protein:** 12 g
- **Fat:** 12 g

Vitamins:

- Rich in Vitamin E and Omega-3 fatty acids from flaxseeds
- Good source of Vitamin B6 and C from apples

Avocado Toast on Sprouted Grain Bread

- **Preparation Time:** 5 minutes
- **Cooking Time:** 2 minutes
- **Servings:** 2

Ingredients:

- 2 slices of sprouted grain bread
- 1 ripe avocado
- Juice of 1/2 a lemon
- Pinch of salt and pepper
- Red pepper flakes (optional for a spicy kick)
- 2 teaspoons of chia seeds (for garnish)

Procedure:

1. Toast the sprouted grain bread slices to your desired crispiness in a toaster or on a skillet over medium heat.
2. In a bowl, mash the ripe avocado with the lemon juice, salt, and pepper until you achieve a creamy, yet slightly chunky consistency.
3. Spread the mashed avocado evenly over the toasted sprouted grain bread. Adjust seasoning to taste, if necessary.
4. Sprinkle with red pepper flakes (if using) and chia seeds for an added crunch and nutrient boost. Serve immediately.

Macronutrients (per serving):

- **Calories:** 300 kcal
- **Carbohydrates:** 30 g
- **Protein:** 9 g
- **Fat:** 17 g

Vitamins:

- High in Vitamin C from lemon juice
- Rich in Omega-3 fatty acids from chia seeds
- Contains Vitamins E, K, and B6 from avocado

Berry Spinach Smoothie Bowl

- **Preparation Time:** 10 minutes
- **Cooking Time:** 0 minutes
- **Servings:** 2

Ingredients:

- 2 cups fresh spinach
- 1 cup frozen mixed berries (blueberries, strawberries, raspberries)
- 1 banana, sliced
- 1/2 cup unsweetened almond milk
- 1 tablespoon chia seeds
- 1 tablespoon flaxseeds
- Toppings: Sliced banana, a handful of fresh berries, and a sprinkle of granola

Procedure:

1. In a blender, combine the spinach, frozen mixed berries, banana, almond milk, chia seeds, and flaxseeds. Blend until smooth and creamy, adjusting the almond milk as needed to reach your desired consistency.
2. Pour the smoothie mixture into two bowls.
3. Decorate the tops of your smoothie bowls with the additional sliced banana, fresh berries, and a sprinkle of granola for added texture and flavor.
4. Serve immediately and enjoy the burst of energy and flavors.

Macronutrients (per serving):

- **Calories:** 290 kcal
- **Carbohydrates:** 45 g
- **Protein:** 8 g
- **Fat:** 9 g

Vitamins:

- High in Vitamin C and antioxidants from berries
- Rich in Vitamin K, A, and iron from spinach
- Omega-3 fatty acids from flaxseeds

Chia Seed Pudding with Kiwi

- **Preparation Time:** 5 minutes (plus at least 4 hours for chilling)
- **Cooking Time:** 0 minutes
- **Servings:** 2

Ingredients:

- 1/4 cup chia seeds
- 1 cup unsweetened almond milk
- 2 kiwis, peeled and sliced
- 1 tablespoon honey or maple syrup (optional for sweetness)
- A pinch of vanilla extract (optional)

Procedure:

1. In a medium bowl, mix the chia seeds and almond milk together. Add the honey (or maple syrup) and vanilla extract if using. Stir well to combine.
2. Cover the bowl with a lid or plastic wrap and refrigerate for at least 4 hours, or overnight, until the pudding achieves a thick and gelatinous consistency.
3. Once set, give the chia pudding a good stir to break up any clumps. If the pudding is too thick, you can add a little more almond milk to adjust the consistency.
4. Divide the pudding into serving bowls or glasses and top with sliced kiwi. Serve chilled.

Macronutrients (per serving):

- **Calories:** 200 kcal
- **Carbohydrates:** 30 g
- **Protein:** 5 g
- **Fat:** 8 g

Vitamins:

- High in Vitamin C and dietary fiber from kiwi
- Rich in Omega-3 fatty acids and Calcium from chia seeds

Coconut Yogurt Parfait with Mango

- **Preparation Time:** 10 minutes
- **Cooking Time:** 0 minutes
- **Servings:** 2

Ingredients:

- 1 cup coconut yogurt
- 1 large mango, peeled and diced
- 1/4 cup granola
- 2 tablespoons shredded coconut
- 2 teaspoons honey or maple syrup (optional)

Procedure:

1. Start by preparing your serving glasses or bowls. Spoon a layer of coconut yogurt at the bottom.
2. Add a layer of diced mango over the yogurt. If you're using honey or maple syrup, drizzle a little over the mango.
3. Sprinkle a layer of granola over the mango, and then add another layer of coconut yogurt.
4. Finish off with a final layer of diced mango and a sprinkle of shredded coconut on top.

Macronutrients (per serving):

- **Calories:** 250 kcal
- **Carbohydrates:** 35 g
- **Protein:** 5 g
- **Fat:** 11 g

Vitamins:

- High in Vitamin C and Vitamin A from mango
- Rich in probiotics and Calcium from coconut yogurt

Energizing Green Juice

- **Preparation Time:** 10 minutes
- **Cooking Time:** 0 minutes
- **Servings:** 2

Ingredients:

- 2 cups spinach
- 1 large cucumber
- 2 green apples, cored and sliced
- 1/2 lemon, peeled
- 1 inch piece of ginger, peeled
- 1 stalk of celery

Procedure:

1. Thoroughly wash all the vegetables and fruits under running water. Chop the cucumber, apples, and celery into pieces small enough to fit through your juicer's feed chute.
2. Start your juicer and begin juicing the spinach, cucumber, celery, green apples, lemon, and ginger, in that order. The soft leaves of spinach benefit from being pressed by the firmer fruits and vegetables that follow.
3. Once all the ingredients have been juiced, stir the juice to combine the flavors evenly.
4. Pour the green juice into two glasses and serve immediately to enjoy the maximum nutritional benefits.

Macronutrients (per serving):

- **Calories:** 120 kcal
- **Carbohydrates:** 30 g
- **Protein:** 2 g
- **Fat:** 0.5 g

Vitamins:

- High in Vitamin C from lemon and apples
- Rich in Vitamin K, A, and iron from spinach
- Contains potassium from cucumber and celery

Flaxseed Pancakes with Blueberry Compote

- **Preparation Time:** 15 minutes
- **Cooking Time:** 20 minutes
- **Servings:** 2

Ingredients:

For the Pancakes:

- 1 cup whole wheat flour
- 2 tablespoons ground flaxseed
- 1 tablespoon baking powder
- 1/4 teaspoon salt
- 1 cup almond milk
- 1 egg (or flax egg for a vegan option: 1 tablespoon ground flaxseed mixed with 3 tablespoons water)
- 2 tablespoons maple syrup
- 1 teaspoon vanilla extract
- Cooking spray or coconut oil (for cooking)

For the Blueberry Compote:

- 1 cup fresh or frozen blueberries
- 2 tablespoons water
- 2 tablespoons maple syrup
- 1 teaspoon lemon juice

Procedure:

1. **Make the Pancake Batter:** In a large bowl, whisk together the whole wheat flour, ground flaxseed, baking powder, and salt. In another bowl, mix the almond milk, egg, maple syrup, and vanilla extract. Combine the wet ingredients with the dry ingredients and stir until just mixed.
2. **Cook the Pancakes:** Heat a non-stick skillet or griddle over medium heat and lightly grease with cooking spray or coconut oil. Pour 1/4 cup of batter for each pancake onto the skillet. Cook until bubbles form on the surface, then flip and cook until golden brown on the other side. Repeat with the remaining batter.
3. **Prepare the Blueberry Compote:** While the pancakes are cooking, combine blueberries, water, maple syrup, and lemon juice in a small saucepan. Bring to a simmer over medium heat, then reduce the heat and cook until the blueberries have burst and the sauce has thickened, about 10 minutes.

4. **Serve:** Stack the pancakes and top with the warm blueberry compote. Serve immediately.

Macronutrients (per serving):
- **Calories:** 425 kcal
- **Carbohydrates:** 75 g
- **Protein:** 12 g
- **Fat:** 9 g

Vitamins:
- High in Omega-3 fatty acids and fiber from flaxseed
- Rich in Vitamin C and antioxidants from blueberries
- Contains iron and calcium from whole wheat flour and almond milk

Golden Turmeric Latte

- **Preparation Time:** 5 minutes
- **Cooking Time:** 5 minutes
- **Servings:** 2

Ingredients:
- 2 cups almond milk
- 1 teaspoon turmeric powder
- 1/2 teaspoon cinnamon
- 1/4 teaspoon ginger powder
- 1 tablespoon honey or maple syrup (adjust to taste)
- Pinch of black pepper (to enhance turmeric absorption)
- 1 teaspoon vanilla extract

Procedure:
1. **Warm the Milk:** In a small saucepan, heat the almond milk over medium heat until it is just simmering.
2. **Add Spices and Sweetener:** Whisk in the turmeric, cinnamon, ginger powder, honey (or maple syrup), and a pinch of black pepper. Continue to heat for another minute, making sure not to let it boil.
3. **Final Touch:** Remove from heat and stir in the vanilla extract.
4. **Serve:** Divide the latte between two mugs, using a frother if you prefer a foamier texture. Serve warm and enjoy the comforting glow.

Macronutrients (per serving):
- **Calories:** 100 kcal
- **Carbohydrates:** 18 g
- **Protein:** 2 g
- **Fat:** 2.5 g

Vitamins:
- Rich in curcumin from turmeric, offering anti-inflammatory benefits.
- Contains calcium and vitamin E from almond milk.

Kale and Mushroom Tofu Scramble

- **Preparation Time:** 10 minutes
- **Cooking Time:** 15 minutes
- **Servings:** 2

Ingredients:

- 1 block (14 oz) firm tofu, pressed and crumbled
- 2 cups kale, chopped
- 1 cup mushrooms, sliced
- 1/2 onion, diced
- 2 cloves garlic, minced
- 1 tablespoon nutritional yeast
- 1/2 teaspoon turmeric
- 1 tablespoon soy sauce or tamari
- 2 tablespoons olive oil
- Salt and pepper to taste

Procedure:

1. **Sauté Vegetables:** Heat the olive oil in a large skillet over medium heat. Add the onion and garlic, sautéing until soft and translucent. Add the mushrooms and cook until they begin to release their moisture and brown slightly.
2. **Add Kale:** Stir in the kale and continue to cook until it starts to wilt, about 3-5 minutes.
3. **Tofu and Seasonings:** Add the crumbled tofu to the skillet along with the turmeric, nutritional yeast, and soy sauce. Cook, stirring frequently, for about 5-7 minutes or until the tofu is heated through and begins to get slightly crispy on the edges. Season with salt and pepper to taste.
4. **Serve:** Divide the scramble between two plates. Enjoy as is or serve with toasted whole grain bread or avocado slices for added flavor and nutrients.

Macronutrients (per serving):

- **Calories:** 330 kcal
- **Carbohydrates:** 15 g
- **Protein:** 25 g
- **Fat:** 20 g

Vitamins:

- High in Vitamin A and C from kale
- Contains calcium, iron, and magnesium from tofu
- Rich in B vitamins from nutritional yeast

Nutty Banana Smoothie

- **Preparation Time:** 5 minutes
- **Cooking Time:** 0 minutes
- **Servings:** 2

Ingredients:

- 2 ripe bananas
- 2 tablespoons almond butter
- 2 cups almond milk
- 1 tablespoon chia seeds
- 1 tablespoon flaxseed meal
- A pinch of cinnamon (optional)
- Ice cubes (optional)

Procedure:

1. **Prepare Ingredients:** Peel the bananas and place them in the blender. Add the almond butter, almond milk, chia seeds, flaxseed meal, and cinnamon if using.
2. **Blend:** Add a handful of ice cubes to the blender if you prefer a colder smoothie. Blend all the ingredients on high until smooth and creamy.
3. **Adjust Consistency:** If the smoothie is too thick, you can add more almond milk to reach your desired consistency. Blend again briefly after any additions.
4. **Serve:** Pour the smoothie into two glasses and enjoy immediately for the freshest taste and maximum nutritional benefits.

Macronutrients (per serving):

- **Calories:** 330 kcal
- **Carbohydrates:** 44 g
- **Protein:** 10 g
- **Fat:** 15 g

Vitamins:

- High in Vitamin E and magnesium from almond butter
- Rich in Omega-3 fatty acids from chia seeds and flaxseed meal
- Good source of Potassium from bananas

Nutty Banana Smoothie

- **Preparation Time:** 5 minutes
- **Cooking Time:** 0 minutes
- **Servings:** 2

Ingredients:

- 2 ripe bananas
- 2 tablespoons of your preferred nut butter (e.g., almond or peanut butter)
- 2 cups unsweetened almond milk
- 2 tablespoons chia seeds
- Ice cubes (optional, adjust to preference)

Procedure:

1. **Blend Smoothie Base:** In a high-speed blender, combine the ripe bananas, nut butter, almond milk, and chia seeds. Add ice cubes if you prefer a chilled smoothie.
2. **Process Until Smooth:** Blend on high until the mixture reaches a smooth and creamy consistency, ensuring no chunks remain.
3. **Adjust Thickness:** If the smoothie is too thick, add a bit more almond milk and blend again. For added sweetness, consider blending in a touch more banana or a drizzle of honey.
4. **Serve Immediately:** Pour the smoothie into glasses, garnishing with a sprinkle of chia seeds or a slice of banana if desired. Enjoy immediately for the best texture and flavor.

Macronutrients (per serving):

- **Calories:** 345 kcal
- **Carbohydrates:** 42 g
- **Protein:** 10 g
- **Fat:** 18 g

Vitamins:

- High in Potassium and Vitamin C from bananas.
- Rich in Vitamin E and Magnesium from nut butter.
- Chia seeds contribute significant amounts of Omega-3 fatty acids and Calcium.

Oatmeal with Pumpkin Seeds and Pears

- **Preparation Time:** 5 minutes
- **Cooking Time:** 10 minutes
- **Servings:** 2

Ingredients:

- 1 cup rolled oats
- 2 cups water or almond milk
- 1 ripe pear, diced
- 1/4 cup pumpkin seeds
- 1 tablespoon honey or maple syrup (optional)
- 1/2 teaspoon cinnamon
- Pinch of salt

Procedure:

1. **Cook the Oats:** In a medium saucepan, bring the water or almond milk to a boil. Add the rolled oats and a pinch of salt, then reduce the heat to low. Simmer, stirring occasionally, until the oats are soft and have absorbed the liquid, about 5 minutes.
2. **Add Flavors:** Stir in the cinnamon and half of the diced pear, cooking for another 2 minutes. The pear will soften slightly and infuse the oatmeal with its sweet flavor.
3. **Sweeten if Desired:** Remove from heat and stir in honey or maple syrup if using, adjusting according to taste.
4. **Serve with Toppings:** Divide the oatmeal between two bowls. Top with the remaining diced pear and sprinkle with pumpkin seeds.

Macronutrients (per serving):

- **Calories:** 290 kcal
- **Carbohydrates:** 45 g
- **Protein:** 10 g
- **Fat:** 8 g

Vitamins:

- High in Vitamin C and fiber from pears.
- Contains Zinc, Magnesium, and other minerals from pumpkin seeds.
- Oats are a good source of B vitamins and iron.

Overnight Oats with Almond Butter and Raspberry

- **Preparation Time:** 10 minutes (plus overnight soaking)
- **Cooking Time:** 0 minutes
- **Servings:** 2

Ingredients:

- 1 cup rolled oats
- 1.5 cups unsweetened almond milk
- 2 tablespoons almond butter
- 1 cup fresh raspberries (plus more for topping)
- 2 tablespoons chia seeds
- 1 tablespoon maple syrup (adjust to taste)
- 1/2 teaspoon vanilla extract

Procedure:

1. **Mix Ingredients:** In a medium bowl, combine rolled oats, almond milk, chia seeds, almond butter, maple syrup, and vanilla extract. Stir well to ensure all ingredients are fully mixed.
2. **Add Raspberries:** Gently fold in the raspberries, being careful not to crush them too much.
3. **Refrigerate Overnight:** Divide the mixture between two mason jars or sealed containers. Place in the refrigerator overnight, allowing the oats to soak and all the flavors to meld together.
4. **Serve:** The next morning, give the oats a good stir. If the mixture is too thick, adjust the consistency by adding a little more almond milk. Top with additional raspberries and a dollop of almond butter before serving.

Macronutrients (per serving):

- **Calories:** 350 kcal
- **Carbohydrates:** 45 g
- **Protein:** 10 g
- **Fat:** 16 g

Vitamins:

- High in Vitamin E and Magnesium from almond butter.
- Rich in Vitamin C and dietary fiber from raspberries.
- Oats and chia seeds provide a good source of B Vitamins, Iron, and Omega-3 fatty acids.

Pineapple and Kale Smoothie

- **Preparation Time:** 5 minutes
- **Cooking Time:** 0 minutes
- **Servings:** 2

Ingredients:

- 2 cups fresh kale, stems removed
- 1 cup pineapple, chopped
- 1 banana, sliced
- 1/2 avocado
- 2 cups unsweetened almond milk
- 1 tablespoon chia seeds
- Ice cubes (optional)

Procedure:

1. **Prep Ingredients:** Ensure the kale is thoroughly washed, and the pineapple is peeled and cored. Slice the banana and scoop out the avocado flesh.
2. **Blend the Greens:** Add the kale and almond milk to the blender first. Blend until the kale is thoroughly processed and the mixture is smooth, ensuring no leafy chunks remain.
3. **Add Fruits and Seeds:** To the kale mixture, add the pineapple, banana, avocado, and chia seeds. If you prefer a colder smoothie, add ice cubes at this stage.
4. **Blend Until Smooth:** Blend all the ingredients until the smoothie reaches your desired consistency. If it's too thick, add a bit more almond milk and blend again.

Macronutrients (per serving):

- **Calories:** 280 kcal
- **Carbohydrates:** 44 g
- **Protein:** 6 g
- **Fat:** 10 g

Vitamins:

- High in Vitamin C and Manganese from pineapple.
- Rich in Vitamin A, K, and Calcium from kale.
- Omega-3 fatty acids from chia seeds and healthy fats from avocado.

Quinoa Breakfast Bowl with Almonds and Berries

- **Preparation Time:** 5 minutes (plus 15 minutes if starting with uncooked quinoa)
- **Cooking Time:** 15 minutes (if cooking quinoa)
- **Servings:** 2

Ingredients:
- 1 cup cooked quinoa (cook according to package instructions if starting uncooked)
- 1/2 cup fresh blueberries
- 1/2 cup fresh strawberries, sliced
- 1/4 cup almonds, roughly chopped
- 2 tablespoons chia seeds
- 1 cup almond milk
- 1 tablespoon honey or maple syrup (optional)
- A pinch of cinnamon (optional)

Procedure:
1. **Prepare Quinoa:** If you haven't pre-cooked your quinoa, rinse 1/2 cup of dry quinoa under cold water, then cook according to package instructions. Generally, combine quinoa with 1 cup of water in a pot, bring to a boil, then simmer covered for about 15 minutes or until the water is absorbed. Fluff with a fork and let cool slightly.
2. **Assemble the Bowl:** Divide the cooked quinoa into two bowls. Pour half a cup of almond milk over each serving of quinoa.
3. **Add Toppings:** Sprinkle the blueberries, strawberries, almonds, and chia seeds evenly over the two bowls. If desired, drizzle with honey or maple syrup and add a pinch of cinnamon for extra flavor.
4. **Serve:** Enjoy your quinoa breakfast bowl immediately, savoring the mix of textures and flavors.

Macronutrients (per serving):
- **Calories:** 380 kcal
- **Carbohydrates:** 54 g
- **Protein:** 12 g
- **Fat:** 15 g

Vitamins:
- High in Vitamin C from berries.
- Rich in Magnesium, Zinc, and Iron from quinoa and almonds.
- Omega-3 fatty acids from chia seeds.

Raspberry Chia Jam on Sprouted Toast

- **Preparation Time:** 10 minutes (plus 1 hour for jam to set)
- **Cooking Time:** 5 minutes
- **Servings:** 2

Ingredients:
- 1 cup fresh or frozen raspberries
- 2 tablespoons chia seeds
- 1 tablespoon honey or maple syrup (adjust to taste)
- 1/2 teaspoon vanilla extract
- 4 slices sprouted grain bread

Procedure:
1. **Make the Chia Jam:** In a small saucepan over medium heat, cook the raspberries until they start to break down and release their juices, about 3-5 minutes. Use a fork or masher to help break them down to your desired consistency.
2. **Add Chia Seeds and Sweetener:** Remove the saucepan from the heat. Stir in the chia seeds, honey (or maple syrup), and vanilla extract. Mix well and let the mixture sit for about an hour to thicken into jam.
3. **Toast the Bread:** While the jam is setting, toast the sprouted grain bread slices to your liking.
4. **Assemble and Serve:** Spread a generous layer of the raspberry chia jam over each slice of toasted bread. Serve immediately and enjoy.

Macronutrients (per serving, including 2 slices of toast):
- **Calories:** 330 kcal
- **Carbohydrates:** 60 g
- **Protein:** 12 g
- **Fat:** 7 g

Vitamins:
- High in Vitamin C and Manganese from raspberries.
- Rich in Omega-3 fatty acids and fiber from chia seeds.
- Contains Iron and B Vitamins from sprouted grain bread.

Spiced Apple Porridge

- **Preparation Time:** 5 minutes
- **Cooking Time:** 15 minutes
- **Servings:** 2

Ingredients:

- 1 cup rolled oats
- 2 cups almond milk
- 1 large apple, peeled and diced
- 2 teaspoons cinnamon
- 1/4 teaspoon nutmeg
- 2 tablespoons maple syrup (or to taste)
- 2 tablespoons chopped walnuts (for topping)
- A pinch of salt

Procedure:

1. **Cook the Oats:** In a medium saucepan, bring the almond milk to a gentle boil. Add the rolled oats and a pinch of salt, then reduce the heat to low. Simmer for about 10 minutes, stirring occasionally, until the oats are soft and the porridge has thickened.
2. **Add Apples and Spices:** Stir in the diced apple, cinnamon, and nutmeg. Continue cooking for another 5 minutes, or until the apples are tender and the porridge is aromatic.
3. **Sweeten:** Remove from heat and stir in the maple syrup, adjusting the amount according to your preference for sweetness.
4. **Serve:** Divide the porridge into bowls, and top with chopped walnuts for an added crunch. Enjoy warm.

Macronutrients (per serving):

- **Calories:** 350 kcal
- **Carbohydrates:** 58 g
- **Protein:** 8 g
- **Fat:** 9 g

Vitamins:

- High in Vitamin E and Omega-3 fatty acids from walnuts.
- Rich in dietary fiber and Vitamin C from apples.
- Contains Iron and Magnesium from oats.

Spinach and Avocado Smoothie

- **Preparation Time:** 5 minutes
- **Cooking Time:** 0 minutes
- **Servings:** 2

Ingredients:

- 2 cups fresh spinach leaves
- 1 ripe avocado, pitted and scooped
- 1 ripe banana
- 1 small apple, cored and sliced
- 2 cups unsweetened almond milk
- 1 tablespoon chia seeds
- Ice cubes (optional)

Procedure:

1. **Blend Greens and Liquid:** In a blender, combine the spinach and almond milk first. Blend until the mixture is smooth, ensuring no spinach leaves are left whole.
2. **Add Fruits and Chia Seeds:** Add the avocado, banana, apple slices, and chia seeds to the blender. If you prefer a colder smoothie, add ice cubes at this stage.
3. **Blend Until Creamy:** Blend all the ingredients together until the smoothie reaches a creamy and smooth consistency. If the smoothie is too thick, you can add a little more almond milk to adjust.
4. **Serve Immediately:** Pour the smoothie into glasses and enjoy immediately to maximize the benefits of the nutrients.

Macronutrients (per serving):

- **Calories:** 330 kcal
- **Carbohydrates:** 44 g
- **Protein:** 6 g
- **Fat:** 17 g

Vitamins:

- High in Vitamin K, A, and C from spinach.
- Rich in Potassium from banana and Vitamin E from avocado.
- Chia seeds provide Omega-3 fatty acids and additional fiber.

Sweet Potato and Black Bean Breakfast Burritos

- **Preparation Time:** 15 minutes
- **Cooking Time:** 20 minutes
- **Servings:** 2

Ingredients:

- 1 medium sweet potato, peeled and diced
- 1 cup black beans, drained and rinsed (canned or cooked)
- 2 large whole wheat or corn tortillas
- 1/2 cup red onion, diced
- 1 clove garlic, minced
- 1 teaspoon ground cumin
- 1/2 teaspoon paprika
- 2 tablespoons olive oil
- Salt and pepper to taste
- 1/2 avocado, sliced
- 1/4 cup fresh cilantro, chopped (optional)
- 2 tablespoons salsa (for serving)

Procedure:

1. **Cook Sweet Potatoes:** In a skillet, heat the olive oil over medium heat. Add the diced sweet potatoes, season with salt, pepper, cumin, and paprika. Cook, stirring occasionally, until the sweet potatoes are tender and slightly browned, about 10-15 minutes.
2. **Add Beans and Seasonings:** Add the red onion and garlic to the skillet with the sweet potatoes. Cook until the onions are soft, about 3 minutes. Stir in the black beans and cook until everything is heated through, about 2 more minutes. Adjust seasoning as needed.
3. **Assemble Burritos:** Warm the tortillas according to package instructions to make them pliable. Divide the sweet potato and black bean mixture between the tortillas. Top each with sliced avocado and a sprinkle of cilantro.
4. **Roll and Serve:** Fold in the sides of each tortilla and roll up tightly. Serve each burrito with a side of salsa.

Macronutrients (per serving):
Calories: 480 kcal; **Carbohydrates:** 65 g; **Protein:** 14 g; **Fat:** 20 g

Vitamins:

- High in Vitamin A from sweet potatoes.
- Rich in Fiber and Iron from black beans.

Zucchini Bread Oatmeal

- **Preparation Time:** 5 minutes
- **Cooking Time:** 10 minutes
- **Servings:** 2

Ingredients:

- 1 cup rolled oats
- 2 cups water or almond milk
- 1 medium zucchini, grated
- 1/2 teaspoon cinnamon
- 1/4 teaspoon nutmeg
- 2 tablespoons chopped walnuts
- 2 tablespoons raisins
- 2 tablespoons maple syrup or honey (optional)
- Pinch of salt

Procedure:

1. **Cook Oats:** In a medium saucepan, bring the water or almond milk to a boil. Add the rolled oats and a pinch of salt, then reduce the heat to a simmer.
2. **Add Zucchini and Spices:** Stir in the grated zucchini, cinnamon, and nutmeg. Cook, stirring occasionally, for about 5-7 minutes or until the oats are soft and the mixture has thickened.
3. **Sweeten and Enhance:** Add the maple syrup or honey (if using) along with the chopped walnuts and raisins. Stir well to combine all the ingredients.
4. **Serve Warm:** Divide the oatmeal into bowls, and if desired, top with a little more cinnamon or a drizzle of maple syrup. Enjoy warm.

Macronutrients (per serving):

- **Calories:** 330 kcal
- **Carbohydrates:** 53 g
- **Protein:** 9 g
- **Fat:** 9 g

Vitamins:

- High in Vitamin C from zucchini.
- Contains Magnesium and Omega-3 fatty acids from walnuts.
- Offers Iron and B vitamins from oat

Chapter 11: Revitalizing Lunches recipes

Avocado Quinoa Salad with Lemon Dressing

- **Preparation Time:** 15 minutes
- **Cooking Time:** 15 minutes (for quinoa)
- **Servings:** 2

Ingredients:

- 1 cup quinoa (uncooked)
- 2 cups water
- 1 ripe avocado, diced
- 1/2 cucumber, diced
- 1/2 red bell pepper, diced
- 1/4 cup red onion, finely chopped
- 1/4 cup fresh cilantro, chopped
- 2 tablespoons olive oil
- Juice of 1 lemon
- Salt and pepper to taste

Procedure:

1. **Cook Quinoa:** Rinse quinoa under cold running water. In a saucepan, combine quinoa with water and bring to a boil. Reduce heat to low, cover, and simmer for about 15 minutes, or until water is absorbed. Fluff with a fork and let cool.
2. **Prepare Vegetables:** While the quinoa is cooling, dice the avocado, cucumber, and red bell pepper. Finely chop the red onion and cilantro.
3. **Make Lemon Dressing:** In a small bowl, whisk together olive oil, lemon juice, salt, and pepper to create the dressing.
4. **Assemble Salad:** In a large bowl, combine the cooled quinoa, diced vegetables, and cilantro. Drizzle with lemon dressing and toss gently to combine. Serve immediately or chill before serving.

Macronutrients (per serving):

- **Calories:** 520 kcal: **Carbohydrates:** 58 g
- **Protein:** 12 g; **Fat:** 28 g

Vitamins:

- High in Vitamin C from lemon and red bell pepper.
- Rich in Vitamin E, K, and folate from avocado.
- Contains magnesium and manganese from quinoa.

Baked Sweet Potato and Hummus Wrap

- **Preparation Time:** 10 minutes
- **Cooking Time:** 25 minutes
- **Servings:** 2

Ingredients:

- 2 medium sweet potatoes, peeled and sliced into thin strips
- 1 tablespoon olive oil
- Salt and pepper to taste
- 4 whole wheat or gluten-free tortillas
- 1/2 cup hummus
- 1 avocado, sliced
- 1 cup spinach leaves
- 1/2 red onion, thinly sliced
- 1 tablespoon lemon juice

Procedure:

1. **Bake Sweet Potatoes:** Preheat the oven to 400°F (200°C). Toss the sweet potato strips with olive oil, salt, and pepper. Spread them on a baking sheet and bake for about 25 minutes, or until tender and slightly crispy.
2. **Prepare Wraps:** Warm the tortillas in the oven for a few minutes or on a skillet over medium heat until they are pliable.
3. **Assemble the Wraps:** Spread hummus evenly over each tortilla. Layer baked sweet potato strips, avocado slices, spinach leaves, and red onion on top of the hummus. Drizzle with lemon juice.
4. **Wrap and Serve:** Roll up the tortillas tightly, tucking in the edges. Slice in half and serve immediately.

Macronutrients (per serving):

- **Calories:** 580 kcal
- **Carbohydrates:** 75 g
- **Protein:** 15 g
- **Fat:** 27 g

Vitamins:

- High in Vitamin A from sweet potatoes.
- Rich in Vitamin C from lemon juice and Vitamin K from spinach.
- Contains healthy fats and Vitamin E from avocado.

Beetroot and Spinach Salad with Walnuts

- **Preparation Time:** 15 minutes
- **Cooking Time:** 0 minutes (assuming pre-cooked beetroots)
- **Servings:** 2

Ingredients:

- 2 medium beetroots, cooked and sliced
- 4 cups baby spinach leaves
- 1/4 cup walnuts, roughly chopped
- 2 tablespoons feta cheese, crumbled (optional)
- 2 tablespoons balsamic vinegar
- 1 tablespoon olive oil
- Salt and pepper to taste
- 1/2 orange, for zest and juice

Procedure:

1. **Prepare the Base:** In a large salad bowl, arrange the baby spinach leaves as the base. Add the sliced beetroots on top of the spinach.
2. **Add Crunch and Flavor:** Sprinkle the chopped walnuts over the beets, and if using, add crumbled feta cheese for a creamy texture and tangy flavor.
3. **Dress the Salad:** In a small bowl, whisk together the balsamic vinegar, olive oil, a pinch of salt, and pepper. Drizzle this dressing over the salad. Add orange zest and a squeeze of orange juice for a citrusy kick.
4. **Toss and Serve:** Gently toss the salad to ensure all the ingredients are evenly coated with the dressing. Serve immediately, enjoying the blend of flavors and textures.

Macronutrients (per serving):

- **Calories:** 250 kcal
- **Carbohydrates:** 20 g
- **Protein:** 6 g
- **Fat:** 17 g

Vitamins:

- High in Vitamin A and C from spinach and orange.
- Rich in Iron and Folate from beetroot.
- Walnuts provide Omega-3 fatty acids and Vitamin E.

Black Bean Taco Salad with Cilantro-Lime Dressing

- **Preparation Time:** 20 minutes
- **Cooking Time:** 0 minutes
- **Servings:** 2

Ingredients:

- 1 cup black beans, drained and rinsed
- 2 cups romaine lettuce, chopped
- 1 cup cherry tomatoes, halved
- 1/2 cup corn kernels (fresh or frozen and thawed)
- 1 avocado, diced
- 1/4 cup red onion, finely chopped
- 1/4 cup cilantro, chopped (plus extra for garnish)
- 2 tablespoons olive oil
- Juice of 1 lime
- 1 garlic clove, minced
- 1 teaspoon honey (optional)
- Salt and pepper to taste
- 1/2 teaspoon ground cumin
- 1/4 cup tortilla strips or crushed tortilla chips (for topping)

Procedure:

1. **Prepare the Salad Base:** In a large salad bowl, combine the black beans, chopped romaine lettuce, cherry tomatoes, corn kernels, diced avocado, and red onion.
2. **Make the Cilantro-Lime Dressing:** In a small bowl, whisk together olive oil, lime juice, minced garlic, honey (if using), chopped cilantro, ground cumin, salt, and pepper until well combined.
3. **Dress the Salad:** Pour the cilantro-lime dressing over the salad ingredients in the bowl. Gently toss to ensure all components are evenly coated with the dressing.
4. **Serve with Garnish:** Divide the salad between two serving plates. Top with tortilla strips and additional cilantro for garnish. Serve immediately to enjoy the fresh flavors.

Macronutrients (per serving): Calories: 420 kcal; **Carbohydrates:** 45 g; **Protein:** 10 g; **Fat:** 24

Vitamins:

- High in Vitamin C from lime and tomatoes.
- Rich in Vitamin K and folate from romaine lettuce.

Broccoli and Almond Soup

- **Preparation Time:** 10 minutes
- **Cooking Time:** 20 minutes
- **Servings:** 2

Ingredients:

- 2 cups broccoli florets
- 1 tablespoon olive oil
- 1 small onion, chopped
- 1 garlic clove, minced
- 3 cups vegetable broth
- 1/4 cup almonds, plus more for garnish
- Salt and pepper to taste
- 1/4 cup almond milk (optional, for creaminess)
- A squeeze of lemon juice (optional, for brightness)

Procedure:

1. **Sauté Vegetables:** In a large pot, heat the olive oil over medium heat. Add the chopped onion and minced garlic, sautéing until soft and translucent, about 3-5 minutes.
2. **Cook Broccoli:** Add the broccoli florets to the pot along with the vegetable broth. Bring to a boil, then reduce the heat and simmer until the broccoli is tender, about 10-15 minutes.
3. **Blend the Soup:** Carefully transfer the soup mixture to a blender, adding the almonds. Blend until smooth. For a creamier texture, add almond milk to the blender. Season with salt and pepper to taste, and add a squeeze of lemon juice if desired.
4. **Serve:** Return the blended soup to the pot to warm through if needed. Serve the soup garnished with chopped almonds.

Macronutrients (per serving):

- **Calories:** 230 kcal
- **Carbohydrates:** 18 g
- **Protein:** 8 g
- **Fat:** 15 g

Vitamins:

- High in Vitamin C and K from broccoli.
- Rich in Vitamin E and magnesium from almonds.
- Contains dietary fiber and antioxidants.

Chickpea and Avocado Sandwich on Sprouted Bread

- **Preparation Time:** 10 minutes
- **Cooking Time:** 0 minutes
- **Servings:** 2

Ingredients:

- 1 can (15 oz) chickpeas, drained and rinsed
- 1 ripe avocado, sliced
- 4 slices sprouted whole grain bread
- Juice of 1/2 a lemon
- 1 tablespoon olive oil
- 1 garlic clove, minced
- Salt and pepper to taste
- 1/2 teaspoon paprika
- Fresh lettuce leaves
- 1 tomato, sliced

Procedure:

1. **Make Chickpea Spread:** In a bowl, mash the chickpeas with a fork or potato masher until mostly smooth. Mix in olive oil, lemon juice, minced garlic, paprika, salt, and pepper until well combined to create a creamy spread.
2. **Prepare the Bread:** Toast the sprouted bread slices if desired for added texture and warmth.
3. **Assemble the Sandwich:** Spread a generous layer of the chickpea mixture on two slices of bread. Layer on avocado slices, tomato slices, and lettuce.
4. **Finish and Serve:** Top with the remaining bread slices, press gently, and cut the sandwiches in half. Serve immediately for the best flavor and freshness.

Macronutrients (per serving):

- **Calories:** 490 kcal
- **Carbohydrates:** 65 g
- **Protein:** 18 g
- **Fat:** 20 g

Vitamins:

- High in Vitamin C from lemon and tomatoes.
- Rich in folate and fiber from chickpeas.
- Contains Vitamin E and healthy fats from avocado.

Cold Lentil Salad with Sun-Dried Tomatoes

- **Preparation Time:** 10 minutes
- **Cooking Time:** 20 minutes (for cooking lentils, if not using precooked)
- **Servings:** 2

Ingredients:

- 1 cup dried green or brown lentils (or 2 cups cooked lentils)
- 1/2 cup sun-dried tomatoes, chopped
- 1/4 cup red onion, finely chopped
- 1/4 cup fresh basil, chopped
- 2 tablespoons olive oil
- 1 tablespoon balsamic vinegar
- Salt and pepper to taste
- 1 garlic clove, minced
- Juice of 1 lemon
- Mixed greens for serving (optional)

Procedure:

1. **Cook Lentils:** If using dried lentils, rinse them under cold water. Bring a pot of water to a boil, add the lentils, and cook for about 20 minutes or until tender. Drain and let cool. Skip this step if using precooked lentils.
2. **Prepare the Dressing:** In a small bowl, whisk together olive oil, balsamic vinegar, lemon juice, minced garlic, salt, and pepper to create the dressing.
3. **Mix Salad Ingredients:** In a large bowl, combine the cooled lentils, sun-dried tomatoes, red onion, and chopped basil. Pour the dressing over the salad and toss well to coat.
4. **Chill and Serve:** Refrigerate the salad for at least 30 minutes to allow the flavors to meld. Serve over a bed of mixed greens if desired.

Macronutrients (per serving):

- **Calories:** 380 kcal
- **Carbohydrates:** 50 g
- **Protein:** 20 g
- **Fat:** 12 g

Vitamins:

- High in Vitamin C from lemon and sun-dried tomatoes.
- Rich in Iron and Folate from lentils.
- Contains Vitamin E from olive oil.

Cucumber Noodle Salad with Peanut Dressing

- **Preparation Time:** 15 minutes
- **Cooking Time:** 0 minutes
- **Servings:** 2

Ingredients:

- 2 large cucumbers
- 1 carrot, peeled
- 1 red bell pepper, thinly sliced
- 1/4 cup cilantro, chopped
- 2 tablespoons green onions, sliced
- 1/4 cup roasted peanuts, chopped

For the Peanut Dressing:

- 3 tablespoons peanut butter
- 1 tablespoon soy sauce
- 1 tablespoon honey or maple syrup
- 1 tablespoon rice vinegar
- 1 teaspoon sesame oil
- 1 small garlic clove, minced
- 1 teaspoon grated ginger
- Water, as needed to thin the dressing

Procedure:

1. **Prepare Vegetables:** Use a spiralizer or vegetable peeler to create noodles from the cucumbers and carrot. Place the cucumber and carrot noodles in a large mixing bowl, add the sliced red bell pepper, cilantro, and green onions.
2. **Make Peanut Dressing:** In a small bowl, whisk together peanut butter, soy sauce, honey or maple syrup, rice vinegar, sesame oil, minced garlic, and grated ginger. Add a little water to achieve a pourable consistency.
3. **Dress the Salad:** Pour the peanut dressing over the vegetable noodles and toss gently until all ingredients are well coated.
4. **Serve:** Divide the salad between two plates, sprinkle with chopped roasted peanuts, and serve immediately.

Macronutrients (per serving): **Calories:** 295 kcal; **Carbohydrates:** 28 g; **Protein:** 10 g; **Fat:** 18 g

Vitamins:

- High in Vitamin A from carrots and Vitamin C from red bell pepper.
- Rich in Vitamin E from peanut butter and Vitamin K from cucumbers.

Curried Cauliflower Rice with Cashews

- **Preparation Time:** 10 minutes
- **Cooking Time:** 15 minutes
- **Servings:** 2

Ingredients:

- 1 large head of cauliflower, grated into rice-sized pieces
- 1 tablespoon coconut oil
- 1 medium onion, finely chopped
- 2 cloves garlic, minced
- 1 tablespoon fresh ginger, grated
- 2 tablespoons curry powder
- 1/2 cup cashews, roasted
- 1/2 cup green peas (frozen and thawed)
- Salt and pepper to taste
- Fresh cilantro for garnish

Procedure:

1. **Prepare Cauliflower Rice:** Wash the cauliflower and pat it dry. Using a food processor or a box grater, grate the cauliflower until it resembles rice grains.
2. **Cook the Aromatics:** In a large skillet, heat the coconut oil over medium heat. Add the chopped onion, garlic, and ginger, sautéing until the onion becomes translucent.
3. **Add Cauliflower and Spices:** Stir in the grated cauliflower and curry powder. Cook for about 10 minutes, stirring frequently, until the cauliflower is tender but still offers a slight crunch. Season with salt and pepper.
4. **Finish and Serve:** Mix in the roasted cashews and green peas, heating through for another 2-3 minutes. Garnish with fresh cilantro before serving.

Macronutrients (per serving):

- **Calories:** 315 kcal
- **Carbohydrates:** 27 g
- **Protein:** 9 g
- **Fat:** 21 g

Vitamins:

- High in Vitamin C from cauliflower.
- Contains Vitamin K and folate from green peas.
- Rich in zinc and magnesium from cashews.

Eggplant and Tomato Stacks with Balsamic Glaze

- **Preparation Time:** 15 minutes
- **Cooking Time:** 30 minutes
- **Servings:** 2

Ingredients:

- 1 large eggplant, sliced into 1/2-inch rounds
- 2 large tomatoes, sliced
- 1/4 cup fresh basil leaves
- 2 tablespoons olive oil
- Salt and pepper to taste
- 1/4 cup balsamic vinegar
- 1 tablespoon honey

Procedure:

1. **Prepare and Cook Eggplant:** Preheat the oven to 400°F (200°C). Brush both sides of the eggplant slices with olive oil and season with salt and pepper. Arrange on a baking sheet and roast in the oven for 25-30 minutes, turning once, until golden and tender.
2. **Make Balsamic Glaze:** While the eggplant is roasting, pour balsamic vinegar and honey into a small saucepan. Simmer over low heat, stirring occasionally, until the mixture reduces to a thick glaze, about 10-15 minutes.
3. **Assemble Stacks:** On each plate, layer an eggplant slice, a tomato slice, and a few basil leaves. Repeat the layering until all ingredients are used, ending with a tomato slice on top.
4. **Serve with Glaze:** Drizzle the balsamic glaze over the stacks before serving. Add a final touch with a sprinkle of fresh basil.

Macronutrients (per serving):

- **Calories:** 290 kcal
- **Carbohydrates:** 35 g
- **Protein:** 4 g
- **Fat:** 16 g

Vitamins:

- High in Vitamin C from tomatoes.
- Contains Vitamin K and antioxidants from eggplant.
- Provides Vitamin E and healthy fats from olive oil.

Grilled Portobello Mushrooms with Quinoa Salad

- **Preparation Time:** 15 minutes
- **Cooking Time:** 20 minutes
- **Servings:** 2

Ingredients:

- 2 large Portobello mushrooms, stems removed
- 1 cup quinoa
- 2 cups water
- 1 small red bell pepper, diced
- 1/4 cup red onion, finely chopped
- 1/4 cup fresh parsley, chopped
- 2 tablespoons olive oil
- Juice of 1 lemon
- Salt and pepper to taste
- 1 clove garlic, minced
- 1 teaspoon balsamic vinegar

Procedure:

1. **Cook Quinoa:** Rinse quinoa under cold water. In a medium saucepan, bring 2 cups of water to a boil. Add quinoa, reduce heat to low, cover, and simmer for 15 minutes or until all water is absorbed. Fluff with a fork and let cool.
2. **Prepare Mushrooms:** While quinoa is cooking, brush the Portobello mushrooms with olive oil, minced garlic, and balsamic vinegar. Season with salt and pepper.
3. **Grill Mushrooms:** Preheat the grill to medium-high heat. Place the mushrooms on the grill, gill side down, and cook for about 5-7 minutes on each side or until they are tender and grill marks appear.
4. **Assemble Salad:** In a large bowl, combine the cooked quinoa, diced red bell pepper, red onion, and chopped parsley. Drizzle with lemon juice and an extra tablespoon of olive oil. Season with salt and pepper to taste. Toss to mix well.

Macronutrients (per serving):

- **Calories:** 410 kcal; **Carbohydrates:** 55 g; **Protein:** 12 g; **Fat:** 18 g

Vitamins:

- High in Vitamin C from red bell pepper and lemon juice.
- Rich in B vitamins from quinoa.
- Contains antioxidants and Vitamin E from olive oil.

Kale and Berry Salad with Poppy Seed Dressing

- **Preparation Time:** 15 minutes
- **Cooking Time:** 0 minutes
- **Servings:** 2

Ingredients:

- 4 cups chopped kale, stems removed
- 1 cup mixed berries (strawberries, blueberries, raspberries)
- 1/4 cup sliced almonds
- 1/4 cup crumbled feta cheese (optional)
- **For the Poppy Seed Dressing:**
  - 2 tablespoons olive oil
  - 1 tablespoon apple cider vinegar
  - 1 tablespoon honey
  - 1 teaspoon poppy seeds
  - Salt and pepper to taste

Procedure:

1. **Prepare the Kale:** Wash the kale thoroughly and chop it into bite-sized pieces. To soften the leaves, massage them with a little olive oil and a pinch of salt for about 2-3 minutes until the kale starts to wilt slightly.
2. **Make the Dressing:** In a small bowl, whisk together olive oil, apple cider vinegar, honey, poppy seeds, and a pinch each of salt and pepper. Adjust the seasoning and sweetness according to your taste.
3. **Assemble the Salad:** In a large mixing bowl, combine the massaged kale, mixed berries, and sliced almonds. Drizzle the poppy seed dressing over the salad and toss gently to coat everything evenly.
4. **Serve:** Divide the salad between two plates, topping each with crumbled feta cheese if using. Serve immediately to enjoy the maximum freshness and crunch.

Macronutrients (per serving):

- **Calories:** 330 kcal
- **Carbohydrates:** 30 g
- **Protein:** 8 g
- **Fat:** 21 g

Vitamins:

- High in Vitamin C from berries and kale.
- Rich in Vitamin K and calcium from kale.
- Contains Vitamin E and healthy fats from olive oil.

Lemon-Garlic Tempeh over Brown Rice

- **Preparation Time:** 10 minutes
- **Cooking Time:** 25 minutes
- **Servings:** 2

Ingredients:

- 1 block (8 oz) tempeh, sliced into 1/2 inch pieces
- 1 cup brown rice
- 2 cups water
- 2 tablespoons olive oil
- Juice and zest of 1 lemon
- 2 cloves garlic, minced
- 1 tablespoon soy sauce
- 1 teaspoon maple syrup
- Salt and pepper to taste
- Fresh parsley, chopped (for garnish)

Procedure:

1. **Cook Brown Rice:** Rinse the brown rice under cold water until the water runs clear. In a medium saucepan, bring 2 cups of water to a boil. Add the rice, reduce heat to low, cover, and simmer for about 25 minutes, or until all the water is absorbed and the rice is tender.
2. **Marinate Tempeh:** In a small bowl, combine the olive oil, lemon juice and zest, minced garlic, soy sauce, maple syrup, salt, and pepper. Place the tempeh slices in the marinade and let sit for at least 10 minutes to absorb the flavors.
3. **Cook Tempeh:** Heat a non-stick skillet over medium heat. Remove tempeh from the marinade (reserve the marinade) and cook for about 3-4 minutes on each side until golden brown and crispy.
4. **Serve:** Spoon the brown rice onto plates, top with the cooked tempeh, and drizzle with the remaining marinade. Garnish with chopped parsley and serve.

Macronutrients (per serving):

- **Calories:** 550 kcal
- **Carbohydrates:** 75 g
- **Protein:** 25 g
- **Fat:** 18 g

Vitamins:

- High in B vitamins from tempeh.
- Rich in Vitamin E from olive oil.
- Contains magnesium and selenium from brown rice.

Mango and Black Bean Quinoa Bowl

- **Preparation Time:** 15 minutes
- **Cooking Time:** 20 minutes
- **Servings:** 2

Ingredients:

- 1 cup quinoa
- 2 cups water
- 1 cup black beans, drained and rinsed (canned or pre-cooked)
- 1 ripe mango, peeled and diced
- 1 avocado, peeled and diced
- 1/2 red bell pepper, diced
- 1/4 cup red onion, finely chopped
- 1/4 cup fresh cilantro, chopped
- Juice of 1 lime
- 2 tablespoons olive oil
- Salt and pepper to taste
- 1 teaspoon chili powder (optional)

Procedure:

1. **Cook Quinoa:** Rinse quinoa under cold running water. In a medium pot, bring 2 cups of water to a boil. Add quinoa, reduce heat to low, cover, and simmer for about 15-20 minutes, or until all water is absorbed and quinoa is fluffy.
2. **Prepare Ingredients:** While the quinoa is cooking, prepare the mango, avocado, red bell pepper, and red onion. In a small bowl, whisk together lime juice, olive oil, salt, pepper, and chili powder (if using) to make the dressing.
3. **Mix the Bowl:** In a large bowl, combine the cooked quinoa, black beans, mango, avocado, red bell pepper, red onion, and cilantro. Drizzle the dressing over the top and gently toss to combine all the ingredients.
4. **Serve:** Divide the mixture between two bowls. Serve immediately, enjoying the fresh, vibrant flavors and textures.

Macronutrients (per serving): Calories: 540 kcal; **Carbohydrates:** 80 g; **Protein:** 16 g; **Fat:** 20 g

Vitamins:

- High in Vitamin C from mango and red bell pepper.
- Rich in Vitamin K and folate from avocado.
- Provides B vitamins from black beans and quinoa.

Mixed Greens with Roasted Pumpkin and Pecans

- **Preparation Time:** 15 minutes
- **Cooking Time:** 30 minutes
- **Servings:** 2

Ingredients:

- 2 cups diced pumpkin
- 1 tablespoon olive oil
- Salt and pepper to taste
- 4 cups mixed greens (such as spinach, arugula, and romaine)
- 1/2 cup pecans, toasted
- 1/4 cup dried cranberries
- 2 tablespoons balsamic vinegar
- 1 teaspoon honey
- 1 teaspoon Dijon mustard

Procedure:

1. **Roast Pumpkin:** Preheat your oven to 400°F (200°C). Toss the diced pumpkin with olive oil, salt, and pepper. Spread on a baking sheet and roast for about 30 minutes or until tender and lightly caramelized.
2. **Prepare Dressing:** While the pumpkin is roasting, whisk together balsamic vinegar, honey, and Dijon mustard in a small bowl. Adjust seasoning with salt and pepper.
3. **Assemble the Salad:** In a large salad bowl, combine the mixed greens, roasted pumpkin, toasted pecans, and dried cranberries.
4. **Serve:** Drizzle the dressing over the salad and toss gently to combine. Serve immediately while the pumpkin is still warm.

Macronutrients (per serving):

- **Calories:** 360 kcal
- **Carbohydrates:** 30 g
- **Protein:** 5 g
- **Fat:** 26 g

Vitamins:

- High in Vitamin A from pumpkin.
- Rich in Vitamin C and Vitamin K from mixed greens.
- Contains antioxidants and essential minerals from pecans.

Roasted Vegetable and Farro Bowl

- **Preparation Time:** 15 minutes
- **Cooking Time:** 30 minutes
- **Servings:** 2

Ingredients:

- 1 cup farro, uncooked
- 2 cups water or vegetable broth
- 1 small zucchini, sliced into half-moons
- 1 red bell pepper, cut into strips
- 1 small red onion, sliced
- 1 carrot, sliced
- 2 tablespoons olive oil
- Salt and pepper to taste
- 2 tablespoons fresh parsley, chopped
- Juice of 1 lemon

Procedure:

1. **Cook Farro:** Rinse farro under cold water. In a medium saucepan, bring water or vegetable broth to a boil. Add farro, reduce heat to low, cover, and simmer for about 25-30 minutes until tender and chewy.
2. **Roast Vegetables:** Preheat your oven to 400°F (200°C). Toss zucchini, red bell pepper, red onion, and carrot with olive oil, salt, and pepper. Spread on a baking sheet in a single layer and roast for 20-25 minutes, stirring halfway through, until vegetables are tender and caramelized.
3. **Assemble Bowls:** Divide the cooked farro between two bowls. Top each with an even distribution of roasted vegetables.
4. **Finish and Serve:** Drizzle lemon juice over each bowl and garnish with chopped parsley. Serve warm.

Macronutrients (per serving):

- **Calories:** 480 kcal
- **Carbohydrates:** 75 g
- **Protein:** 12 g
- **Fat:** 16 g

Vitamins:

- High in Vitamin C from red bell pepper and lemon.
- Rich in fiber and B vitamins from farro.
- Contains beta-carotene from carrots.

Spiced Chickpea Stew with Coconut Milk

- **Preparation Time:** 10 minutes
- **Cooking Time:** 30 minutes
- **Servings:** 2

Ingredients:

- 1 can (15 oz) chickpeas, drained and rinsed
- 1 can (14 oz) coconut milk
- 1 large onion, chopped
- 2 cloves garlic, minced
- 1 tablespoon ginger, grated
- 1 large tomato, diced
- 1 teaspoon turmeric
- 1 teaspoon cumin
- 1/2 teaspoon coriander
- 1/2 teaspoon chili powder
- 2 tablespoons olive oil
- Salt and pepper to taste
- Fresh cilantro, chopped (for garnish)
- Juice of 1 lime

Procedure:

1. **Sauté Aromatics:** In a large pot, heat olive oil over medium heat. Add chopped onion, garlic, and ginger, and sauté until the onion becomes translucent. Stir in turmeric, cumin, coriander, and chili powder, cooking for about 1 minute until fragrant.
2. **Add Chickpeas and Tomatoes:** Incorporate the chickpeas and diced tomatoes into the pot. Cook for about 5 minutes, stirring occasionally, allowing the tomatoes to break down slightly.
3. **Simmer with Coconut Milk:** Pour in the coconut milk and bring the mixture to a gentle simmer. Reduce heat and let simmer for 20 minutes, stirring occasionally. Season with salt and pepper to taste.
4. **Finish and Serve:** Remove from heat, stir in fresh lime juice, and garnish with chopped cilantro. Serve hot, ideally over cooked rice or with a side of naan bread.

Macronutrients (per serving):
Calories: 560 kcal; **Carbohydrates:** 45 g; **Protein:** 15 g; **Fat:** 37 g
Vitamins:
High in Vitamin C from tomatoes and lime juice. Rich in iron and magnesium from chickpeas.

Spinach and Strawberry Salad with Almonds

This Spinach and Strawberry Salad with Almonds combines crisp, fresh spinach with juicy strawberries and crunchy almonds, all tossed in a light vinaigrette. It's a vibrant salad that's not only pleasing to the eye but also packed with nutrients like vitamin C, iron, and healthy fats, making it a perfect choice for a refreshing, health-boosting meal.

- **Preparation Time:** 10 minutes
- **Cooking Time:** 0 minutes
- **Servings:** 2

Ingredients:

- 4 cups fresh spinach, washed and dried
- 1 cup strawberries, sliced
- 1/4 cup almonds, toasted and roughly chopped
- 2 tablespoons olive oil
- 1 tablespoon balsamic vinegar
- 1 teaspoon honey
- Salt and pepper to taste
- Optional: 1/4 cup crumbled feta cheese or goat cheese

Procedure:

1. **Prepare the Dressing:** In a small bowl, whisk together olive oil, balsamic vinegar, honey, salt, and pepper until well combined.
2. **Combine the Salad Ingredients:** In a large salad bowl, place the spinach leaves. Add the sliced strawberries and toasted almonds.
3. **Toss the Salad:** Drizzle the dressing over the spinach, strawberries, and almonds. Toss gently to ensure all ingredients are evenly coated with the dressing.
4. **Serve:** Divide the salad between two plates, optionally topping each with crumbled feta or goat cheese for added flavor and richness. Serve immediately.

Macronutrients (per serving):
Calories: 280 kcal; **Carbohydrates:** 18 g; **Protein:** 6 g; **Fat:** 21 g
Vitamins:

- High in Vitamin C from strawberries.
- Rich in Vitamin E and magnesium from almonds.
- Contains Vitamin A and iron from spinach.

Sweet Potato and Kale Buddha Bowl

- **Preparation Time:** 15 minutes
- **Cooking Time:** 25 minutes
- **Servings:** 2

Ingredients:

- 2 medium sweet potatoes, peeled and cubed
- 2 cups kale, washed and roughly chopped
- 1 cup quinoa
- 2 cups vegetable broth
- 1 avocado, sliced
- 1/4 cup pumpkin seeds, toasted
- 2 tablespoons olive oil
- Salt and pepper to taste

For the dressing:

- 2 tablespoons tahini
- 1 tablespoon lemon juice
- 1 teaspoon maple syrup
- Water to thin, as needed
- Salt to taste

Procedure:

1. **Cook Quinoa:** Rinse the quinoa under cold water. In a pot, bring the vegetable broth to a boil, add the quinoa, reduce to a simmer, cover, and cook for about 15 minutes until the broth is absorbed and quinoa is fluffy.
2. **Roast Sweet Potatoes:** Preheat the oven to 400°F (200°C). Toss sweet potato cubes with 1 tablespoon olive oil, salt, and pepper. Spread on a baking sheet and roast for 25 minutes, or until tender and lightly browned.
3. **Sauté Kale:** In a skillet over medium heat, add the remaining tablespoon of olive oil. Add the kale and sauté until wilted and slightly crispy, about 5-7 minutes. Season with salt and pepper.
4. **Prepare the Dressing and Assemble:** Whisk together tahini, lemon juice, maple syrup, and enough water to achieve a pourable consistency. Season with salt. Divide the quinoa, roasted sweet potatoes, and sautéed kale between two bowls. Top each bowl with sliced avocado and pumpkin seeds. Drizzle with tahini dressing.

Macronutrients (per serving):

- **Calories:** 560 kcal
- **Carbohydrates:** 75 g
- **Protein:** 15 g
- **Fat:** 25 g

Vitamins:

- High in Vitamin A and C from sweet potatoes and kale.
- Rich in healthy fats and Vitamin E from avocado and olive oil.
- Provides magnesium and zinc from pumpkin seeds.

Zucchini Ribbon Salad with Avocado and Pine Nuts

Indulge in the freshness of Zucchini Ribbon Salad with Avocado and Pine Nuts, a light yet satisfying dish perfect for a nutritious lunch. This salad blends the crispness of thinly sliced zucchini with the creaminess of avocado and the crunch of pine nuts, offering a delightful texture and flavor profile. It's packed with essential nutrients, promoting heart health and providing anti-inflammatory benefits.

- **Preparation Time:** 10 minutes
- **Cooking Time:** 0 minutes
- **Servings:** 2

Ingredients:

- 2 large zucchinis
- 1 ripe avocado, diced
- 1/4 cup pine nuts, toasted
- 2 tablespoons olive oil
- Juice of 1 lemon
- Salt and pepper to taste
- A handful of fresh basil leaves, torn

Procedure:

1. **Prepare Zucchini Ribbons:** Use a vegetable peeler or a mandoline slicer to slice the zucchinis into thin, long ribbons. Place the ribbons in a large salad bowl.
2. **Make the Dressing:** In a small bowl, whisk together the olive oil, lemon juice, salt, and pepper until well combined.
3. **Assemble the Salad:** Add the diced avocado and toasted pine nuts to the zucchini ribbons. Drizzle the dressing over the salad and gently toss to coat all the ingredients evenly.
4. **Serve:** Garnish with torn basil leaves just before serving to add a fresh, herby flavor.

Macronutrients (per serving):

- **Calories:** 350 kcal
- **Carbohydrates:** 18 g
- **Protein:** 5 g
- **Fat:** 30 g

Vitamins:

- High in Vitamin C from lemon and zucchini.
- Rich in Vitamin E and magnesium from pine nuts.
- Contains healthy fats and Vitamin K from avocado.

Benefits:

This Zucchini Ribbon Salad is not only visually appealing but also loaded with vitamins and healthy fats. The zucchini provides a high amount of vitamin C, which supports immune function and skin health. Avocado offers healthy monounsaturated fats that are good for heart health and maintaining healthy cholesterol levels. Additionally, pine nuts contribute vitamin E and antioxidants that help protect the body's cells from damag

Almond-Crusted Baked Tofu

- **Preparation Time:** 15 minutes
- **Cooking Time:** 25 minutes
- **Servings:** 2

Ingredients:

- 1 block (14 oz) firm tofu, pressed and cut into slices
- 1/2 cup finely ground almonds
- 2 tablespoons nutritional yeast
- 1 teaspoon garlic powder
- 1 teaspoon onion powder
- 1/2 teaspoon paprika
- Salt and pepper to taste
- 2 tablespoons olive oil
- 1 tablespoon soy sauce or tamari

Procedure:

1. **Preheat Oven and Prepare Tofu:** Preheat your oven to 375°F (190°C). After pressing the tofu to remove excess water, slice it into 1/2-inch thick pieces.
2. **Prepare Almond Coating:** In a shallow dish, mix together the ground almonds, nutritional yeast, garlic powder, onion powder, paprika, salt, and pepper.
3. **Coat Tofu:** Brush each tofu slice with a thin layer of olive oil and soy sauce, then dredge in the almond mixture, pressing gently to adhere the coating on all sides.
4. **Bake:** Arrange the coated tofu slices on a baking sheet lined with parchment paper. Bake in the preheated oven for 25 minutes, turning halfway through, until the coating is golden and crispy.

Macronutrients (per serving):

- **Calories:** 520 kcal
- **Carbohydrates:** 15 g
- **Protein:** 30 g
- **Fat:** 39 g

Vitamins:

- High in Vitamin E and magnesium from almonds.
- Contains B vitamins from nutritional yeast.
- Provides iron and calcium from tofu.

Barley and Vegetable Stew

- **Preparation Time:** 15 minutes
- **Cooking Time:** 45 minutes
- **Servings:** 2

Ingredients:

- 1/2 cup pearl barley, rinsed
- 4 cups vegetable broth
- 1 carrot, diced
- 1 celery stalk, diced
- 1 small onion, chopped
- 2 cloves garlic, minced
- 1/2 cup diced potatoes
- 1/2 cup chopped green beans
- 1/2 teaspoon dried thyme
- 1/2 teaspoon dried rosemary
- Salt and pepper to taste
- 2 tablespoons olive oil
- Optional: 1/4 cup chopped parsley for garnish

Procedure:

1. **Sauté Vegetables:** In a large pot, heat the olive oil over medium heat. Add the onion, garlic, carrot, and celery, and sauté for about 5 minutes until the vegetables start to soften.
2. **Cook Barley:** Add the rinsed barley to the pot along with the vegetable broth, thyme, and rosemary. Bring to a boil, then reduce heat to a simmer, cover, and cook for 30 minutes.
3. **Add Remaining Vegetables:** Add the potatoes and green beans to the pot. Continue to simmer, covered, for an additional 15 minutes, or until the barley and vegetables are tender.
4. **Season and Serve:** Season the stew with salt and pepper to taste. Serve hot, garnished with chopped parsley if desired.

Macronutrients (per serving):
Calories: 350 kcal; **Carbohydrates:** 58 g; Protein: 8 g; **Fat:** 10 g

Vitamins:

- High in Vitamin A from carrots.
- Contains Vitamin C from green beans and potatoes.

Broccoli Almond Stir-Fry

- **Preparation Time:** 10 minutes
- **Cooking Time:** 10 minutes
- **Servings:** 2

Ingredients:

- 2 cups broccoli florets
- 1/4 cup almonds, slivered and toasted
- 1 tablespoon olive oil
- 2 cloves garlic, minced
- 1 tablespoon ginger, minced
- 2 tablespoons soy sauce
- 1 tablespoon sesame oil
- 1 teaspoon honey
- Salt and pepper to taste
- Optional: sesame seeds for garnish

Procedure:

1. **Prepare Ingredients:** Wash and cut the broccoli into florets. Toast the slivered almonds in a dry pan until they're golden brown and set them aside.
2. **Sauté Aromatics:** Heat olive oil in a large skillet or wok over medium heat. Add minced garlic and ginger, and sauté for about 1 minute until fragrant.
3. **Cook Broccoli:** Increase the heat to high and add the broccoli florets to the skillet. Stir-fry for about 5-7 minutes until the broccoli is tender but still crisp.
4. **Finish the Dish:** Lower the heat to medium. Add the soy sauce, sesame oil, and honey to the skillet, stirring to coat the broccoli. Season with salt and pepper. Stir in the toasted almonds, cook for another minute, then remove from heat. Serve hot, garnished with sesame seeds if desired.

Macronutrients (per serving):

- **Calories:** 290 kcal
- **Carbohydrates:** 18 g
- **Protein:** 8 g
- **Fat:** 22 g

Vitamins:

- High in Vitamin C from broccoli.
- Contains Vitamin E and healthy fats from almonds and sesame oil.
- Provides iron and fiber.

Butternut Squash Soup with Sage

- **Preparation Time:** 15 minutes
- **Cooking Time:** 30 minutes
- **Servings:** 2

Ingredients:

- 1 medium butternut squash, peeled, seeded, and cubed
- 1 tablespoon olive oil
- 1 small onion, chopped
- 2 cloves garlic, minced
- 4 cups vegetable broth
- 6 fresh sage leaves, plus more for garnish
- Salt and pepper to taste
- Optional: a dollop of cream or a drizzle of coconut milk for serving

Procedure:

1. **Sauté Aromatics:** In a large pot, heat the olive oil over medium heat. Add the onion and garlic, and sauté until the onion is translucent, about 5 minutes.
2. **Cook Squash:** Add the cubed butternut squash to the pot along with the vegetable broth and sage leaves. Bring to a boil, then reduce the heat and simmer for about 20-25 minutes, or until the squash is tender.
3. **Blend the Soup:** Remove the sage leaves. Use an immersion blender to purée the soup directly in the pot until smooth. Alternatively, carefully transfer the soup to a blender and blend until smooth, then return to the pot.
4. **Season and Serve:** Season the soup with salt and pepper to taste. Serve hot, garnished with fresh sage leaves and a dollop of cream or a drizzle of coconut milk if desired.

Macronutrients (per serving):

- **Calories:** 200 kcal
- **Carbohydrates:** 35 g
- **Protein:** 3 g
- **Fat:** 7 g

Vitamins:

- High in Vitamin A from butternut squash.
- Contains Vitamin C.
- Provides fiber and potassium.

Cauliflower Steaks with Herb Sauce

- **Preparation Time:** 10 minutes
- **Cooking Time:** 25 minutes
- **Servings:** 2

Ingredients:

- 1 large head of cauliflower
- 2 tablespoons olive oil
- Salt and pepper to taste
- **For the Herb Sauce:**
    - 1/4 cup fresh parsley, chopped
    - 1/4 cup fresh basil, chopped
    - 2 tablespoons chives, chopped
    - 1 clove garlic, minced
    - Juice of 1 lemon
    - 1/3 cup olive oil
    - Salt and pepper to taste

Procedure:

1. **Prepare Cauliflower:** Preheat your oven to 400°F (200°C). Remove the leaves from the cauliflower and cut the head into two 1-inch thick slices (steaks), keeping the stem intact to hold the steaks together. Brush both sides of each steak with olive oil and season with salt and pepper.
2. **Roast Cauliflower Steaks:** Place the cauliflower steaks on a baking sheet lined with parchment paper. Roast in the preheated oven for about 25 minutes, turning halfway through, until golden brown and tender.
3. **Make Herb Sauce:** While the cauliflower is roasting, combine parsley, basil, chives, minced garlic, lemon juice, and olive oil in a blender or food processor. Blend until smooth. Season with salt and pepper to taste.
4. **Serve:** Plate the roasted cauliflower steaks and generously drizzle with the herb sauce. Serve immediately.

Macronutrients (per serving):

- **Calories:** 395 kcal
- **Carbohydrates:** 14 g
- **Protein:** 5 g
- **Fat:** 36 g

Vitamins:

- High in Vitamin C from cauliflower and lemon juice.
- Rich in Vitamin K from cauliflower.
- Contains antioxidants from fresh herbs.

Chickpea and Spinach Curry

- **Preparation Time:** 10 minutes
- **Cooking Time:** 20 minutes
- **Servings:** 2

Ingredients:

- 1 can (15 oz) chickpeas, drained and rinsed
- 2 cups fresh spinach, washed
- 1 large onion, finely chopped
- 2 cloves garlic, minced
- 1 tablespoon grated ginger
- 1 large tomato, diced
- 1 tablespoon olive oil
- 1 teaspoon cumin seeds
- 1 teaspoon turmeric powder
- 1 teaspoon coriander powder
- 1/2 teaspoon garam masala
- 1/2 teaspoon chili powder (adjust to taste)
- Salt to taste
- 1 cup coconut milk
- Fresh cilantro for garnish

Procedure:

1. **Sauté Aromatics:** In a large skillet or saucepan, heat the olive oil over medium heat. Add the cumin seeds and let them sizzle for a few seconds. Then add the chopped onion, garlic, and ginger, sautéing until the onions turn translucent and slightly golden.
2. **Add Spices and Tomato:** Stir in the turmeric, coriander, garam masala, and chili powder, cooking for about 1 minute until fragrant. Add the diced tomato and cook until the tomatoes soften and release their juices.
3. **Incorporate Chickpeas and Spinach:** Add the chickpeas to the pan along with the fresh spinach. Cook until the spinach wilts, about 3-4 minutes.
4. **Simmer with Coconut Milk:** Pour in the coconut milk and bring the mixture to a gentle simmer. Season with salt and let it cook for another 10 minutes until the curry slightly thickens. Garnish with fresh cilantro before serving.

Macronutrients (per serving): **Calories:** 435 kcal; **Carbohydrates:** 45 g; **Protein:** 14 g; **Fat:** 23
Vitamins:

- High in Vitamin A from spinach.
- Rich in Vitamin C from tomatoes.

Eggplant Lasagna with Cashew Ricotta

- **Preparation Time:** 20 minutes
- **Cooking Time:** 45 minutes
- **Servings:** 2

Ingredients:

- 1 large eggplant, sliced lengthwise into thin strips
- 1 cup raw cashews, soaked for 4 hours or overnight
- 1/4 cup nutritional yeast
- 1 lemon, juiced
- 1 garlic clove
- Salt and pepper to taste
- 2 cups marinara sauce
- 1 tablespoon olive oil
- Fresh basil leaves for garnish

Procedure:

1. **Prepare Eggplant:** Preheat the oven to 375°F (190°C). Brush eggplant slices with olive oil and season with salt and pepper. Arrange slices in a single layer on a baking sheet and bake for 20-25 minutes until tender and slightly browned.
2. **Make Cashew Ricotta:** Drain and rinse the soaked cashews. In a food processor, combine cashews, nutritional yeast, lemon juice, garlic, and a pinch of salt. Blend until smooth and creamy, adding a little water if needed to achieve a ricotta-like consistency.
3. **Assemble Lasagna:** In a baking dish, spread a thin layer of marinara sauce. Layer baked eggplant slices, followed by a layer of cashew ricotta. Repeat the layers until all ingredients are used, finishing with a layer of marinara sauce on top.
4. **Bake and Serve:** Bake the lasagna in the preheated oven for 20 minutes. Let it cool slightly before garnishing with fresh basil and serving.

Macronutrients (per serving):

Calories: 600 kcal; **Carbohydrates:** 51 g; **Protein:** 20 g; **Fat:** 37 g

Vitamins:

- High in Vitamin C from lemon and marinara sauce.
- Contains Vitamin E from olive oil.
- Provides B vitamins from nutritional yeast and fiber from eggplant.

Garlic Lemon Lentil Salad

- **Preparation Time:** 10 minutes
- **Cooking Time:** 20 minutes
- **Servings:** 2

Ingredients:

- 1 cup dried green lentils
- 2 cups water
- 1 large garlic clove, minced
- Juice and zest of 1 lemon
- 2 tablespoons olive oil
- 1/2 cucumber, diced
- 1 red bell pepper, diced
- 1/4 cup fresh parsley, chopped
- Salt and pepper to taste

Procedure:

1. **Cook Lentils:** Rinse the lentils under cold water. In a medium pot, bring 2 cups of water to a boil, add lentils, reduce heat, and simmer for about 15-20 minutes or until lentils are tender but not mushy. Drain any excess water and let cool.
2. **Make Dressing:** In a small bowl, whisk together minced garlic, lemon juice, lemon zest, olive oil, salt, and pepper to create a zesty dressing.
3. **Prepare Vegetables:** Dice the cucumber and red bell pepper, and chop the parsley.
4. **Assemble Salad:** In a large bowl, combine the cooked lentils, diced cucumber, bell pepper, and parsley. Pour the dressing over the salad and toss to combine thoroughly. Serve chilled or at room temperature.

Macronutrients (per serving):

- **Calories:** 360 kcal
- **Carbohydrates:** 50 g
- **Protein:** 18 g
- **Fat:** 10 g

Vitamins:

- High in Vitamin C from lemon and red bell pepper.
- Rich in iron and folate from lentils.
- Contains Vitamin A from red bell pepper and Vitamin E from olive oil.

Grilled Asparagus and Quinoa Salad

- **Preparation Time:** 10 minutes
- **Cooking Time:** 20 minutes
- **Servings:** 2

Ingredients:

- 1 cup quinoa
- 2 cups water
- 1 bunch asparagus, trimmed
- 1 tablespoon olive oil
- Salt and pepper to taste
- Juice and zest of 1 lemon
- 1/4 cup sliced almonds, toasted
- 1/4 cup feta cheese, crumbled (optional)
- 1 tablespoon fresh parsley, chopped

Procedure:

1. **Cook Quinoa:** Rinse quinoa under cold running water. In a medium saucepan, bring 2 cups of water to a boil. Add quinoa, reduce heat to low, cover, and simmer for about 15 minutes, or until all water is absorbed and quinoa is fluffy. Remove from heat and let it cool slightly.
2. **Grill Asparagus:** Preheat a grill or grill pan to medium-high heat. Toss asparagus with olive oil, salt, and pepper. Grill the asparagus for about 5-7 minutes, turning occasionally, until tender and charred. Let it cool and then cut into 1-inch pieces.
3. **Prepare Dressing:** In a small bowl, whisk together lemon juice, lemon zest, and additional olive oil. Season with salt and pepper to taste.
4. **Assemble Salad:** In a large bowl, mix the cooked quinoa, grilled asparagus, toasted almonds, and parsley. Drizzle with the lemon dressing and toss to combine. Sprinkle with crumbled feta cheese if using. Serve immediately or chill before serving.

Macronutrients (per serving):

- **Calories:** 450 kcal
- **Carbohydrates:** 55 g
- **Protein:** 16 g
- **Fat:** 20 g

Vitamins:

- High in Vitamin C and K from asparagus and lemon.
- Contains B vitamins and magnesium from quinoa.
- Rich in Vitamin E from almonds.

Herbed Mushroom and Quinoa Risotto

- **Preparation Time:** 10 minutes
- **Cooking Time:** 25 minutes
- **Servings:** 2

Ingredients:

- 1 cup quinoa, rinsed
- 2 cups vegetable broth
- 1 cup mushrooms, sliced
- 1 small onion, finely chopped
- 2 cloves garlic, minced
- 1 tablespoon olive oil
- 1/4 cup white wine (optional)
- 1 tablespoon fresh thyme, chopped
- 1 tablespoon fresh parsley, chopped
- Salt and pepper to taste
- 1/4 cup grated Parmesan cheese (optional for a vegan alternative, use nutritional yeast)

Procedure:

1. **Cook Quinoa:** In a medium saucepan, bring the vegetable broth to a boil. Add quinoa, reduce heat to low, cover, and cook for about 15 minutes, or until the liquid is absorbed and quinoa is tender.
2. **Sauté Vegetables:** While the quinoa is cooking, heat olive oil in a large skillet over medium heat. Add the onion and garlic, and sauté until the onion becomes translucent. Add the mushrooms and cook until they are soft and browned.
3. **Combine Ingredients:** Once the quinoa is cooked, stir it into the skillet with the mushrooms. If using, deglaze the pan with white wine and let the alcohol cook off. Add the fresh thyme, parsley, and season with salt and pepper. Cook together for a few minutes until everything is well combined.
4. **Finish and Serve:** Stir in the Parmesan cheese or nutritional yeast until melted and creamy. Adjust seasoning as needed. Serve the risotto garnished with additional fresh herbs.

Macronutrients (per serving):

- **Calories:** 380 kcal
- **Carbohydrates:** 54 g

- **Protein:** 16 g
- **Fat:** 12 g

Vitamins:
- High in Vitamin B from mushrooms and quinoa.
- Rich in antioxidants and Vitamin C from parsley.
- Provides iron and magnesium from quinoa.

Kale and Sweet Potato Sauté

- **Preparation Time:** 10 minutes
- **Cooking Time:** 20 minutes
- **Servings:** 2

Ingredients:
- 1 large sweet potato, peeled and diced
- 2 cups kale, stems removed and leaves chopped
- 1 medium onion, diced
- 2 cloves garlic, minced
- 2 tablespoons olive oil
- Salt and pepper to taste
- 1/2 teaspoon paprika
- Optional: sprinkle of crushed red pepper for heat

Procedure:
1. **Prepare Ingredients:** Heat olive oil in a large skillet over medium heat. Add the diced onion and garlic, and sauté until the onion becomes translucent and fragrant, about 3-5 minutes.
2. **Cook Sweet Potato:** Add the diced sweet potato to the skillet, season with salt, pepper, and paprika. Cover and cook for about 10 minutes, stirring occasionally, until the sweet potatoes are nearly tender.
3. **Add Kale:** Add the chopped kale to the skillet, stirring well to combine with the sweet potatoes. Continue to cook for another 5-7 minutes, until the kale has wilted and the sweet potatoes are fully tender.
4. **Season and Serve:** Adjust the seasoning with additional salt and pepper if needed. If desired, add a sprinkle of crushed red pepper for a bit of heat. Serve hot as a nutritious side dish or a light main course.

Macronutrients (per serving): Calories: 280 kcal; **Carbohydrates:** 38 g; **Protein:** 5 g; **Fat:** 14 g

Vitamins:
- High in Vitamin A and C from sweet potatoes and kale.
- Contains Vitamin K and calcium from kale.
- Provides potassium and manganese from sweet potatoes.

Lentil Bolognese with Zucchini Noodles

- **Preparation Time:** 15 minutes
- **Cooking Time:** 30 minutes
- **Servings:** 2

Ingredients:

- 1 cup dried red lentils
- 2 cups vegetable broth
- 2 large zucchinis, spiralized into noodles
- 1 small onion, finely chopped
- 2 cloves garlic, minced
- 1 can (14 oz) crushed tomatoes
- 2 tablespoons tomato paste
- 1 tablespoon olive oil
- 1 teaspoon dried oregano
- 1 teaspoon dried basil
- Salt and pepper to taste
- Fresh basil for garnish

Procedure:

1. **Cook Lentils:** Rinse lentils under cold water. In a medium saucepan, bring vegetable broth to a boil, add lentils, reduce heat, and simmer for 15-20 minutes until lentils are tender but not mushy. Drain any excess liquid and set aside.
2. **Prepare Sauce:** Heat olive oil in a large skillet over medium heat. Add onion and garlic, and sauté until onion is translucent. Stir in crushed tomatoes, tomato paste, oregano, and basil. Let the sauce simmer for about 10 minutes to combine the flavors.
3. **Combine Lentils and Sauce:** Add the cooked lentils to the tomato sauce in the skillet. Stir well and season with salt and pepper. Cook together for another 5 minutes, allowing the flavors to meld.
4. **Serve:** Divide spiralized zucchini noodles between plates and top with the hot lentil Bolognese. Garnish with fresh basil leaves before serving.

Macronutrients (per serving):

- **Calories:** 410 kcal
- **Carbohydrates:** 65 g
- **Protein:** 25 g
- **Fat:** 8 g

Vitamins:

- High in Vitamin C from tomatoes and zucchini.
- Rich in folate and iron from lentils.
- Contains antioxidants from herbs and garlic.

Miso-Glazed Brussels Sprouts

- **Preparation Time:** 10 minutes
- **Cooking Time:** 20 minutes
- **Servings:** 2

Ingredients:

- 400 grams (about 14 ounces) Brussels sprouts, trimmed and halved
- 1 tablespoon olive oil
- Salt and pepper to taste
- 2 tablespoons miso paste
- 1 tablespoon honey
- 1 tablespoon rice vinegar
- 1 teaspoon sesame oil
- 1 tablespoon water
- Optional: sesame seeds for garnish

Procedure:

1. **Prepare Brussels Sprouts:** Preheat the oven to 400°F (200°C). Toss the Brussels sprouts with olive oil, salt, and pepper. Spread them on a baking sheet, cut side down, and roast in the oven for about 20 minutes, or until they are tender and the edges are caramelized.
2. **Make Miso Glaze:** While the Brussels sprouts are roasting, whisk together miso paste, honey, rice vinegar, sesame oil, and water in a small bowl until smooth.
3. **Glaze Brussels Sprouts:** Once the Brussels sprouts are roasted, remove them from the oven and immediately toss them with the miso glaze while they are still hot.
4. **Serve:** Plate the Brussels sprouts and sprinkle with sesame seeds if desired. Serve warm as a side dish.

Macronutrients (per serving):

- **Calories:** 250 kcal
- **Carbohydrates:** 30 g
- **Protein:** 8 g
- **Fat:** 12 g

Vitamins:

- High in Vitamin C and K from Brussels sprouts.
- Contains B vitamins from miso.
- Provides dietary fiber, iron, and antioxidants.

Portobello Mushroom Fajitas

- **Preparation Time:** 15 minutes
- **Cooking Time:** 10 minutes
- **Servings:** 2

Ingredients:

- 2 large Portobello mushrooms, sliced
- 1 red bell pepper, sliced
- 1 green bell pepper, sliced
- 1 onion, sliced
- 2 tablespoons olive oil
- 1 teaspoon chili powder
- 1 teaspoon cumin
- 1/2 teaspoon smoked paprika
- Salt and pepper to taste
- 4 whole wheat or corn tortillas
- Optional toppings: lime wedges, fresh cilantro, avocado slices, salsa

Procedure:

1. **Prep and Cook Vegetables:** In a large skillet, heat the olive oil over medium-high heat. Add the sliced mushrooms, bell peppers, and onion. Sauté for about 5-7 minutes or until the vegetables are tender and slightly charred.
2. **Season:** Sprinkle the chili powder, cumin, smoked paprika, salt, and pepper over the vegetables while they cook, stirring frequently to ensure even coating and flavor distribution.
3. **Warm Tortillas:** While the vegetables are cooking, warm the tortillas in a dry pan or in the microwave for a few seconds until they are pliable.
4. **Assemble and Serve:** Divide the vegetable mixture among the warmed tortillas. Serve with optional toppings like lime wedges, fresh cilantro, avocado slices, and salsa.

Macronutrients (per serving):
Calories: 350 kcal; **Carbohydrates:** 45 g; **Protein:** 8 g; **Fat:** 16 g

Vitamins:

- High in Vitamin C from bell peppers.
- Contains B vitamins from whole wheat tortillas.
- Provides dietary fiber and iron from mushrooms.

Pumpkin and Chickpea Tagine

- **Preparation Time:** 15 minutes
- **Cooking Time:** 40 minutes
- **Servings:** 2

Ingredients:

- 1 cup diced pumpkin
- 1 can (15 oz) chickpeas, drained and rinsed
- 1 large onion, chopped
- 2 cloves garlic, minced
- 1 tablespoon olive oil
- 2 teaspoons ground cumin
- 1 teaspoon ground cinnamon
- 1/2 teaspoon ground ginger
- 1/4 teaspoon ground turmeric
- 2 cups vegetable broth
- 1/4 cup raisins
- Salt and pepper to taste
- Fresh cilantro, chopped, for garnish

Procedure:

1. **Sauté Aromatics:** In a tagine or large pot, heat olive oil over medium heat. Add the chopped onion and garlic, sautéing until the onion becomes translucent. Stir in cumin, cinnamon, ginger, and turmeric, cooking for another minute until fragrant.
2. **Add Main Ingredients:** Add the diced pumpkin, chickpeas, and raisins to the pot. Stir to coat the ingredients with the spices.
3. **Simmer:** Pour in the vegetable broth, bring to a boil, then reduce the heat to low. Cover and let simmer for about 30-35 minutes, or until the pumpkin is tender and the flavors have melded together.
4. **Serve:** Season with salt and pepper to taste. Garnish with chopped cilantro before serving. Serve hot, ideally with couscous or crusty bread for a complete meal.

Macronutrients (per serving): Calories: 380 kcal; **Carbohydrates:** 65 g; **Protein:** 13 g; **Fat:** 9 g

Vitamins:

- High in Vitamin A from pumpkin.
- Contains Vitamin C from raisins.
- Provides significant amounts of fiber and iron from chickpeas.

Quinoa Stuffed Bell Peppers

- **Preparation Time:** 15 minutes
- **Cooking Time:** 30 minutes
- **Servings:** 2

Ingredients:

- 2 large bell peppers, any color, halved and seeded
- 1/2 cup quinoa
- 1 cup vegetable broth
- 1 small onion, finely chopped
- 1 clove garlic, minced
- 1/2 cup chopped mushrooms
- 1/2 cup frozen corn, thawed
- 1/2 cup black beans, drained and rinsed
- 1 teaspoon olive oil
- 1/2 teaspoon cumin
- 1/2 teaspoon paprika
- Salt and pepper to taste
- Fresh parsley or cilantro, chopped, for garnish

Procedure:

1. **Cook Quinoa:** Rinse quinoa under cold water. In a small pot, bring the vegetable broth to a boil, add quinoa, reduce heat, cover, and simmer for about 15 minutes, or until all liquid is absorbed and quinoa is fluffy.
2. **Prepare Vegetable Mixture:** While quinoa is cooking, heat olive oil in a skillet over medium heat. Add onion and garlic, and sauté until softened. Stir in mushrooms, corn, and black beans, cooking until mushrooms are soft. Season with cumin, paprika, salt, and pepper.
3. **Stuff the Peppers:** Preheat the oven to 375°F (190°C). Mix the cooked quinoa into the skillet with the vegetable mixture. Spoon the filling evenly into the halved bell peppers.
4. **Bake and Serve:** Place the stuffed peppers in a baking dish and cover with foil. Bake in the preheated oven for about 15-20 minutes, until the peppers are tender. Remove the foil and bake for another 5 minutes to slightly char the

tops. Garnish with fresh parsley or cilantro before serving.

Macronutrients (per serving):
- **Calories:** 320 kcal
- **Carbohydrates:** 55 g
- **Protein:** 12 g
- **Fat:** 7 g

Vitamins:
- High in Vitamin C from bell peppers.
- Contains Vitamin A and several B vitamins from quinoa.
- Provides iron and magnesium.

Roasted Beet and Walnut Salad

- **Preparation Time:** 10 minutes
- **Cooking Time:** 30 minutes
- **Servings:** 2

Ingredients:
- 3 medium beets, peeled and diced
- 1/2 cup walnuts, roughly chopped
- 4 cups mixed salad greens (such as arugula and spinach)
- 1/4 cup crumbled goat cheese (optional)
- 2 tablespoons olive oil
- 1 tablespoon balsamic vinegar
- 1 teaspoon honey
- Salt and pepper to taste

Procedure:
1. **Roast Beets:** Preheat your oven to 400°F (200°C). Toss the diced beets with 1 tablespoon of olive oil, salt, and pepper. Spread them on a baking sheet and roast in the oven for about 30 minutes, or until tender and slightly caramelized, stirring halfway through the cooking time.
2. **Prepare Dressing:** In a small bowl, whisk together the remaining olive oil, balsamic vinegar, and honey. Season with salt and pepper to taste.
3. **Assemble Salad:** In a large salad bowl, combine the mixed salad greens, roasted beets, walnuts, and crumbled goat cheese if using.
4. **Serve:** Drizzle the dressing over the salad and toss gently to combine. Serve immediately, enjoying the blend of flavors and textures.

Macronutrients (per serving):
- **Calories:** 385 kcal
- **Carbohydrates:** 24 g
- **Protein:** 10 g
- **Fat:** 29 g

Vitamins:
- High in Vitamin C and folate from beets.
- Contains Vitamin E and omega-3 fatty acids from walnuts.
- Provides calcium from goat cheese (if used).

Spiced Cauliflower and Green Beans

- **Preparation Time:** 10 minutes
- **Cooking Time:** 20 minutes
- **Servings:** 2

Ingredients:

- 1 medium head cauliflower, cut into florets
- 2 cups green beans, trimmed
- 2 tablespoons olive oil
- 1 teaspoon cumin seeds
- 1 teaspoon ground turmeric
- 1/2 teaspoon ground coriander
- 1/4 teaspoon chili powder (adjust to taste)
- Salt and pepper to taste
- Fresh cilantro, chopped, for garnish

Procedure:

1. **Preheat and Prep:** Preheat your oven to 400°F (200°C). In a large bowl, toss the cauliflower florets and green beans with olive oil, cumin seeds, turmeric, coriander, chili powder, salt, and pepper until well coated.
2. **Roast Vegetables:** Spread the seasoned cauliflower and green beans in a single layer on a baking sheet. Roast in the preheated oven for about 20 minutes, or until the vegetables are tender and starting to brown, stirring halfway through for even cooking.
3. **Check Seasoning:** Once roasted, taste the vegetables and adjust the seasoning if needed, adding more salt or pepper as desired.
4. **Serve:** Transfer the roasted vegetables to a serving dish, sprinkle with chopped cilantro for a fresh flavor boost, and serve warm.

Macronutrients (per serving): Calories: 210 kcal; **Carbohydrates:** 18 g; **Protein:** 6 g; **Fat:** 14 g

Vitamins:

- High in Vitamin C and K from cauliflower and green beans.
- Contains Vitamin A and iron.
- Provides a good source of antioxidants from turmeric and other spices.

Sweet Corn and Black Bean Tacos

- **Preparation Time:** 10 minutes
- **Cooking Time:** 10 minutes
- **Servings:** 2

Ingredients:

- 1 cup canned black beans, drained and rinsed
- 1 cup sweet corn kernels, fresh or frozen
- 4 small corn tortillas
- 1/2 red onion, finely chopped
- 1 ripe avocado, sliced
- 1 small tomato, diced
- 1 jalapeño, seeded and finely chopped (optional)
- Juice of 1 lime
- 1 tablespoon olive oil
- Salt and pepper to taste
- Fresh cilantro, chopped, for garnish
- Optional: 1/4 cup shredded cheese or vegan cheese alternative

Procedure:

1. **Sauté Vegetables:** In a skillet, heat the olive oil over medium heat. Add the corn, black beans, and jalapeño (if using). Cook for about 5-7 minutes until the corn is lightly charred and the beans are heated through.
2. **Warm Tortillas:** While the filling cooks, warm the tortillas in a dry skillet over medium heat for about 30 seconds on each side or until they are pliable and slightly toasted.
3. **Assemble Tacos:** Distribute the bean and corn mixture evenly among the warmed tortillas. Top each taco with sliced avocado, diced tomato, and red onion.
4. **Serve:** Sprinkle with fresh lime juice, cilantro, and optional cheese. Serve immediately.

Macronutrients (per serving):

Calories: 380 kcal; **Carbohydrates:** 52 g; **Protein:** 12 g; **Fat:** 18 g

Vitamins:

High in Vitamin C from lime and tomatoes.

Contains good amounts of Vitamin A and K from avocado.

Provides B vitamins and iron from black beans.

Tomato Basil Spaghetti Squash

- **Preparation Time:** 10 minutes
- **Cooking Time:** 40 minutes
- **Servings:** 2

Ingredients:

- 1 medium spaghetti squash
- 1 cup cherry tomatoes, halved
- 1/4 cup fresh basil leaves, chopped
- 2 cloves garlic, minced
- 2 tablespoons olive oil
- Salt and pepper to taste
- Optional: grated Parmesan cheese or nutritional yeast for topping

Procedure:

1. **Roast Spaghetti Squash:** Preheat the oven to 400°F (200°C). Halve the spaghetti squash lengthwise and scoop out the seeds. Drizzle with 1 tablespoon of olive oil, and season with salt and pepper. Place cut-side down on a baking sheet and roast for about 30-40 minutes, or until the flesh is tender and can be shredded into strands with a fork.
2. **Prepare Tomato Basil Mixture:** While the squash is roasting, heat the remaining olive oil in a skillet over medium heat. Add the minced garlic and sauté for 1-2 minutes until fragrant. Add the cherry tomatoes and cook until they are soft and bursting, about 5-7 minutes. Remove from heat and stir in the chopped basil.
3. **Assemble the Dish:** Once the squash is cooked, use a fork to scrape the inside to create spaghetti-like strands. Transfer these strands to a serving dish.
4. **Serve:** Spoon the tomato basil mixture over the spaghetti squash strands. Toss gently to combine. Serve warm, topped with grated Parmesan cheese or nutritional yeast if desired.

Macronutrients (per serving):

- **Calories:** 200 kcal
- **Carbohydrates:** 30 g
- **Protein:** 2 g
- **Fat:** 10 g

Vitamins:

- High in Vitamin C and Vitamin A from tomatoes and spaghetti squash.
- Contains several B vitamins and minerals like potassium and magnesium.

Benefits:

This Tomato Basil Spaghetti Squash dish is a fantastic source of dietary fiber and antioxidants, particularly beta-carotene and Vitamin C, which help to protect against oxidative stress and support immune function. The olive oil not only adds flavor but also provides heart-healthy monounsaturated fats. This meal is ideal for those managing their carbohydrate intake while still enjoying a satisfying and delicious dish.

Chapter 13: Healthy snacks and sides

Almond Butter Stuffed Dates

- **Preparation Time:** 10 minutes
- **Cooking Time:** 0 minutes
- **Servings:** 2 (about 6 stuffed dates each)

Ingredients:

- 12 Medjool dates
- 1/4 cup almond butter
- Optional toppings: chopped almonds, coconut flakes, or dark chocolate shavings

Procedure:

1. **Prepare Dates:** Carefully slit each date down the middle to remove the pit, creating a pocket but not cutting all the way through.
2. **Stuff Dates:** Using a small spoon or a piping bag, fill each date with about a teaspoon of almond butter.
3. **Add Toppings:** If using, sprinkle the stuffed dates with your choice of chopped almonds, coconut flakes, or dark chocolate shavings for extra flavor and texture.
4. **Serve:** Arrange the stuffed dates on a plate and serve immediately, or chill in the refrigerator for a firmer texture before serving.

Macronutrients (per serving):

Calories: 350 kcal; **Carbohydrates:** 58 g; **Protein:** 6 g; **Fat:** 14 g

Vitamins:

- High in Vitamin E from almond butter.
- Contains potassium and magnesium from dates.
- Provides B vitamins, especially niacin and folate.

Baked Kale Chips

- **Preparation Time:** 10 minutes
- **Cooking Time:** 10 minutes
- **Servings:** 2

Ingredients:

- 1 bunch of kale, washed and dried
- 1 tablespoon olive oil
- Salt to taste
- Optional seasonings: paprika, garlic powder, or nutritional yeast

Procedure:

1. **Preheat Oven & Prepare Kale:** Preheat your oven to 350°F (175°C). Remove the kale leaves from the stems and tear them into bite-sized pieces.
2. **Season Kale:** Place the kale pieces in a large bowl. Drizzle with olive oil and sprinkle with salt and any other seasonings you like. Toss well to evenly coat all the pieces.
3. **Bake:** Spread the kale in a single layer on a baking sheet lined with parchment paper. Bake in the preheated oven for about 10 minutes, or until the edges are brown but not burnt.
4. **Serve:** Let the kale chips cool slightly (they will crisp up more as they cool), then serve immediately for the best texture.

Macronutrients (per serving): Calories: 150 kcal; **Carbohydrates:** 10 g; **Protein:** 4 g; **Fat:** 10 g

Vitamins:

- High in Vitamin K, which is essential for blood clotting and bone health.
- Rich in Vitamin A, important for vision and immune function.
- Provides Vitamin C, necessary for the growth, development, and repair of all body tissues.

Carrot and Hummus Roll-Ups

- **Preparation Time:** 10 minutes
- **Cooking Time:** 0 minutes
- **Servings:** 2

Ingredients:

- 2 large whole wheat tortillas
- 1/2 cup hummus
- 2 medium carrots, julienned
- 1/4 cup red bell pepper, julienned
- 1/4 cup cucumber, julienned
- 1 handful of fresh spinach leaves
- Optional: sprinkle of sesame seeds or crushed red pepper for extra flavor

Procedure:

1. **Prepare Ingredients:** Lay out the whole wheat tortillas on a flat surface. Spread a generous layer of hummus over each tortilla, covering them almost completely.
2. **Add Vegetables:** Arrange a line of julienned carrots, red bell pepper, and cucumber along with a few spinach leaves horizontally across the center of each tortilla.
3. **Roll Them Up:** Carefully roll up the tortillas tightly around the vegetables, ensuring that the filling stays in place. If necessary, you can add a light smear of hummus at the edge of the tortilla to help seal the roll.
4. **Serve:** Cut each roll into 1 to 2-inch pieces, similar to sushi rolls, and serve immediately. Optionally, sprinkle sesame seeds or crushed red pepper on top for added taste.

Macronutrients (per serving):

- **Calories:** 250 kcal
- **Carbohydrates:** 38 g
- **Protein:** 8 g
- **Fat:** 8 g

Vitamins:

- High in Vitamin A from carrots, which supports vision and immune health.
- Rich in Vitamin C from red bell peppers, essential for the growth, development, and repair of body tissues.
- Contains folate and iron from spinach.

Cauliflower Buffalo Wings

- **Preparation Time:** 15 minutes
- **Cooking Time:** 20 minutes
- **Servings:** 2

Ingredients:

- 1 head cauliflower, cut into bite-sized florets
- 1/2 cup all-purpose flour (or chickpea flour for gluten-free option)
- 1/2 cup water
- 1 teaspoon garlic powder
- Salt and pepper to taste
- 1/2 cup buffalo sauce or hot sauce
- 1 tablespoon olive oil or melted butter
- Optional: 1/4 cup blue cheese or ranch dressing for dipping

Procedure:

1. **Prepare Batter:** In a large bowl, mix the flour, water, garlic powder, salt, and pepper until smooth. Dip each cauliflower floret into the batter, ensuring each piece is evenly coated. Shake off the excess batter.
2. **Bake Cauliflower:** Preheat the oven to 450°F (230°C). Place the battered cauliflower on a baking sheet lined with parchment paper, spreading them out in a single layer. Bake for about 20 minutes, flipping halfway through, until the cauliflower is crispy and golden.
3. **Toss with Sauce:** In a separate bowl, combine the buffalo sauce with olive oil or melted butter. Toss the baked cauliflower in the sauce until well coated.
4. **Serve:** Return the cauliflower to the oven and bake for an additional 5 minutes to set the sauce. Serve hot with blue cheese or ranch dressing for dipping, if desired.

Macronutrients (per serving): Calories: 290 kcal; **Carbohydrates:** 35 g; **Protein:** 7 g; **Fat:** 15 g (varies with sauce and dressing)

Vitamins:

- High in Vitamin C from cauliflower.
- Contains Vitamin K.
- Provides B vitamins depending on the type of flour used.

Chia Seed Pudding with Berries

- **Preparation Time:** 10 minutes (plus several hours or overnight for setting)
- **Cooking Time:** 0 minutes
- **Servings:** 2

Ingredients:

- 1/4 cup chia seeds
- 1 cup unsweetened almond milk (or any other plant-based milk)
- 1 tablespoon honey or maple syrup (optional, for sweetness)
- 1/2 teaspoon vanilla extract
- 1/2 cup mixed berries (such as strawberries, blueberries, and raspberries)
- Optional toppings: additional berries, mint leaves, or a sprinkle of coconut flakes

Procedure:

1. **Mix Pudding Base:** In a bowl, combine chia seeds, almond milk, honey (if using), and vanilla extract. Stir thoroughly to mix.
2. **Refrigerate:** Cover the bowl and refrigerate for at least 4 hours, preferably overnight, until the mixture achieves a pudding-like consistency.
3. **Prepare Berries:** Wash and prepare the berries by slicing any larger ones, like strawberries, into smaller pieces to match the size of other berries.
4. **Serve:** Stir the pudding to ensure the texture is uniform and spoon into serving dishes. Top with mixed berries and any additional desired toppings before serving.

Macronutrients (per serving): Calories: 180 kcal; Carbohydrates: 24 g; Protein: 5 g; Fat: 9 g
Vitamins:

- High in Vitamin C and antioxidants from the berries.
- Provides significant amounts of calcium and Vitamin D if fortified almond milk is used.
- Rich in Omega-3 fatty acids from chia seeds.

Cinnamon Baked Apples

- **Preparation Time:** 10 minutes
- **Cooking Time:** 30 minutes
- **Servings:** 2

Ingredients:

- 2 large apples (such as Granny Smith or Honeycrisp)
- 2 tablespoons brown sugar or honey
- 1/2 teaspoon ground cinnamon
- 1/4 teaspoon nutmeg
- 2 teaspoons butter (or coconut oil for a vegan option)
- Optional: 1/4 cup chopped walnuts or pecans

Procedure:

1. **Prepare Apples:** Preheat your oven to 375°F (190°C). Core the apples and slice off the very top or bottom just enough to allow them to sit flat in a baking dish.
2. **Mix Filling:** In a small bowl, mix the brown sugar (or honey), cinnamon, and nutmeg. If using, add chopped nuts to the mixture for extra crunch and flavor.
3. **Stuff Apples:** Place the apples in a baking dish. Divide the sugar and spice mixture between the apples, filling the cores, and top each with a teaspoon of butter or coconut oil.
4. **Bake:** Cover the dish with foil and bake in the preheated oven for 20 minutes. Remove the foil and continue baking for another 10 minutes, or until the apples are soft and the filling is bubbling.

Macronutrients (per serving):

- **Calories:** 200 kcal
- **Carbohydrates:** 40 g
- **Protein:** 1 g
- **Fat:** 5 g

Vitamins:

- High in Vitamin C from apples.
- Contains a good amount of dietary fiber.
- Provides a variety of antioxidants from cinnamon and nutmeg.

Coconut Yogurt Parfait

- **Preparation Time:** 10 minutes
- **Cooking Time:** 0 minutes
- **Servings:** 2

Ingredients:

- 1 cup coconut yogurt (unsweetened)
- 1/2 cup granola (preferably homemade or low-sugar)
- 1/2 cup fresh berries (such as strawberries, blueberries, or raspberries)
- 2 tablespoons honey or maple syrup (optional)
- Optional toppings: shredded coconut, chia seeds, or a sprinkle of cinnamon

Procedure:

1. **Layer Ingredients:** Begin by placing a layer of coconut yogurt at the bottom of two serving glasses or bowls. Add a layer of granola on top of the yogurt, then a layer of fresh berries.
2. **Repeat Layers:** Repeat the layering process until the glasses are filled, ending with a layer of berries on top for a visually appealing presentation.
3. **Add Sweetener and Toppings:** Drizzle honey or maple syrup over the top layer if a sweeter taste is desired. Sprinkle with optional toppings such as shredded coconut, chia seeds, or cinnamon for extra flavor and nutrients.
4. **Serve:** Serve immediately or refrigerate until ready to enjoy. The parfait can be chilled for an hour before serving to enhance the flavors and firm up the yogurt layers.

Macronutrients (per serving):

- **Calories:** 280 kcal
- **Carbohydrates:** 36 g
- **Protein:** 6 g
- **Fat:** 12 g

Vitamins:

- High in Vitamin C from fresh berries.
- Provides a variety of B vitamins from granola.
- Contains dietary fiber, calcium, and probiotics from coconut yogurt.

Cucumber Tomato Salad with Herbs

- **Preparation Time:** 10 minutes
- **Cooking Time:** 0 minutes
- **Servings:** 2

Ingredients:

- 1 large cucumber, diced
- 2 large ripe tomatoes, diced
- 1/4 cup red onion, finely sliced
- 1/4 cup fresh parsley, chopped
- 1/4 cup fresh basil, chopped
- 2 tablespoons olive oil
- 1 tablespoon red wine vinegar
- Salt and pepper to taste
- Optional: crumbled feta cheese or black olives

Procedure:

1. **Prepare Vegetables:** In a large mixing bowl, combine the diced cucumbers, tomatoes, and thinly sliced red onions.
2. **Add Herbs:** Stir in chopped parsley and basil to the vegetable mix, blending well to distribute evenly.
3. **Dress the Salad:** Whisk together olive oil, red wine vinegar, salt, and pepper in a small bowl. Drizzle this dressing over the salad and toss gently to coat all the ingredients.
4. **Serve:** Serve the salad immediately, or chill it in the refrigerator for 30 minutes before serving to enhance the flavors. Optionally, top with crumbled feta cheese or black olives for added taste and texture.

Macronutrients (per serving):

- **Calories:** 180 kcal
- **Carbohydrates:** 14 g
- **Protein:** 3 g
- **Fat:** 14 g

Vitamins:

- High in Vitamin C from tomatoes and cucumbers.
- Contains Vitamin K and Vitamin A from fresh herbs.
- Provides dietary fiber and a range of minerals like potassium.

Flaxseed and Banana Smoothie

- **Preparation Time:** 5 minutes
- **Cooking Time:** 0 minutes
- **Servings:** 2

Ingredients:

- 2 ripe bananas
- 2 tablespoons ground flaxseed
- 1 cup unsweetened almond milk (or any plant-based milk)
- 1/2 cup Greek yogurt (or plant-based yogurt for a vegan option)
- 1 tablespoon honey (optional, for sweetness)
- 1/2 teaspoon vanilla extract
- Ice cubes (optional, for a chilled smoothie)

Procedure:

1. **Prepare Ingredients:** Peel the bananas and place them in a blender. Add the ground flaxseed.
2. **Add Liquids:** Pour in the almond milk and add the Greek yogurt to the blender. If using honey, add it along with the vanilla extract for extra flavor.
3. **Blend:** Blend all the ingredients on high until smooth. If you prefer a colder smoothie, add a handful of ice cubes to the blender before mixing.
4. **Serve:** Pour the smoothie into two glasses and serve immediately for the freshest taste and best texture.

Macronutrients (per serving):

- **Calories:** 240 kcal
- **Carbohydrates:** 38 g
- **Protein:** 8 g
- **Fat:** 7 g

Vitamins:

- High in Vitamin B6 and C from bananas.
- Provides a good source of calcium and Vitamin D if fortified milk is used.
- Rich in omega-3 fatty acids and fiber from flaxseeds.

Garlic Roasted Chickpeas

- **Preparation Time:** 5 minutes
- **Cooking Time:** 30 minutes
- **Servings:** 2

Ingredients:

- 1 can (15 oz) chickpeas, drained, rinsed, and patted dry
- 2 tablespoons olive oil
- 1 teaspoon garlic powder
- 1/2 teaspoon salt
- 1/4 teaspoon black pepper
- Optional: pinch of cayenne pepper or paprika for extra spice

Procedure:

1. **Preheat Oven:** Preheat your oven to 400°F (200°C).
2. **Season Chickpeas:** In a bowl, toss the dried chickpeas with olive oil, garlic powder, salt, black pepper, and any additional spices if using. Ensure that all chickpeas are evenly coated with the seasoning.
3. **Bake:** Spread the chickpeas in a single layer on a baking sheet lined with parchment paper. Bake in the preheated oven for about 25-30 minutes, stirring halfway through, until golden and crispy.
4. **Cool and Serve:** Remove the chickpeas from the oven and let them cool on the baking sheet for a few minutes to further crisp up. Serve warm or at room temperature as a snack or salad topping.

Macronutrients (per serving):

- **Calories:** 280 kcal
- **Carbohydrates:** 35 g
- **Protein:** 10 g
- **Fat:** 12 g

Vitamins:

- High in Vitamin B6 and folate from chickpeas.
- Contains iron and magnesium.
- Provides antioxidants from garlic powder and olive oil.

Green Bean Almondine

- **Preparation Time:** 10 minutes
- **Cooking Time:** 15 minutes
- **Servings:** 2

Ingredients:

- 1 pound fresh green beans, trimmed
- 1/4 cup sliced almonds
- 2 tablespoons olive oil
- 2 cloves garlic, minced
- Salt and pepper to taste
- Lemon zest (from 1 lemon) for garnish

Procedure:

1. **Cook Green Beans:** Bring a large pot of salted water to a boil. Add the green beans and cook for about 3-5 minutes until they are bright green and tender but still crisp. Drain and plunge into ice water to stop the cooking process and retain the vibrant color.
2. **Toast Almonds:** In a dry skillet over medium heat, toast the sliced almonds, stirring frequently, until they are golden brown and fragrant. Remove from the skillet and set aside.
3. **Sauté Garlic:** In the same skillet, heat the olive oil over medium heat. Add the minced garlic and sauté for about 1 minute until fragrant but not browned.
4. **Combine and Serve:** Add the drained green beans to the skillet with the garlic, tossing to coat. Season with salt and pepper. Serve the green beans topped with toasted almonds and a sprinkle of fresh lemon zest.

Macronutrients (per serving):

- **Calories:** 250 kcal
- **Carbohydrates:** 14 g
- **Protein:** 6 g
- **Fat:** 20 g

Vitamins:

- High in Vitamin C and Vitamin K from green beans.
- Contains Vitamin E from almonds.
- Provides dietary fiber, iron, and calcium.

Grilled Zucchini with Lemon Salt

- **Preparation Time:** 10 minutes
- **Cooking Time:** 10 minutes
- **Servings:** 2

Ingredients:

- 2 medium zucchinis, sliced lengthwise
- 1 tablespoon olive oil
- 1 lemon, zested and juiced
- 1 teaspoon coarse sea salt
- Freshly ground black pepper to taste

Procedure:

1. **Prepare Lemon Salt:** In a small bowl, mix the lemon zest with coarse sea salt. Set aside for garnishing.
2. **Preheat Grill:** Preheat your grill or grill pan over medium-high heat.
3. **Grill Zucchini:** Brush the zucchini slices with olive oil and season with a little black pepper. Place them on the hot grill and cook for about 4-5 minutes on each side, or until tender and grill marks appear.
4. **Serve:** Arrange the grilled zucchini on a serving platter. Sprinkle the lemon salt over the zucchini and drizzle with a little fresh lemon juice before serving.

Macronutrients (per serving):

- **Calories:** 100 kcal
- **Carbohydrates:** 8 g
- **Protein:** 2 g
- **Fat:** 7 g

Vitamins:

- High in Vitamin C from lemon and zucchini.
- Contains potassium, essential for blood pressure regulation and kidney health.
- Provides a good amount of Vitamin A and magnesium.

Homemade Almond Granola

- **Preparation Time:** 10 minutes
- **Cooking Time:** 20 minutes
- **Servings:** 2

Ingredients:

- 1 cup rolled oats
- 1/2 cup raw almonds, chopped
- 1/4 cup pumpkin seeds
- 2 tablespoons honey or maple syrup
- 2 tablespoons coconut oil, melted
- 1/2 teaspoon vanilla extract
- 1/4 teaspoon salt
- 1/2 teaspoon cinnamon

Procedure:

1. **Preheat Oven and Mix Dry Ingredients:** Preheat your oven to 300°F (150°C). In a large bowl, combine the rolled oats, chopped almonds, pumpkin seeds, salt, and cinnamon.
2. **Combine Wet Ingredients and Mix:** In a small bowl, whisk together the melted coconut oil, honey (or maple syrup), and vanilla extract. Pour this mixture over the dry ingredients and stir until everything is well coated.
3. **Bake:** Spread the granola mixture in an even layer on a baking sheet lined with parchment paper. Bake in the preheated oven for about 20 minutes, stirring halfway through to ensure even cooking and to prevent burning.
4. **Cool and Store:** Remove the granola from the oven and let it cool completely on the baking sheet. The granola will become crunchier as it cools. Once cooled, store in an airtight container at room temperature.

Macronutrients (per serving): Calories: 400 kcal; **Carbohydrates:** 34 g; **Protein:** 10 g; **Fat:** 26 g

Vitamins:

- High in Vitamin E from almonds.
- Contains several B vitamins, especially from oats and pumpkin seeds.
- Provides a good source of magnesium and zinc.

Lemon Pepper Edamame

- **Preparation Time:** 5 minutes
- **Cooking Time:** 10 minutes
- **Servings:** 2

Ingredients:

- 2 cups frozen edamame in pods
- 1 tablespoon olive oil
- Zest of 1 lemon
- 1/2 teaspoon black pepper
- 1/2 teaspoon salt

Procedure:

1. **Cook Edamame:** Bring a pot of water to a boil and add the frozen edamame. Cook for about 5 minutes, or until the edamame are warmed through and tender. Drain and pat dry.
2. **Season:** In a mixing bowl, toss the cooked edamame with olive oil, lemon zest, black pepper, and salt.
3. **Heat:** In a skillet over medium heat, sauté the seasoned edamame for about 3-5 minutes, just until the pods are slightly charred and the flavors are well blended.
4. **Serve:** Serve the Lemon Pepper Edamame warm, either as a snack or as a side dish.

Macronutrients (per serving):

- **Calories:** 190 kcal
- **Carbohydrates:** 14 g
- **Protein:** 12 g
- **Fat:** 10 g

Vitamins:

- High in Vitamin C from lemon zest.
- Rich in Vitamin K and folate from edamame.
- Contains iron and magnesium.

Mixed Nuts and Dried Fruit Trail Mix

- **Preparation Time:** 5 minutes
- **Cooking Time:** 0 minutes
- **Servings:** 2

Ingredients:

- 1/4 cup almonds
- 1/4 cup walnuts
- 1/4 cup cashews
- 1/4 cup dried cranberries
- 1/4 cup raisins
- 1/4 cup dried apricots, chopped
- Optional: sprinkle of sea salt or cinnamon for extra flavor

Procedure:

1. **Select Ingredients:** Choose a variety of nuts and dried fruits for a balanced mix of flavors and textures. Ensure that all nuts are unsalted and raw for the healthiest option, and look for unsweetened or lightly sweetened dried fruits.
2. **Mix Ingredients:** In a large bowl, combine the almonds, walnuts, cashews, dried cranberries, raisins, and chopped dried apricots. Toss them together until evenly mixed.
3. **Add Flavor:** If desired, add a sprinkle of sea salt or cinnamon and mix again to distribute the flavor throughout the trail mix.
4. **Serve or Store:** Serve immediately for a quick snack, or store the trail mix in an airtight container or individual snack bags for easy portability and freshness.

Macronutrients (per serving):

- **Calories:** 350 kcal
- **Carbohydrates:** 45 g
- **Protein:** 8 g
- **Fat:** 18 g

Vitamins:

- High in Vitamin E from nuts.
- Rich in iron and magnesium from dried fruits and nuts.
- Contains antioxidants from dried cranberries and vitamin A from apricots.

Oven-Baked Sweet Potato Fries

- **Preparation Time:** 10 minutes
- **Cooking Time:** 25 minutes
- **Servings:** 2

Ingredients:

- 2 large sweet potatoes, peeled and cut into 1/4-inch thick fries
- 2 tablespoons olive oil
- 1/2 teaspoon paprika
- 1/4 teaspoon garlic powder
- Salt and pepper to taste

Procedure:

1. **Preheat Oven and Prepare Potatoes:** Preheat your oven to 425°F (220°C). In a large bowl, toss the sweet potato fries with olive oil, paprika, garlic powder, salt, and pepper until evenly coated.
2. **Arrange Fries:** Spread the fries in a single layer on a baking sheet lined with parchment paper, ensuring they aren't touching too much so they can crisp up properly.
3. **Bake:** Place in the preheated oven and bake for about 25 minutes, turning the fries halfway through the cooking time, until they are golden and crisp.
4. **Serve:** Remove the fries from the oven and let them cool slightly on the baking sheet for a few minutes to further crisp up. Serve warm.

Macronutrients (per serving):

- **Calories:** 290 kcal
- **Carbohydrates:** 47 g
- **Protein:** 3 g
- **Fat:** 10 g

Vitamins:

- High in Vitamin A from sweet potatoes.
- Contains Vitamin C.
- Provides potassium and dietary fiber.

Pea and Mint Dip

- **Preparation Time:** 10 minutes
- **Cooking Time:** 5 minutes
- **Servings:** 2

Ingredients:

- 1 cup frozen peas
- 1/4 cup fresh mint leaves
- 1 clove garlic, minced
- 2 tablespoons Greek yogurt (use plant-based yogurt for a vegan option)
- 1 tablespoon lemon juice
- 1 tablespoon olive oil
- Salt and pepper to taste

Procedure:

1. **Cook Peas:** Bring a small pot of water to a boil. Add the frozen peas and cook for about 3-5 minutes until they are tender. Drain and rinse under cold water to cool down quickly.
2. **Blend Ingredients:** In a food processor or blender, combine the cooked peas, fresh mint leaves, minced garlic, Greek yogurt, lemon juice, and olive oil. Blend until smooth.
3. **Season:** Taste the dip and season with salt and pepper as needed. Adjust the consistency by adding a little water or more yogurt if it's too thick.
4. **Chill and Serve:** Transfer the dip to a bowl and chill in the refrigerator for at least 30 minutes to enhance the flavors. Serve with a drizzle of olive oil on top and a side of raw vegetables or whole-grain crackers.

Macronutrients (per serving):

- **Calories:** 150 kcal
- **Carbohydrates:** 13 g
- **Protein:** 5 g
- **Fat:** 8 g

Vitamins:

- High in Vitamin C and Vitamin K from peas.
- Contains Vitamin A from mint.
- Provides calcium from Greek yogurt.

Raw Veggie Sticks with Avocado Dip

- **Preparation Time:** 10 minutes
- **Cooking Time:** 0 minutes
- **Servings:** 2

Ingredients:

- **For the Veggie Sticks:**
  - 1 carrot, peeled and cut into sticks
  - 1 cucumber, cut into sticks
  - 1 red bell pepper, cut into sticks
  - 1 celery stalk, cut into sticks
- **For the Avocado Dip:**
  - 1 ripe avocado
  - Juice of 1 lime
  - 1 clove garlic, minced
  - Salt and pepper to taste
  - Optional: a pinch of chili powder or cumin for extra flavor

Procedure:

1. **Prepare Vegetables:** Wash, peel (where necessary), and cut the vegetables into stick shapes for easy dipping.
2. **Make Avocado Dip:** In a medium bowl, mash the ripe avocado with a fork until smooth. Add lime juice, minced garlic, and season with salt, pepper, and optional spices like chili powder or cumin. Mix well until combined.
3. **Serve:** Arrange the vegetable sticks on a plate or in a serving dish. Place the bowl of avocado dip in the center for sharing.
4. **Enjoy:** Dip the vegetable sticks into the avocado mixture and enjoy a fresh, satisfying snack.

Macronutrients (per serving):

- **Calories:** 250 kcal
- **Carbohydrates:** 22 g
- **Protein:** 4 g
- **Fat:** 18 g

Vitamins:

- High in Vitamin C from red bell pepper and lime juice.
- Rich in Vitamin A from carrots.
- Contains Vitamin E and K from avocado.

Spicy Pumpkin Seeds

- **Preparation Time:** 5 minutes
- **Cooking Time:** 15 minutes
- **Servings:** 2

Ingredients:

- 1 cup raw pumpkin seeds
- 1 tablespoon olive oil
- 1/2 teaspoon chili powder
- 1/4 teaspoon garlic powder
- 1/4 teaspoon smoked paprika
- Salt to taste
- Optional: a pinch of cayenne pepper for extra heat

Procedure:

1. **Preheat Oven:** Preheat your oven to 350°F (175°C).
2. **Season Seeds:** In a bowl, toss the pumpkin seeds with olive oil, chili powder, garlic powder, smoked paprika, salt, and cayenne pepper if using. Mix well to ensure all seeds are evenly coated.
3. **Bake:** Spread the seasoned pumpkin seeds in a single layer on a baking sheet lined with parchment paper. Bake in the preheated oven for about 15 minutes, stirring occasionally, until the seeds are golden and crunchy.
4. **Cool and Serve:** Remove the seeds from the oven and let them cool on the baking sheet. This will help them crisp up further. Once cool, serve as a snack or store in an airtight container.

Macronutrients (per serving):

- **Calories:** 318 kcal
- **Carbohydrates:** 4 g
- **Protein:** 18 g
- **Fat:** 27 g

Vitamins:

- High in Zinc, which supports immune function and skin health.
- Rich in Magnesium, important for muscle and nerve function.
- Provides a good source of Iron and Vitamin K.

Zucchini Muffins

- **Preparation Time:** 15 minutes
- **Cooking Time:** 20 minutes
- **Servings:** 2 (6 muffins total)

Ingredients:

- 1 cup grated zucchini (about 1 medium zucchini)
- 1 cup all-purpose flour
- 1/2 cup whole wheat flour
- 1/4 cup sugar
- 1/4 cup vegetable oil
- 1 large egg
- 1/2 cup unsweetened applesauce
- 1 teaspoon baking powder
- 1/2 teaspoon baking soda
- 1/2 teaspoon salt
- 1 teaspoon cinnamon
- Optional: 1/4 cup chopped walnuts or raisins

Procedure:

1. **Prepare Ingredients:** Preheat your oven to 350°F (175°C). Line a muffin tin with paper liners or grease with a little oil. Squeeze the grated zucchini in a clean cloth to remove excess moisture.
2. **Mix Dry Ingredients:** In a large bowl, combine both flours, sugar, baking powder, baking soda, salt, and cinnamon.
3. **Combine Wet Ingredients and Zucchini:** In another bowl, whisk together the egg, vegetable oil, and applesauce. Stir in the grated zucchini. Add the wet ingredients to the dry ingredients, stirring just until combined. Fold in walnuts or raisins if using.
4. **Bake:** Divide the batter evenly among the muffin cups. Bake for about 20 minutes, or until a toothpick inserted into the center of a muffin comes out clean. Let the muffins cool in the pan for a few minutes before transferring to a wire rack to cool completely.

Macronutrients (per serving, 3 muffins):
Calories: 460 kcal; **Carbohydrates:** 60 g; **Protein:** 8 g; **Fat:** 22 g
Vitamins: High in Vitamin C from zucchini. Contains Vitamin E from vegetable

Chapter 14: Wholesome desserts

Almond Joy Energy Bites

- **Preparation Time:** 15 minutes
- **Cooking Time:** 0 minutes (needs chilling)
- **Servings:** 2 (about 6 bites each)

Ingredients:

- 1 cup raw almonds
- 1 cup dates, pitted
- 1/2 cup shredded unsweetened coconut
- 1/4 cup cocoa powder
- 1 teaspoon vanilla extract
- A pinch of salt
- Water (if needed, to help blend)

Procedure:

1. **Blend Ingredients:** In a food processor, combine the almonds, dates, shredded coconut, cocoa powder, vanilla extract, and a pinch of salt. Process until the mixture is finely ground and sticks together when pinched. If the mixture is too dry, add a teaspoon of water at a time until it reaches the desired consistency.
2. **Form Bites:** Scoop out tablespoon-sized amounts of the mixture and roll them into balls using your hands.
3. **Chill:** Place the energy bites on a baking sheet lined with parchment paper and refrigerate for at least 30 minutes to firm up.
4. **Serve or Store:** Serve chilled. Store any leftovers in an airtight container in the refrigerator for up to a week or in the freezer for longer storage.

Macronutrients (per serving, about 6 bites):

- **Calories:** 300 kcal
- **Carbohydrates:** 35 g
- **Protein:** 8 g
- **Fat:** 18 g

Vitamins:

- High in Vitamin E from almonds.
- Provides significant amounts of magnesium and potassium from dates and almonds.

Apple Cinnamon Baked Oatmeal Cups

- **Preparation Time:** 10 minutes
- **Cooking Time:** 25 minutes
- **Servings:** 2 (6 cups total)

Ingredients:

- 1 cup rolled oats
- 1 medium apple, peeled and diced
- 1 cup unsweetened almond milk
- 1 egg
- 1/4 cup honey or maple syrup
- 1 teaspoon cinnamon
- 1/2 teaspoon baking powder
- 1/4 teaspoon salt
- Optional: 1/4 cup raisins or walnuts for added texture and flavor

Procedure:

1. **Preheat and Prepare:** Preheat your oven to 375°F (190°C). Grease a 6-cup muffin tin or line it with paper liners.
2. **Mix Ingredients:** In a large bowl, combine the rolled oats, cinnamon, baking powder, and salt. In another bowl, whisk together the almond milk, egg, and honey. Add the wet ingredients to the dry ingredients and mix until combined. Stir in the diced apple and optional raisins or walnuts.
3. **Fill Muffin Tin:** Divide the oatmeal mixture evenly among the prepared muffin cups, filling each nearly to the top.
4. **Bake and Serve:** Bake in the preheated oven for 25 minutes, or until the tops are golden and set. Let them cool for 5 minutes before removing from the tin. Serve warm or store in the refrigerator for up to a week.

Macronutrients (per serving, 3 cups):

- **Calories:** 320 kcal
- **Carbohydrates:** 60 g
- **Protein:** 7 g
- **Fat:** 5 g

Vitamins:

- High in Vitamin E from almonds (if using almond milk).
- Contains significant amounts of Vitamin C from apples.
- Provides B vitamins from oats and a good amount of dietary fiber.

Avocado Chocolate Mousse

- **Preparation Time:** 10 minutes
- **Cooking Time:** 0 minutes (plus chilling time)
- **Servings:** 2

Ingredients:

- 2 ripe avocados, peeled and pitted
- 1/4 cup unsweetened cocoa powder
- 1/4 cup honey or maple syrup (adjust to taste)
- 1/2 teaspoon vanilla extract
- A pinch of salt
- Optional: 1 tablespoon almond milk or any plant-based milk for smoother consistency

Procedure:

1. **Blend Ingredients:** In a blender or food processor, combine the avocados, cocoa powder, honey (or maple syrup), vanilla extract, and salt. Blend until the mixture is smooth and creamy. If the mousse is too thick, add a tablespoon of almond milk to adjust the consistency.
2. **Taste and Adjust:** Taste the mousse and adjust the sweetness if needed by adding a little more honey or syrup.
3. **Chill:** Transfer the mousse to serving dishes and refrigerate for at least 30 minutes to allow it to set and develop flavors.
4. **Serve:** Serve chilled, optionally garnished with fresh berries, a sprinkle of cocoa powder, or shaved dark chocolate.

Macronutrients (per serving):

- **Calories:** 380 kcal
- **Carbohydrates:** 40 g
- **Protein:** 4 g
- **Fat:** 25 g

Vitamins:

- High in Vitamin E from avocados.
- Contains significant amounts of Vitamin C and Vitamin K.
- Provides potassium and magnesium.

Banana Coconut Ice Cream

- **Preparation Time:** 10 minutes (plus freezing time)
- **Cooking Time:** 0 minutes
- **Servings:** 2

Ingredients:

- 3 ripe bananas, sliced and frozen
- 1/2 cup coconut milk (full-fat for creamier texture)
- 1 teaspoon vanilla extract
- Optional: 2 tablespoons shredded coconut for extra flavor and texture

Procedure:

1. **Prepare Bananas:** Prior to preparation, peel and slice the bananas, then freeze them until solid, preferably overnight.
2. **Blend Ingredients:** In a food processor or high-powered blender, combine the frozen banana slices, coconut milk, and vanilla extract. Blend until the mixture is smooth and creamy. You may need to pause and stir occasionally to ensure even blending.
3. **Add Coconut:** If using shredded coconut, add it towards the end of blending and pulse a few times to mix it into the ice cream.
4. **Freeze and Serve:** For a soft-serve texture, serve immediately. For a firmer consistency, transfer the ice cream to an airtight container and freeze for 2-3 hours before serving.

Macronutrients (per serving):

- **Calories:** 280 kcal
- **Carbohydrates:** 44 g
- **Protein:** 3 g
- **Fat:** 12 g

Vitamins:

- High in Vitamin C from bananas.
- Contains significant amounts of Vitamin B6 and magnesium.
- Provides a good source of iron and healthy fats from coconut milk.

Carrot Cake Balls

- **Preparation Time:** 20 minutes
- **Cooking Time:** 0 minutes (requires chilling)
- **Servings:** 2 (about 6 balls each)

Ingredients:

- 1 cup finely grated carrots
- 1 cup rolled oats
- 1/4 cup raisins
- 1/4 cup finely chopped walnuts
- 1/4 cup coconut flakes
- 1/4 cup honey or maple syrup
- 1 teaspoon cinnamon
- 1/2 teaspoon nutmeg
- 1/4 teaspoon ground ginger
- 2 tablespoons cream cheese or coconut cream for binding (use coconut cream for a vegan option)

Procedure:

1. **Mix Ingredients:** In a large bowl, combine the grated carrots, oats, raisins, walnuts, coconut flakes, spices, and honey or maple syrup. Mix thoroughly until all components are evenly distributed.
2. **Bind Mixture:** Add cream cheese or coconut cream to the mixture. Use your hands or a spoon to blend until the mixture is sticky and holds together when pressed.
3. **Form Balls:** Scoop tablespoon-sized amounts of the mixture and roll them into balls between your palms. If the mixture is too sticky, slightly wet your hands with water or dust them with oat flour.
4. **Chill and Serve:** Place the carrot cake balls on a tray lined with parchment paper and refrigerate for at least an hour to firm up. Serve chilled, or store in an airtight container in the refrigerator for up to a week.

Macronutrients (per serving, about 6 balls):
Calories: 350 kcal; **Carbohydrates:** 50 g; **Protein:** 6 g; **Fat:** 15 g

Vitamins:

- High in Vitamin A from carrots.
- Contains Vitamin E from walnuts.
- Provides B vitamins from oats

Chia Seed Coconut Pudding

- **Preparation Time:** 10 minutes
- **Cooking Time:** 0 minutes (requires several hours of refrigeration)
- **Servings:** 2

Ingredients:

- 1/3 cup chia seeds
- 1 cup coconut milk (full-fat for a creamier texture)
- 2 tablespoons honey or maple syrup
- 1/2 teaspoon vanilla extract
- Optional toppings: sliced bananas, berries, or shredded coconut

Procedure:

1. **Mix Ingredients:** In a medium bowl, combine the chia seeds, coconut milk, honey (or maple syrup), and vanilla extract. Stir well to mix everything thoroughly.
2. **Refrigerate:** Cover the bowl with plastic wrap or a lid and refrigerate for at least 4 hours, or overnight, until the mixture thickens and the chia seeds have absorbed the liquid, forming a gel-like texture.
3. **Stir and Adjust:** After chilling, stir the pudding to check the consistency. If it's too thick, add a little more coconut milk to reach your desired texture.
4. **Serve:** Spoon the pudding into serving bowls or glasses, and top with your choice of sliced bananas, berries, or a sprinkle of shredded coconut for added flavor and decoration.

Macronutrients (per serving):

- **Calories:** 340 kcal
- **Carbohydrates:** 30 g
- **Protein:** 6 g
- **Fat:** 24 g

Vitamins:

- High in Omega-3 fatty acids from chia seeds.
- Rich in iron and calcium from chia seeds.
- Provides a good source of Vitamin C if served with berries, and potassium if served with bananas.

Cinnamon Baked Pears

- **Preparation Time:** 10 minutes
- **Cooking Time:** 30 minutes
- **Servings:** 2

Ingredients:

- 2 large ripe pears (such as Bartlett or Anjou), halved and cored
- 2 teaspoons honey (or maple syrup for a vegan option)
- 1/2 teaspoon ground cinnamon
- A pinch of nutmeg
- Optional: a dollop of Greek yogurt or whipped coconut cream for serving

Procedure:

1. **Preheat Oven and Prepare Pears:** Preheat your oven to 350°F (175°C). Place the pear halves cut-side up on a baking dish. If the pears wobble, slice a small piece off the rounded side to make them sit flat.
2. **Season Pears:** Drizzle each pear half with honey and sprinkle evenly with cinnamon and nutmeg.
3. **Bake:** Cover the baking dish with foil and bake in the preheated oven for about 20-25 minutes. Remove the foil and continue baking for another 5-10 minutes, or until the pears are tender and caramelized.
4. **Serve:** Serve the baked pears warm with a dollop of Greek yogurt or whipped coconut cream if desired.

Macronutrients (per serving):

- **Calories:** 150 kcal
- **Carbohydrates:** 38 g
- **Protein:** 1 g
- **Fat:** 0.3 g

Vitamins:

- High in Vitamin C and K.
- Provides a good amount of dietary fiber.
- Contains small amounts of B vitamins.

Date and Nut Bars

- **Preparation Time:** 15 minutes
- **Cooking Time:** 0 minutes (requires chilling)
- **Servings:** 2 (about 6 bars total)

Ingredients:

- 1 cup pitted Medjool dates
- 1/2 cup raw almonds
- 1/2 cup walnuts
- 1/4 cup shredded unsweetened coconut
- 1 tablespoon chia seeds
- 1 teaspoon vanilla extract
- Pinch of salt

Procedure:

1. **Process Ingredients:** In a food processor, combine the dates, almonds, walnuts, shredded coconut, chia seeds, vanilla extract, and a pinch of salt. Process until the mixture becomes sticky and holds together when pinched. You may need to stop and scrape down the sides a few times to ensure everything is evenly mixed.
2. **Press Mixture:** Line a small baking dish or loaf pan with parchment paper. Transfer the date and nut mixture to the pan, pressing it firmly into an even layer using the back of a spoon or your hands.
3. **Chill to Set:** Place the dish in the refrigerator for at least 1 hour to allow the bars to set and harden.
4. **Slice and Serve:** Remove the mixture from the dish, lifting out the parchment paper. Cut into bars or squares. Store the bars in an airtight container in the refrigerator for up to a week.

Macronutrients (per serving, 3 bars): Calories: 400 kcal; Carbohydrates: 50 g; Protein: 8 g; Fat: 20 g

Vitamins:

- High in Vitamin E from almonds and walnuts.
- Contains significant amounts of magnesium, potassium, and iron.
- Provides B vitamins and omega-3 fatty acids from chia seeds.

Fig and Walnut Bites

- **Preparation Time:** 10 minutes
- **Cooking Time:** 0 minutes (requires chilling)
- **Servings:** 2 (about 8 bites each)

Ingredients:

- 1 cup dried figs, stems removed
- 1/2 cup walnuts
- 1/4 cup rolled oats
- 1 teaspoon cinnamon
- A pinch of sea salt
- Optional: 1 tablespoon honey or maple syrup for extra sweetness

Procedure:

1. **Blend Ingredients:** In a food processor, combine the dried figs, walnuts, rolled oats, cinnamon, and sea salt. Pulse until the mixture is well combined and begins to stick together. If the mixture is too dry, add honey or maple syrup to help it bind.
2. **Form Bites:** Scoop out tablespoon-sized amounts of the mixture and roll into balls between your palms. If the mixture sticks to your hands, slightly wet them with water or lightly oil them.
3. **Chill to Set:** Place the formed bites on a plate or tray lined with parchment paper. Refrigerate for at least 30 minutes to firm up and make them easier to handle.
4. **Serve or Store:** Serve the fig and walnut bites chilled. Store any leftovers in an airtight container in the refrigerator for up to a week.

Macronutrients (per serving, 8 bites):

- **Calories:** 350 kcal
- **Carbohydrates:** 45 g
- **Protein:** 6 g
- **Fat:** 18 g

Vitamins:

- High in dietary fiber and Vitamin B6 from figs.
- Contains significant amounts of Vitamin E and omega-3 fatty acids from walnuts.
- Provides iron, magnesium, and potassium.

Ginger Peach Sorbet

- **Preparation Time:** 10 minutes (plus freezing time)
- **Cooking Time:** 0 minutes
- **Servings:** 2

Ingredients:

- 4 ripe peaches, peeled and sliced
- 1/4 cup freshly squeezed orange juice
- 2 tablespoons honey or agave syrup
- 1 tablespoon freshly grated ginger
- 1 teaspoon lemon juice

Procedure:

1. **Prepare the Fruit:** In a blender, combine the sliced peaches, orange juice, honey (or agave syrup), grated ginger, and lemon juice. Blend until the mixture is completely smooth.
2. **Freeze:** Pour the blended mixture into a shallow dish or ice cream maker. If using a dish, place it in the freezer. Freeze for about 1-2 hours, then stir it vigorously with a fork. Repeat this process every hour until the sorbet is firm but scoopable.
3. **Serve:** Once the sorbet is ready, scoop it into bowls or glasses.
4. **Garnish and Enjoy:** Optionally, garnish with fresh peach slices or a sprinkle of ground ginger for an extra flavor boost.

Macronutrients (per serving):

- **Calories:** 200 kcal
- **Carbohydrates:** 50 g
- **Protein:** 2 g
- **Fat:** 0 g

Vitamins:

- High in Vitamin C from peaches, orange juice, and lemon juice.
- Contains Vitamin A from peaches.
- Provides a good amount of dietary fiber and potassium.

Lemon Basil Sorbet

- **Preparation Time:** 10 minutes (plus freezing time)
- **Cooking Time:** 0 minutes
- **Servings:** 2

Ingredients:

- 1 cup fresh lemon juice (about 4-5 large lemons)
- 2 teaspoons lemon zest
- 1 cup water
- 3/4 cup granulated sugar (or honey for a natural alternative)
- 1/4 cup fresh basil leaves, finely chopped

Procedure:

1. **Prepare Syrup:** In a small saucepan over medium heat, combine water and sugar (or honey). Heat until the sugar has completely dissolved into a syrup. Remove from heat and allow to cool slightly.
2. **Infuse Basil:** Add the chopped basil leaves to the syrup while it is still warm, letting them steep for about 5 minutes to infuse the flavor.
3. **Mix and Strain:** Stir in the lemon juice and zest into the basil syrup. Strain the mixture through a fine sieve to remove the basil pieces and zest, ensuring a smooth sorbet base.
4. **Freeze:** Pour the strained mixture into an ice cream maker and churn according to the manufacturer's instructions. If you don't have an ice cream maker, pour the mixture into a shallow container and freeze, stirring vigorously every 30 minutes to break up ice crystals until frozen (about 2-3 hours).

Macronutrients (per serving):

- **Calories:** 180 kcal
- **Carbohydrates:** 47 g (if using sugar; varies if using honey)
- **Protein:** 0 g
- **Fat:** 0 g

Vitamins:

- High in Vitamin C from lemon juice.
- Provides small amounts of iron and antioxidants from basil.

Mango Lime Chia Pudding

- **Preparation Time:** 15 minutes
- **Cooking Time:** 0 minutes (requires at least 4 hours of refrigeration)
- **Servings:** 2

Ingredients:

- 1 ripe mango, peeled and cubed
- 1 cup unsweetened coconut milk
- 1/4 cup chia seeds
- Juice and zest of 1 lime
- 2 tablespoons honey or agave syrup (adjust to taste)

Procedure:

1. **Prepare Mango Puree:** In a blender, combine the cubed mango, lime juice, and honey (or agave syrup). Blend until smooth.
2. **Mix with Chia:** Pour the mango mixture into a bowl, add the chia seeds and half of the lime zest, and mix well. The chia seeds will begin to absorb the liquid and thicken the mixture.
3. **Refrigerate:** Divide the mixture into serving glasses or bowls, cover, and refrigerate for at least 4 hours, or overnight, until the chia pudding has set and is thick.
4. **Serve:** Once set, garnish with the remaining lime zest and additional mango cubes or coconut flakes if desired before serving.

Macronutrients (per serving):

- **Calories:** 280 kcal
- **Carbohydrates:** 45 g
- **Protein:** 5 g
- **Fat:** 10 g

Vitamins:

- High in Vitamin C from mango and lime.
- Provides a good source of Vitamin A from mango.
- Contains omega-3 fatty acids and fiber from chia seeds.

Mixed Berry Compote

- **Preparation Time:** 5 minutes
- **Cooking Time:** 10 minutes
- **Servings:** 2

Ingredients:

- 1 cup fresh or frozen mixed berries (such as strawberries, blueberries, raspberries, and blackberries)
- 2 tablespoons honey or maple syrup (adjust to taste)
- 1 teaspoon lemon juice
- 1/4 teaspoon vanilla extract

Procedure:

1. **Cook Berries:** In a small saucepan over medium heat, combine the mixed berries and honey (or maple syrup). Cook, stirring occasionally, until the berries begin to release their juices, about 5 minutes.
2. **Simmer:** Reduce heat to low and continue to simmer the mixture for another 5 minutes, stirring frequently until the berries break down and the mixture thickens slightly.
3. **Add Flavors:** Stir in the lemon juice and vanilla extract, and cook for an additional minute.
4. **Cool and Serve:** Remove from heat and let the compote cool slightly. It can be served warm or chilled, depending on your preference.

Macronutrients (per serving):

- **Calories:** 120 kcal
- **Carbohydrates:** 30 g
- **Protein:** 1 g
- **Fat:** 0 g

Vitamins:

- High in Vitamin C, particularly from strawberries and raspberries.
- Provides a good source of Vitamin K from blueberries.
- Contains antioxidants and dietary fiber.

Oatmeal Raisin Cookies (Sugar-Free)

- **Preparation Time:** 15 minutes
- **Cooking Time:** 12 minutes
- **Servings:** 2 (6 cookies each)

Ingredients:

- 1 cup rolled oats
- 1/2 cup whole wheat flour
- 1/3 cup unsweetened applesauce
- 1/4 cup raisins
- 2 tablespoons melted coconut oil
- 1 egg
- 1 teaspoon vanilla extract
- 1 teaspoon cinnamon
- 1/2 teaspoon baking soda
- A pinch of salt

Procedure:

1. **Mix Dry Ingredients:** In a large bowl, combine the rolled oats, whole wheat flour, cinnamon, baking soda, and salt.
2. **Combine Wet Ingredients:** In another bowl, whisk together the unsweetened applesauce, melted coconut oil, egg, and vanilla extract.
3. **Combine Mixtures and Add Raisins:** Add the wet ingredients to the dry ingredients and mix until just combined. Fold in the raisins.
4. **Bake Cookies:** Preheat your oven to 350°F (175°C). Line a baking sheet with parchment paper. Drop tablespoon-sized portions of the cookie dough onto the sheet, spacing them about 2 inches apart. Flatten them slightly. Bake for 10-12 minutes or until the edges are golden brown. Let them cool on the baking sheet for 5 minutes before transferring to a wire rack to cool completely.

Macronutrients (per serving, 6 cookies): Calories: 320 kcal; **Carbohydrates:** 48 g; **Protein:** 8 g; **Fat:** 12 g

Vitamins:

- High in Vitamin E from coconut oil.
- Contains B vitamins from whole wheat flour and oats.
- Provides iron and antioxidants from raisins.

Pumpkin Spice Energy Balls

- **Preparation Time:** 15 minutes
- **Cooking Time:** 0 minutes (requires chilling)
- **Servings:** 2 (about 6 balls each)

Ingredients:

- 1 cup rolled oats
- 1/2 cup pumpkin puree
- 1/4 cup almond butter
- 1/4 cup ground flaxseed
- 2 tablespoons honey or maple syrup
- 1 teaspoon vanilla extract
- 1/2 teaspoon cinnamon
- 1/4 teaspoon nutmeg
- 1/4 teaspoon ground ginger
- A pinch of cloves
- Optional: 1/4 cup chopped pecans or walnuts for added texture

Procedure:

1. **Mix Ingredients:** In a large bowl, combine all ingredients: rolled oats, pumpkin puree, almond butter, ground flaxseed, honey, vanilla extract, cinnamon, nutmeg, ginger, and cloves. Stir until everything is thoroughly mixed. If using, fold in the chopped nuts.
2. **Chill Mixture:** Cover the bowl and refrigerate for at least 30 minutes. This chilling time helps the mixture firm up, making it easier to shape.
3. **Form Balls:** Once chilled, use a tablespoon to scoop the mixture and roll into balls between the palms of your hands.
4. **Store or Serve:** Place the energy balls on a baking sheet lined with parchment paper. You can serve them immediately or store them in an airtight container in the refrigerator for up to a week.

Macronutrients (per serving, 6 balls): Calories: 300 kcal; **Carbohydrates:** 35 g; **Protein:** 8 g; **Fat:** 15 g

Vitamins: High in Vitamin A from pumpkin puree. Contains Vitamin E from almond butter and ground flaxseed. Provides omega-3 fatty acids from flaxseed

Raw Cacao Truffles

- **Preparation Time:** 15 minutes
- **Cooking Time:** 0 minutes (requires chilling)
- **Servings:** 2 (about 8 truffles each)

Ingredients:

- 1 cup Medjool dates, pitted
- 1/2 cup raw almonds
- 1/3 cup raw cacao powder, plus extra for rolling
- 1 tablespoon coconut oil
- 1/4 teaspoon sea salt
- Optional: 1 teaspoon vanilla extract or a pinch of cinnamon for extra flavor

Procedure:

1. **Blend Ingredients:** In a food processor, blend the pitted dates and almonds until they form a sticky, crumbly mixture. Add the raw cacao powder, coconut oil, sea salt, and optional vanilla extract or cinnamon. Process until the mixture is well combined and sticks together when pressed.
2. **Form Truffles:** Scoop out tablespoon-sized portions of the mixture. Roll between your palms to form smooth balls.
3. **Coat Truffles:** Roll each truffle in additional cacao powder to coat. This adds an extra layer of chocolate flavor and a gourmet finish.
4. **Chill and Serve:** Place the truffles on a plate or baking sheet lined with parchment paper. Refrigerate for at least 30 minutes to firm up before serving. Store any leftovers in an airtight container in the refrigerator.

Macronutrients (per serving, about 8 truffles):
Calories: 320 kcal; **Carbohydrates:** 45 g; Protein: 5 g; **Fat:** 16 g

Vitamins: High in magnesium from raw cacao, which is essential for over 300 biochemical reactions in the body. Contains iron and antioxidants from raw cacao and almonds. Provides Vitamin E and healthy fats from almonds and coconut oil.

Spiced Roasted Chickpeas

- **Preparation Time:** 5 minutes
- **Cooking Time:** 30 minutes
- **Servings:** 2 (about 1 cup each)

Ingredients:

- 1 can (15 oz) chickpeas, drained, rinsed, and patted dry
- 2 tablespoons olive oil
- 1 teaspoon ground cumin
- 1 teaspoon paprika
- 1/2 teaspoon garlic powder
- 1/4 teaspoon cayenne pepper (adjust to taste)
- Salt to taste

Procedure:

1. **Preheat Oven and Prepare Chickpeas:** Preheat your oven to 400°F (200°C). Ensure the chickpeas are thoroughly dried after rinsing to achieve maximum crunchiness.
2. **Season Chickpeas:** In a bowl, toss the dried chickpeas with olive oil, cumin, paprika, garlic powder, cayenne pepper, and salt until evenly coated.
3. **Roast:** Spread the seasoned chickpeas in a single layer on a baking sheet. Roast in the preheated oven for about 25-30 minutes, shaking the pan or stirring the chickpeas halfway through to ensure even cooking.
4. **Cool and Serve:** Remove the chickpeas from the oven and let them cool on the baking sheet for a few minutes to further crisp up. Serve warm or at room temperature.

Macronutrients (per serving):

- **Calories:** 282 kcal
- **Carbohydrates:** 35 g
- **Protein:** 10 g
- **Fat:** 12 g

Vitamins:

- High in Vitamin B6 and folate from chickpeas.
- Contains iron and magnesium.
- Provides antioxidants from garlic powder and paprika.

Strawberry Banana Soft Serve

- **Preparation Time:** 10 minutes (plus time for freezing the fruits)
- **Cooking Time:** 0 minutes
- **Servings:** 2

Ingredients:

- 2 large bananas, sliced and frozen
- 1 cup strawberries, hulled and frozen
- Optional: 1 tablespoon honey or maple syrup for extra sweetness
- Optional: a splash of almond milk for smoother blending

Procedure:

1. **Prepare Fruit:** Prior to preparation, peel and slice the bananas, and hull the strawberries. Freeze them until they are solid, ideally overnight.
2. **Blend Ingredients:** Place the frozen banana slices and strawberries into a food processor or high-powered blender. Blend on high until the mixture reaches a smooth and creamy consistency, resembling soft serve. Use a tablespoon or two of almond milk if necessary to facilitate blending.
3. **Add Sweetener (Optional):** If you prefer a sweeter taste, add honey or maple syrup during the blending process.
4. **Serve Immediately:** Once blended to the right consistency, serve the soft serve immediately for the best texture, or freeze it for a few hours for a firmer consistency.

Macronutrients (per serving):

- **Calories:** 180 kcal
- **Carbohydrates:** 45 g
- **Protein:** 2 g
- **Fat:** 0.5 g

Vitamins:

- High in Vitamin C from strawberries.
- Provides a good amount of potassium and dietary fiber from bananas.
- Contains several other essential nutrients such as Vitamin B6 and manganese.

Sweet Potato Brownies

- **Preparation Time:** 15 minutes
- **Cooking Time:** 25 minutes
- **Servings:** 2 (about 6 brownies each)

Ingredients:

- 1 cup mashed cooked sweet potato (about 1 medium sweet potato)
- 1/2 cup almond butter or peanut butter
- 1/4 cup cocoa powder
- 1/4 cup honey or maple syrup
- 1 egg
- 1 teaspoon vanilla extract
- 1/2 teaspoon baking soda
- Pinch of salt

Procedure:

1. **Prepare Sweet Potato:** Preheat your oven to 350°F (175°C). Peel and cube the sweet potato, then boil or steam until tender. Mash thoroughly until smooth.
2. **Mix Ingredients:** In a large mixing bowl, combine the mashed sweet potato, almond butter, cocoa powder, honey, egg, vanilla extract, baking soda, and a pinch of salt. Stir well until the mixture is completely smooth and evenly mixed.
3. **Bake:** Line an 8x8 inch baking dish with parchment paper. Pour the brownie mixture into the dish, spreading evenly. Bake in the preheated oven for 20-25 minutes, or until a toothpick inserted into the center comes out mostly clean.
4. **Cool and Serve:** Allow the brownies to cool in the pan for at least 10 minutes before slicing into squares. Serve warm or at room temperature.

Macronutrients (per serving, about 6 brownies):

- **Calories:** 350 kcal
- **Carbohydrates:** 40 g
- **Protein:** 10 g
- **Fat:** 18 g

Vitamins:

- High in Vitamin A from sweet potatoes.
- Provides iron and magnesium from cocoa powder.
- Contains good amounts of Vitamin E and healthy fats from almond butter.

Zucchini Bread (Sugar-Free)

- **Preparation Time:** 15 minutes
- **Cooking Time:** 50 minutes
- **Servings:** 2 (about 6 slices each)

Ingredients:

- 1.5 cups grated zucchini (about 1 medium zucchini)
- 2 cups whole wheat flour
- 1/2 cup unsweetened applesauce
- 2 eggs
- 1/4 cup olive oil
- 1 teaspoon vanilla extract
- 1 teaspoon baking soda
- 1/2 teaspoon salt
- 2 teaspoons cinnamon
- Optional: 1/2 cup chopped nuts (e.g., walnuts, almonds) or seeds for added texture and nutrients

Procedure:

1. **Prepare Ingredients:** Preheat your oven to 350°F (175°C). Grease a 9x5 inch loaf pan or line it with parchment paper. Squeeze the grated zucchini with a towel to remove excess moisture.
2. **Mix Wet and Dry Ingredients:** In one bowl, mix the whole wheat flour, baking soda, salt, and cinnamon. In another larger bowl, whisk together the eggs, applesauce, olive oil, and vanilla extract. Stir in the grated zucchini.
3. **Combine and Add Nuts/Seeds:** Add the dry ingredients to the wet ingredients and stir until just combined. Fold in nuts or seeds if using.
4. **Bake:** Pour the batter into the prepared loaf pan. Bake for about 50 minutes, or until a toothpick inserted into the center comes out clean. Let the bread cool in the pan for 10 minutes, then turn out onto a wire rack to cool completely.

Macronutrients (per serving, about 6 slices):

- **Calories:** 320 kcal
- **Carbohydrates:** 38 g
- **Protein:** 8 g
- **Fat:** 16 g

Vitamins:

High in Vitamin A and C from zucchini.

- Contains several B vitamins from whole wheat flour.

Chapter 15: Healing beverages

Almond Ginger Smoothie

- **Preparation Time:** 5 minutes
- **Cooking Time:** 0 minutes
- **Servings:** 2

Ingredients:

- 1 cup unsweetened almond milk
- 1 banana, sliced and frozen
- 1 tablespoon almond butter
- 1/2 teaspoon freshly grated ginger
- 1 tablespoon honey (optional, for sweetness)
- Ice cubes (optional, for a thicker consistency)

Procedure:

1. **Blend Ingredients:** In a blender, combine the almond milk, frozen banana, almond butter, and freshly grated ginger. Add honey if desired for extra sweetness.
2. **Adjust Consistency:** Add a few ice cubes if you prefer a thicker smoothie; blend until smooth.
3. **Taste and Adjust:** Taste the smoothie and adjust the sweetness or ginger according to your preference by adding more honey or ginger and blending again.
4. **Serve Immediately:** Pour the smoothie into glasses and serve immediately for the freshest flavor and best texture.

Macronutrients (per serving):

- **Calories:** 180 kcal
- **Carbohydrates:** 27 g
- **Protein:** 4 g
- **Fat:** 7 g

Vitamins:

- High in Vitamin E from almond butter.
- Provides a good amount of potassium from bananas.
- Contains calcium and Vitamin D if the almond milk is fortified.

Beetroot and Carrot Juice

- **Preparation Time:** 10 minutes
- **Cooking Time:** 0 minutes
- **Servings:** 2

Ingredients:

- 2 medium beetroots, peeled and chopped
- 4 large carrots, peeled and chopped
- 1 inch piece of fresh ginger, peeled
- 1 lemon, peeled
- Optional: 1 apple for added sweetness

Procedure:

1. **Prepare Ingredients:** Wash, peel, and chop the beetroots and carrots. Peel the ginger and lemon. If using an apple, core and cut it into pieces.
2. **Juice Ingredients:** Using a juicer, process the beetroots, carrots, ginger, lemon, and optional apple. Make sure to alternate between the harder vegetables (beets and carrots) and the softer ones (lemon, ginger, and apple) to maximize juice extraction.
3. **Stir and Check Flavor:** Once all the ingredients are juiced, stir the mixture thoroughly. Taste and adjust by adding more lemon or apple according to your preference.
4. **Serve Immediately:** Pour the juice into glasses and serve immediately to enjoy its full nutritional benefits. Optionally, you can strain the juice for a smoother texture.

Macronutrients (per serving): **Calories:** 120 kcal; **Carbohydrates:** 28 g; **Protein:** 3 g; **Fat:** 0.5 g

Vitamins:

- High in Vitamin A from carrots.
- Rich in Vitamin C from lemon and beetroots.
- Provides folate, potassium, and magnesium.

Celery Cucumber Cleanse Juice

- **Preparation Time:** 10 minutes
- **Cooking Time:** 0 minutes
- **Servings:** 2

Ingredients:

- 5 stalks of celery, washed and chopped
- 1 large cucumber, washed and chopped
- 1 green apple, cored and sliced (optional for sweetness)
- Juice of 1 lemon
- 1 inch piece of fresh ginger, peeled

Procedure:

1. **Prepare Ingredients:** Ensure all vegetables are thoroughly washed. Chop the celery and cucumber into manageable pieces for juicing. Slice the green apple if using, and peel the ginger.
2. **Juicing:** Feed the celery, cucumber, apple, and ginger through a juicer. Alternate between the softer ingredients (cucumber and apple) and the firmer ones (celery and ginger) to maximize juice extraction.
3. **Add Lemon Juice:** Once all the ingredients are juiced, stir in the fresh lemon juice to enhance flavor and add an extra vitamin boost.
4. **Serve Chilled:** Pour the juice into glasses and serve immediately to enjoy the maximum nutritional benefits. For an extra refreshing drink, serve over ice.

Macronutrients (per serving):

- **Calories:** 80 kcal
- **Carbohydrates:** 18 g
- **Protein:** 2 g
- **Fat:** 0 g

Vitamins:

- High in Vitamin K from celery.
- Rich in Vitamin C from cucumber, apple, and lemon.
- Provides good amounts of potassium and folate.

Chamomile Lavender Tea

- **Preparation Time:** 5 minutes
- **Cooking Time:** 10 minutes
- **Servings:** 2

Ingredients:

- 2 tablespoons dried chamomile flowers
- 1 tablespoon dried lavender flowers
- 2 cups boiling water
- Optional: honey or lemon for flavor

Procedure:

1. **Heat Water:** Bring 2 cups of water to a boil in a small pot or kettle.
2. **Prepare Tea:** Place the dried chamomile and lavender flowers in a tea infuser or directly into a teapot.
3. **Steep:** Pour the boiling water over the chamomile and lavender. Cover and let steep for 8-10 minutes, allowing the flavors and properties of the herbs to fully infuse the water.
4. **Serve:** Strain the tea into cups if you've used loose flowers. Optionally, sweeten with honey or add a slice of lemon for extra flavor. Serve hot.

Macronutrients (per serving):

- **Calories:** 2 kcal
- **Carbohydrates:** 0.5 g
- **Protein:** 0 g
- **Fat:** 0 g

Vitamins:

- Provides small amounts of Vitamin C if lemon is added.
- Contains trace minerals such as magnesium and potassium from the herbs.

Cinnamon Turmeric Latte

- **Preparation Time:** 5 minutes
- **Cooking Time:** 5 minutes
- **Servings:** 2

Ingredients:

- 2 cups almond milk (or any other plant-based milk)
- 1 teaspoon turmeric powder
- 1/2 teaspoon cinnamon powder
- 1/4 teaspoon ginger powder
- 1 tablespoon honey or maple syrup (optional, for sweetness)
- Pinch of black pepper (to enhance turmeric absorption)
- Optional: 1 teaspoon coconut oil (for richness and added health benefits)

Procedure:

1. **Heat Ingredients:** In a small saucepan, combine the almond milk, turmeric, cinnamon, ginger, and a pinch of black pepper. Heat over medium heat while stirring constantly to prevent the spices from settling at the bottom.
2. **Add Sweeteners and Fats:** Once the mixture is hot but not boiling, reduce the heat and add honey (or maple syrup) and coconut oil if using. Stir well until everything is fully integrated and the coconut oil has melted.
3. **Simmer:** Allow the mixture to simmer for another minute to let the flavors meld together, stirring occasionally.
4. **Serve:** Pour the latte into mugs through a strainer if desired to remove any undissolved spices. Serve hot and enjoy immediately.

Macronutrients (per serving): Calories: 70 kcal; **Carbohydrates:** 12 g; **Protein:** 2 g; **Fat:** 2.5 g (varies if coconut oil is added)

Vitamins:

- Provides a good source of Vitamin B from almond milk.
- Contains antioxidants from turmeric, cinnamon, and ginger.
- Includes dietary fiber from spices, if not strained.

Coconut Water Electrolyte Drink

- **Preparation Time:** 5 minutes
- **Cooking Time:** 0 minutes
- **Servings:** 2

Ingredients:

- 2 cups pure coconut water
- Juice of 1 lime
- 1/4 teaspoon Himalayan pink salt (rich in minerals)
- 1 tablespoon honey (optional, for sweetness)
- A few mint leaves (for added flavor)

Procedure:

1. **Mix Ingredients:** In a jug or bottle, combine the coconut water, freshly squeezed lime juice, and Himalayan pink salt. Stir well to dissolve the salt completely.
2. **Add Sweetener:** If you prefer a sweeter taste, stir in the honey until well combined.
3. **Enhance Flavor:** Add a few mint leaves to the mixture, and give it another good stir. This adds a refreshing flavor that complements the lime.
4. **Serve Chilled:** Refrigerate for at least 30 minutes or serve over ice immediately to enjoy a chilled, refreshing electrolyte drink.

Macronutrients (per serving):

- **Calories:** 60 kcal
- **Carbohydrates:** 15 g
- **Protein:** 1 g
- **Fat:** 0 g

Vitamins:

- High in Vitamin C from lime juice.
- Provides a significant amount of potassium and magnesium from coconut water.
- Contains trace amounts of sodium and calcium.

Detox Green Tea

- **Preparation Time:** 5 minutes
- **Cooking Time:** 5 minutes
- **Servings:** 2

Ingredients:

- 2 cups water
- 2 teaspoons green tea leaves or 2 green tea bags
- 1/2 lemon, sliced
- 1 inch ginger root, thinly sliced
- Optional: honey or fresh mint leaves for additional flavor

Procedure:

1. **Boil Water:** Bring 2 cups of water to a boil in a small saucepan.
2. **Add Ingredients:** Add the green tea leaves (or bags), sliced lemon, and ginger to the boiling water. Reduce the heat and let it simmer for about 3-5 minutes. This allows the flavors and nutrients to infuse the water.
3. **Steep:** Remove the saucepan from the heat and let the tea steep for an additional 2-3 minutes. The longer it steeps, the stronger the flavors and benefits.
4. **Serve:** Strain the tea into cups, discarding the leaves, lemon, and ginger. If desired, sweeten with a little honey or add fresh mint leaves for a refreshing touch. Serve the tea warm or chilled.

Macronutrients (per serving):

- **Calories:** 2 kcal (more if honey is added)
- **Carbohydrates:** 0.5 g
- **Protein:** 0 g
- **Fat:** 0 g

Vitamins:

- High in Vitamin C from lemon.
- Contains antioxidants, notably EGCG (epigallocatechin gallate), from green tea, which are known for their cancer-fighting properties.
- Provides a modest amount of potassium.

Energizing Spirulina Smoothie

- **Preparation Time:** 5 minutes
- **Cooking Time:** 0 minutes
- **Servings:** 2

Ingredients:

- 1 banana, preferably frozen for creaminess
- 1 cup fresh spinach leaves
- 1 tablespoon spirulina powder
- 1 cup unsweetened almond milk (or any other plant-based milk)
- 1/2 cup pineapple chunks (can be fresh or frozen)
- Optional: 1 tablespoon honey or agave syrup for sweetness

Procedure:

1. **Prepare Ingredients:** If not using a frozen banana, consider adding a few ice cubes to the blender to chill and thicken your smoothie.
2. **Blend:** In a blender, combine the banana, spinach leaves, spirulina powder, almond milk, and pineapple chunks. Blend on high until smooth.
3. **Sweeten if Desired:** Taste the smoothie and add honey or agave syrup if a sweeter taste is desired. Blend again to mix thoroughly.
4. **Serve Immediately:** Pour the smoothie into glasses and serve immediately to enjoy the maximum nutritional benefits and best flavor.

Macronutrients (per serving):

- **Calories:** 150 kcal
- **Carbohydrates:** 30 g
- **Protein:** 5 g
- **Fat:** 2 g

Vitamins:

- High in Vitamin C from pineapple.
- Rich in Vitamin A and iron from spinach.
- Contains Vitamin B12 and essential amino acids from spirulina.

Fennel Digestive Tea

- **Preparation Time:** 5 minutes
- **Cooking Time:** 10 minutes
- **Servings:** 2

Ingredients:

- 2 teaspoons of fennel seeds
- 2 cups of water
- Optional: honey or lemon slices to taste

Procedure:

1. **Crush the Seeds:** Lightly crush the fennel seeds with a mortar and pestle to release their oils, which contain the active ingredients that aid digestion.
2. **Boil Water:** Bring two cups of water to a boil in a small saucepan.
3. **Steep the Fennel Seeds:** Add the crushed fennel seeds to the boiling water, reduce the heat, and let it simmer for 8-10 minutes. This allows the flavors and beneficial compounds to infuse the water.
4. **Strain and Serve:** Strain the tea into cups, discarding the seeds. If desired, sweeten with honey or add a slice of lemon to enhance the flavor before serving.

Macronutrients (per serving):

- **Calories:** 2 kcal
- **Carbohydrates:** 0.5 g
- **Protein:** 0.1 g
- **Fat:** 0.1 g

Vitamins:

- Provides a small amount of Vitamin C if lemon is added.
- Contains minerals such as iron, calcium, and magnesium, which are crucial for overall health.

Ginger Lemonade

- **Preparation Time:** 10 minutes
- **Cooking Time:** 0 minutes
- **Servings:** 2

Ingredients:

- 4 cups of water
- Juice of 2 large lemons
- 2 tablespoons of freshly grated ginger
- 2 tablespoons of honey or to taste (optional, for sweetness)
- Ice cubes
- Mint leaves for garnish (optional)

Procedure:

1. **Prepare Ginger Infusion:** In a small saucepan, combine 1 cup of water and the freshly grated ginger. Bring to a simmer, remove from heat, and let it steep for about 5 minutes.
2. **Strain and Cool:** Strain the ginger-infused water into a pitcher to remove the ginger pieces. Allow it to cool for a few minutes.
3. **Mix Lemonade:** Add the freshly squeezed lemon juice and the remaining 3 cups of water to the pitcher. Stir in honey to sweeten, adjusting according to your taste.
4. **Serve:** Fill glasses with ice, pour the ginger lemonade over the ice, and garnish with mint leaves if using. Serve immediately for a refreshing drink.

Macronutrients (per serving):

- **Calories:** 50 kcal
- **Carbohydrates:** 14 g
- **Protein:** 0 g
- **Fat:** 0 g

Vitamins:

- High in Vitamin C from lemon juice.
- Provides a small amount of magnesium and potassium.

Golden Milk

- **Preparation Time:** 5 minutes
- **Cooking Time:** 10 minutes
- **Servings:** 2

Ingredients:

- 2 cups of almond milk (or any plant-based milk)
- 1 teaspoon turmeric powder
- 1/2 teaspoon cinnamon powder
- 1/4 teaspoon ginger powder
- 1 pinch of black pepper (enhances absorption of curcumin)
- 1 tablespoon honey or maple syrup (optional, for sweetness)

Procedure:

1. **Heat Ingredients:** In a small saucepan, combine the almond milk, turmeric, cinnamon, ginger, and black pepper. Heat the mixture over medium heat until it is hot but not boiling, stirring occasionally to prevent sticking and to ensure even mixing of the spices.
2. **Simmer:** Reduce heat to low and let the mixture simmer for about 10 minutes. This allows the flavors to meld and the spices to fully infuse the milk.
3. **Sweeten:** Remove from heat and stir in honey or maple syrup, adjusting according to your taste preference.
4. **Serve:** Strain the mixture through a fine mesh sieve to remove any large particles of spice. Serve the golden milk warm, ideally before bedtime or during a relaxing moment.

Macronutrients (per serving):

- **Calories:** 60 kcal
- **Carbohydrates:** 9 g
- **Protein:** 1 g
- **Fat:** 2.5 g (varies depending on the type of milk used)

Vitamins:

- High in Vitamin B12 and Vitamin D if using fortified almond milk.
- Provides a significant amount of calcium (also dependent on milk fortification).
- Contains curcumin from turmeric, known for its anti-inflammatory effects.

Hibiscus and Rosehip Tea

- **Preparation Time:** 5 minutes
- **Cooking Time:** 10 minutes
- **Servings:** 2

Ingredients:

- 2 tablespoons dried hibiscus flowers
- 2 tablespoons dried rosehips
- 4 cups of water
- Optional: honey or lemon slices for additional flavor

Procedure:

1. **Boil Water:** Bring 4 cups of water to a boil in a kettle or saucepan.
2. **Steep Tea:** Add the dried hibiscus flowers and rosehips to the boiling water. Remove from heat and allow to steep for about 10 minutes. This will extract the flavors and beneficial compounds from the herbs.
3. **Strain and Serve:** Strain the tea through a fine mesh sieve into a teapot or directly into cups, discarding the solids.
4. **Flavor as Desired:** If you prefer a sweeter taste, stir in honey to your liking. You can also add a slice of lemon to each cup for an extra burst of flavor and Vitamin C.

Macronutrients (per serving):

- **Calories:** 5 kcal
- **Carbohydrates:** 1 g
- **Protein:** 0 g
- **Fat:** 0 g

Vitamins:

- High in Vitamin C, especially from the rosehips, which are among the richest plant sources of this vitamin.
- Contains antioxidants such as anthocyanins and flavonoids from hibiscus flowers, which have health-promoting properties.

Kale and Apple Green Juice

- **Preparation Time:** 10 minutes
- **Cooking Time:** 0 minutes
- **Servings:** 2

Ingredients:

- 4 large kale leaves, stems removed
- 2 medium green apples, cored and quartered
- 1 cucumber, chopped
- 1 lemon, peeled
- 1 inch piece of fresh ginger, peeled
- Optional: A handful of fresh mint leaves for additional flavor

Procedure:

1. **Prepare Ingredients:** Wash all the fruits and vegetables thoroughly. Remove the stems from the kale and core the apples. Peel the lemon and ginger.
2. **Juice the Ingredients:** Feed the kale leaves, green apples, cucumber, lemon, and ginger through a juicer. Alternate the softer ingredients (like kale and cucumber) with harder ones (like apples) to maximize juice extraction.
3. **Enhance Flavor:** If desired, add some fresh mint leaves at the end of the juicing process for a refreshing taste.
4. **Serve Immediately:** Stir the juice well and serve immediately to enjoy the maximum nutritional benefits. Pour over ice if preferred chilled.

Macronutrients (per serving):

- **Calories:** 120 kcal
- **Carbohydrates:** 30 g
- **Protein:** 2 g
- **Fat:** 0.5 g

Vitamins:

- High in Vitamin A and Vitamin C from kale and apples.
- Contains significant amounts of Vitamin K from kale.
- Provides potassium from cucumber and magnesium from apples.

Lemon Balm and Mint Tea

- **Preparation Time:** 5 minutes
- **Cooking Time:** 10 minutes
- **Servings:** 2

Ingredients:

- 2 tablespoons fresh or dried lemon balm leaves
- 2 tablespoons fresh or dried mint leaves
- 4 cups of water
- Optional: honey or a slice of lemon for additional flavor

Procedure:

1. **Boil Water:** Bring 4 cups of water to a boil in a kettle or saucepan.
2. **Add Herbs:** Once the water reaches a boil, remove it from the heat and add the lemon balm and mint leaves. Use a spoon to gently bruise the leaves in the water, releasing more of their oils and flavor.
3. **Steep the Tea:** Cover the pot and allow the herbs to steep for about 10 minutes. The longer you steep, the stronger the flavor and herbal benefits.
4. **Strain and Serve:** Strain the tea into cups, discarding the leaves. If desired, sweeten with honey or add a slice of lemon to each cup. Serve hot.

Macronutrients (per serving):

- **Calories:** 0 kcal (add calories for honey or lemon if used)
- **Carbohydrates:** 0 g (add for honey if used)
- **Protein:** 0 g
- **Fat:** 0 g

Vitamins:

- Provides small amounts of Vitamin C if lemon is added.
- Contains trace minerals and antioxidants from the herbs.

Moringa Leaf Tea

- **Preparation Time:** 5 minutes
- **Cooking Time:** 10 minutes
- **Servings:** 2

Ingredients:

- 2 teaspoons dried moringa leaves
- 4 cups of boiling water
- Optional: honey or lemon slices for additional flavor

Procedure:

1. **Boil Water:** Bring 4 cups of water to a boil in a kettle or saucepan.
2. **Steep the Tea:** Place the dried moringa leaves in a tea infuser or directly into the boiling water. Remove the water from heat and allow the leaves to steep for about 5 to 10 minutes, depending on how strong you prefer the tea.
3. **Strain and Serve:** If you added the leaves without an infuser, strain the tea through a fine mesh sieve into cups. Discard the leaves.
4. **Flavor as Desired:** Add honey or a slice of lemon to each cup if desired for additional flavor. Stir well and enjoy the tea either hot or chilled.

Macronutrients (per serving):

- **Calories:** 5 kcal
- **Carbohydrates:** 1 g
- **Protein:** 0.3 g
- **Fat:** 0 g

Vitamins:

- High in Vitamin A, Vitamin C, and iron.
- Contains significant amounts of calcium, potassium, and protein.
- Provides antioxidants such as chlorogenic acid and quercetin.

Parsley and Lemon Detox Water

- **Preparation Time:** 5 minutes
- **Cooking Time:** 0 minutes
- **Servings:** 2

Ingredients:

- 1 large lemon, thinly sliced
- 1/4 cup fresh parsley leaves, roughly chopped
- 4 cups of water
- Ice cubes (optional)

Procedure:

1. **Prepare Ingredients:** Wash the lemon and parsley thoroughly. Slice the lemon into thin rounds and roughly chop the parsley leaves.
2. **Combine in Pitcher:** In a large pitcher, add the sliced lemon and chopped parsley. If you prefer your drink chilled, add ice cubes to the pitcher.
3. **Add Water:** Pour cold water over the lemon and parsley. Stir gently to combine all the ingredients.
4. **Refrigerate:** Allow the mixture to infuse in the refrigerator for at least 2 hours or overnight to enhance the flavors and extract the beneficial oils and compounds from the lemon and parsley.

Macronutrients (per serving):

- **Calories:** 10 kcal
- **Carbohydrates:** 3 g
- **Protein:** 0.4 g
- **Fat:** 0 g

Vitamins:

- High in Vitamin C from lemon.
- Contains Vitamin A and iron from parsley.
- Provides antioxidants and essential oils from both ingredients.

Pumpkin Spice Smoothie

- **Preparation Time:** 5 minutes
- **Cooking Time:** 0 minutes
- **Servings:** 2

Ingredients:

- 1 cup canned pumpkin puree (ensure it's 100% pumpkin)
- 1 banana, frozen
- 1 1/2 cups almond milk (or any plant-based milk)
- 1/4 cup Greek yogurt (use coconut yogurt for a vegan option)
- 2 tablespoons maple syrup
- 1 teaspoon pumpkin pie spice
- 1/2 teaspoon vanilla extract
- Ice cubes (optional for a thicker texture)

Procedure:

1. **Blend Ingredients:** In a blender, combine the pumpkin puree, frozen banana, almond milk, Greek yogurt, maple syrup, pumpkin pie spice, and vanilla extract. Add a handful of ice cubes if you prefer a thicker smoothie.
2. **Process Until Smooth:** Blend on high until all the ingredients are thoroughly combined and the texture is smooth and creamy.
3. **Taste and Adjust:** Taste the smoothie and adjust the sweetness by adding more maple syrup if needed. If the smoothie is too thick, add a little more almond milk to reach your desired consistency.
4. **Serve Immediately:** Pour the smoothie into glasses and serve immediately for the best flavor and nutrient retention.

Macronutrients (per serving):

- **Calories:** 280 kcal
- **Carbohydrates:** 50 g
- **Protein:** 8 g
- **Fat:** 6 g

Vitamins:

- High in Vitamin A from pumpkin.
- Provides a good amount of calcium and Vitamin D if using fortified almond milk.
- Contains potassium from the banana and additional probiotics from Greek yogurt.

Red Raspberry Leaf Tea

- **Preparation Time:** 5 minutes
- **Cooking Time:** 10 minutes
- **Servings:** 2

Ingredients:

- 2 tablespoons dried red raspberry leaves
- 4 cups of water
- Optional: honey or lemon for taste

Procedure:

1. **Boil Water:** Bring 4 cups of water to a rolling boil in a kettle or saucepan.
2. **Steep the Leaves:** Add the dried red raspberry leaves to the boiling water. Remove from heat and allow the leaves to steep for about 10 minutes. The longer you steep, the stronger and more beneficial the tea.
3. **Strain the Tea:** Strain the tea into cups or a teapot, removing the raspberry leaves.
4. **Add Flavor:** If desired, enhance the flavor with a little honey or a squeeze of lemon. This can also help soften the naturally astringent taste of the tea.

Macronutrients (per serving):

- **Calories:** Nearly negligible unless honey or lemon is added
- **Carbohydrates:** 0 g (add for honey if used)
- **Protein:** 0 g
- **Fat:** 0 g

Vitamins:

- Rich in Vitamin C, especially when lemon is added.
- Contains magnesium, potassium, iron, and B vitamins.

Soothing Peppermint Tea

- **Preparation Time:** 5 minutes
- **Cooking Time:** 10 minutes
- **Servings:** 2

Ingredients:

- 2 tablespoons of fresh or dried peppermint leaves
- 4 cups of water
- Optional: honey or lemon slices for added flavor

Procedure:

1. **Boil Water:** Bring 4 cups of water to a boil in a kettle or saucepan.
2. **Steep the Tea:** Add the peppermint leaves to the boiled water. Remove from heat and let them steep for about 10 minutes. The longer the steep, the stronger the flavor and digestive benefits.
3. **Strain and Serve:** Strain the tea through a fine mesh sieve into teacups, discarding the leaves.
4. **Enhance Flavor:** If desired, add honey for sweetness or a slice of lemon for a tangy twist. Serve the tea warm to enjoy its soothing effects.

Macronutrients (per serving):

- **Calories:** Negligible unless honey or lemon is added
- **Carbohydrates:** 0 g (add for honey or lemon if used)
- **Protein:** 0 g
- **Fat:** 0 g

Vitamins:

- Peppermint leaves are a good source of Vitamin A and Vitamin C, particularly if fresh leaves are used.
- Contains small amounts of minerals such as manganese.

Watermelon Basil Hydration Juice

- **Preparation Time:** 10 minutes
- **Cooking Time:** 0 minutes
- **Servings:** 2

Ingredients:

- 4 cups cubed watermelon (seedless or seeds removed)
- 1/2 cup fresh basil leaves
- Juice of 1 lime
- Ice cubes (optional for serving)

Procedure:

1. **Blend Ingredients:** In a blender, combine the cubed watermelon, basil leaves, and lime juice. Blend until smooth.
2. **Strain (Optional):** For a smoother juice, strain the mixture through a fine mesh sieve to remove pulp and basil leaves. Otherwise, skip this step for a fuller texture.
3. **Chill:** Refrigerate the juice for at least 30 minutes to enhance the flavors or serve immediately over ice for instant refreshment.
4. **Serve:** Pour the chilled or iced juice into glasses and garnish with a sprig of basil or a slice of lime if desired.

Macronutrients (per serving):

- **Calories:** 80 kcal
- **Carbohydrates:** 20 g
- **Protein:** 2 g
- **Fat:** 0 g

Vitamins:

- High in Vitamin C from watermelon and lime.
- Provides a good amount of Vitamin A from watermelon.
- Contains antioxidants and trace amounts of various minerals such as magnesi

Part III: Implementing Wellness into Everyday Life

Part III of this book focuses on seamlessly integrating wellness practices into your daily routine to promote sustainable health improvements. It goes beyond nutrition and recipes, delving into the broader aspects of wellness, including physical activity, mental health, and environmental factors that influence overall well-being.

The 30-Day Meal Plan for Optimal Health

This comprehensive 30-day meal plan is designed to help individuals achieve optimal health by incorporating a variety of nutritious recipes that balance macros and micros, focus on whole foods, and maintain around 1800 kcal per day. Each day is structured to include breakfast, a snack, lunch, a dessert, and dinner, ensuring a well-rounded intake of nutrients. Below, we detail a sample day from the meal plan, utilizing recipes previously developed.

Day 1: Balanced and Nutritious

Breakfast: Almond Butter and Banana Oatmeal
- **Calories:** 460 kcal
- Rich in fiber and protein, this oatmeal is topped with banana and almond butter, offering a hearty and satisfying start to the day.

Snack: Carrot and Hummus Roll-Ups
- **Calories:** 150 kcal
- Crunchy carrot sticks wrapped in creamy hummus provide a light, nutritious snack rich in vitamins and protein.

Lunch: Avocado Quinoa Salad with Lemon Dressing
- **Calories:** 400 kcal
- This salad combines the richness of avocado with the protein-packed quinoa, dressed in a zesty lemon vinaigrette for a refreshing midday meal.

Dessert: Cinnamon Baked Pears
- **Calories:** 150 kcal
- A sweet and spicy dessert featuring tender baked pears sprinkled with cinnamon, perfect for satisfying sweet cravings healthily.

Dinner: Kale and Sweet Potato Sauté
- **Calories:** 500 kcal
- A warm, comforting dinner that pairs nutrient-dense kale and sweet potatoes, sautéed to perfection, providing a filling and fiber-rich end to the day.

Daily Total: 1660 kcal

Day 2: Nutrient-Dense and Energizing

Breakfast: Berry Spinach Smoothie Bowl
- **Calories:** 350 kcal
- A vibrant blend of berries and spinach, topped with seeds for extra nutrients, this smoothie bowl is an antioxidant powerhouse that kickstarts your morning.

Snack: Cucumber Noodle Salad with Peanut Dressing
- **Calories:** 120 kcal
- Light and refreshing, this salad is perfect for a mid-morning snack, offering hydration and a protein boost from the peanut dressing.

Lunch: Grilled Portobello Mushrooms with Quinoa Salad
- **Calories:** 400 kcal
- Hearty portobello mushrooms served with a side of protein-rich quinoa salad make a filling and nutritious midday meal.

Dessert: Mango Lime Chia Pudding
- **Calories:** 180 kcal
- This tropical chia pudding is not only delicious but also packed with fiber and healthy fats, making it a perfect post-lunch treat.

Dinner: Lentil Bolognese with Zucchini Noodles
- **Calories:** 500 kcal
- A comforting and hearty dinner option that packs plenty of plant-based protein and fiber without skimping on flavor.

Daily Total: 1550 kcal

Day 3: Refreshing and Satisfying

Breakfast: Nutty Banana Smoothie
- **Calories:** 400 kcal
- A creamy smoothie made with bananas, nut butter, and oats, providing a balanced mix of carbs, protein, and healthy fats.

Snack: Homemade Almond Granola
- **Calories:** 150 kcal
- Crunchy and sweet, this homemade granola is a great mid-morning snack, providing energy through its oats and nuts content.

Lunch: Chickpea and Avocado Sandwich on Sprouted Bread
- **Calories:** 400 kcal
- A filling sandwich that combines the creaminess of avocado with the heartiness of chickpeas, packed with fiber and protein.

Dessert: Apple Cinnamon Baked Oatmeal Cups
- **Calories:** 150 kcal
- Warm and comforting, these oatmeal cups are a sweet treat that's also good for your health, perfect for an afternoon pick-me-up.

Dinner: Butternut Squash Soup with Sage
- **Calories:** 300 kcal
- A creamy and soothing soup that's light yet satisfying, ideal for ending the day on a warm note.

Daily Total: 1400 kcal

Day 4: High Energy Day

Breakfast: Energizing Green Juice
- **Calories:** 150 kcal
- Start your day with a refreshing juice made from kale, apple, cucumber, and a touch of ginger to wake up your senses and boost your metabolism.

Snack: Greek Yogurt with Honey and Almonds
- **Calories:** 200 kcal
- A perfect combination of protein-rich Greek yogurt, honey for a touch of sweetness, and almonds for a crunch that will keep you full and energized until lunch.

Lunch: Quinoa and Black Bean Salad
- **Calories:** 450 kcal
- A protein-packed salad with quinoa, black beans, tomatoes, and avocado, dressed in a lime and cilantro vinaigrette for a refreshing midday meal.

Dessert: Dark Chocolate and Nut Clusters
- **Calories:** 100 kcal
- Indulge in a small portion of dark chocolate combined with nuts for an antioxidant-rich treat that satisfies your sweet tooth.

Dinner: Chicken Stir-Fry with Vegetables and Brown Rice
- **Calories:** 500 kcal
- A hearty and healthy stir-fry with lean chicken, a variety of vegetables, and a side of whole grain brown rice to replenish your energy after a long day.

Daily Total: 1400 kcal

Day 5: Relaxation and Digestion

Breakfast: Chia Seed Pudding with Kiwi
- **Calories:** 300 kcal
- A soothing start to the day with omega-3 rich chia seeds soaked in almond milk and topped with fresh, vitamin C-rich kiwi.

Snack: Baked Kale Chips
- **Calories:** 100 kcal
- Crunchy and light, these kale chips are not only delicious but also packed with fiber and micronutrients.

Lunch: Turkey and Spinach Wrap
- **Calories:** 400 kcal
- A whole-grain wrap filled with lean turkey, spinach, and a light cream cheese spread to keep things light and nutritious.

Dessert: Baked Apple with Cinnamon
- **Calories:** 120 kcal
- A comforting dessert of warm baked apples sprinkled with cinnamon, perfect for soothing digestion and boosting fiber intake.

Dinner: Salmon with Steamed Broccoli and Quinoa
- **Calories:** 480 kcal
- Omega-3 rich salmon served with fiber-packed broccoli and quinoa, a meal that supports heart health and digestion.

Daily Total: 1400 kcal

Day 6: Detox Focus

Breakfast: Avocado Toast on Sprouted Grain Bread
- **Calories:** 250 kcal
- Start your detox day with healthy fats from avocado and fiber from sprouted grain bread to kickstart your metabolism.

Snack: Raw Carrot Sticks with Hummus
- **Calories:** 150 kcal
- A light, crunchy snack that's perfect for detoxification, thanks to the fiber in carrots and protein in hummus.

Lunch: Beetroot and Carrot Juice
- **Calories:** 120 kcal
- Cleanse your system with a juice rich in betaine from beets, aiding liver function and improving blood flow.

Dessert: Fresh Fruit Salad
- **Calories:** 100 kcal
- A mix of your favorite fruits, providing essential vitamins and antioxidants to support the body's natural detox processes.

Dinner: Ginger Turmeric Chicken with Steamed Greens
- **Calories:** 400 kcal
- Turmeric and ginger provide anti-inflammatory benefits, while lean chicken and greens make this dinner both detoxifying and filling.

Daily Total: 1020 kcal

Day 7: Heart Health Day

Breakfast: Oatmeal with Pumpkin Seeds and Pears
- **Calories:** 350 kcal
- A warm bowl of oatmeal topped with heart-healthy pumpkin seeds and slices of pear, providing fiber and essential minerals.

Snack: Walnuts and Dark Chocolate
- **Calories:** 200 kcal
- A heart-friendly snack featuring walnuts known for omega-3 fatty acids and antioxidant-rich dark chocolate.

Lunch: Tomato Basil Mozzarella Salad
- **Calories:** 300 kcal
- Fresh tomatoes, basil, and mozzarella make a light and refreshing salad, drizzled with olive oil for healthy fats.

Dessert: Greek Yogurt with Blueberries
- **Calories:** 150 kcal
- Creamy Greek yogurt topped with blueberries, offering protein and antioxidants that support cardiovascular health.

Dinner: Grilled Salmon with Asparagus
- **Calories:** 500 kcal
- Omega-3 rich salmon grilled to perfection, served with fiber-rich asparagus, an ideal dinner for heart health.

Daily Total: 1500 kcal

Day 8: Brain Boosting Day

Breakfast: Blueberry Spinach Smoothie
- **Calories:** 300 kcal
- A nutrient-packed smoothie with blueberries and spinach, both known for their brain-boosting antioxidants.

Snack: Avocado and Whole-Grain Crackers
- **Calories:** 200 kcal
- Healthy fats from avocado spread on fiber-rich whole-grain crackers, perfect for maintaining cognitive function.

Lunch: Walnut and Beet Salad with Citrus Vinaigrette
- **Calories:** 350 kcal
- Beets and walnuts topped with a citrus dressing, providing nutrients essential for brain health.

Dessert: Dark Chocolate Square
- **Calories:** 100 kcal
- A small portion of dark chocolate to satisfy sweet cravings and boost serotonin levels.

Dinner: Baked Trout with Quinoa Pilaf
- **Calories:** 550 kcal
- Trout, a great source of omega-3 for brain health, served with quinoa pilaf rich in proteins and B vitamins.

Daily Total: 1500 kcal

Day 9: Muscle Maintenance Day

Breakfast: Greek Yogurt with Mixed Nuts and Honey
- **Calories:** 400 kcal
- High-protein Greek yogurt mixed with nuts for healthy fats and honey for a touch of sweetness.

Snack: Cottage Cheese with Pineapple
- **Calories:** 200 kcal
- Cottage cheese is rich in protein, paired with pineapple for an enzyme boost that helps in digestion.

Lunch: Chicken and Avocado Wrap
- **Calories:** 450 kcal
- A protein-rich wrap filled with chicken and avocado, providing both protein and healthy fats.

Dessert: Apple Slices with Almond Butter
- **Calories:** 150 kcal
- Crisp apple slices with a spread of almond butter for a satisfying post-lunch treat.

Dinner: Beef Stir-Fry with Broccoli and Bell Peppers
- **Calories:** 500 kcal
- Lean beef and vegetables stir-fried in a light sauce, providing iron and protein necessary for muscle repair.

Daily Total: 1700 kcal

Day 10: Sustainable Energy Day

Breakfast: Energizing Green Juice
- **Calories:** 150 kcal
- A refreshing juice made from kale, apple, cucumber, and ginger to kickstart your day with a burst of nutrients.

Snack: Trail Mix with Nuts and Dried Fruits
- **Calories:** 200 kcal
- A handy snack packed with healthy fats and natural sugars for a quick energy boost.

Lunch: Turkey and Spinach Salad with Avocado
- **Calories:** 450 kcal
- Lean turkey breast on a bed of spinach, topped with avocado slices for a balance of protein, iron, and healthy fats.

Dessert: Baked Pear with Cinnamon
- **Calories:** 100 kcal
- A warm, lightly sweetened pear baked with a sprinkle of cinnamon, perfect for a mid-afternoon treat.

Dinner: Grilled Chicken with Sweet Potato Fries
- **Calories:** 600 kcal
- Grilled chicken breast served with a side of baked sweet potato fries, providing a perfect mix of protein and complex carbs for evening satiety.

Daily Total: 1500 kcal

Day 11: Mental Clarity Day

Breakfast: Avocado Toast with Poached Egg
- **Calories:** 300 kcal
- Creamy avocado and a poached egg atop whole-grain toast, offering healthy fats and protein to support brain function.

Snack: Greek Yogurt with Walnuts and Honey
- **Calories:** 250 kcal
- A serving of Greek yogurt mixed with walnuts and a drizzle of honey for enhanced cognitive performance.

Lunch: Quinoa Salad with Blueberries and Almonds
- **Calories:** 400 kcal
- Quinoa mixed with fresh blueberries, almonds, and a light vinaigrette, rich in antioxidants and healthy fats.

Dessert: Dark Chocolate Square
- **Calories:** 100 kcal
- A small portion of dark chocolate, known for improving focus and mood.

Dinner: Salmon with Asparagus
- **Calories:** 450 kcal
- Oven-baked salmon with steamed asparagus, providing omega-3 fatty acids and vitamins for brain health.

Daily Total: 1500 kcal

Day 12: Balanced Mood Day

Breakfast: Berry Spinach Smoothie
- **Calories:** 300 kcal
- A smoothie made with a variety of berries and fresh spinach to start the day with mood-enhancing nutrients.

Snack: Hummus with Carrot and Celery Sticks
- **Calories:** 150 kcal
- Freshly cut vegetables dipped in protein-rich hummus for a satisfying crunch.

Lunch: Lentil Soup with Whole-Grain Bread
- **Calories:** 350 kcal
- A hearty bowl of lentil soup served with a slice of whole-grain bread, rich in fiber and B vitamins.

Dessert: Fresh Fruit Salad
- **Calories:** 150 kcal
- A mix of seasonal fruits, providing natural sweetness and essential micronutrients.

Dinner: Turkey Meatballs with Zucchini Noodles
- **Calories:** 450 kcal
- Baked turkey meatballs served over a bed of zucchini noodles, offering a light yet protein-packed meal.

Daily Total: 1400 kcal

Day 13: Gut Health Day

Breakfast: Coconut Yogurt Parfait with Mango
- **Calories:** 300 kcal
- Probiotic-rich coconut yogurt layered with mango for a fiber boost, promoting digestive health.

Snack: Kefir with a Dash of Cinnamon
- **Calories:** 150 kcal
- A glass of kefir sprinkled with cinnamon to aid digestion and add anti-inflammatory properties.

Lunch: Grilled Chicken Salad with Mixed Greens and Avocado
- **Calories:** 500 kcal
- Lean chicken breast atop a bed of mixed greens and avocado, dressed with olive oil and lemon, offering healthy fats and fiber.

Dessert: Chia Seed Pudding with Kiwi
- **Calories:** 200 kcal
- Chia seeds soaked in almond milk and topped with kiwi, enhancing gut motility and providing omega-3 fatty acids.

Dinner: Baked Salmon with Roasted Brussels Sprouts
- **Calories:** 550 kcal
- Omega-3 rich salmon with fiber-loaded Brussels sprouts to support overall digestive health.

Daily Total: 1700 kcal

Day 14: Immune Boosting Day

Breakfast: Oatmeal with Sliced Almonds and Blueberries
- **Calories:** 350 kcal
- Hearty oatmeal packed with antioxidants from blueberries and healthy fats from almonds.

Snack: Turmeric and Ginger Tea
- **Calories:** 10 kcal
- A warming beverage known for its immune-boosting and anti-inflammatory effects.

Lunch: Spinach and Strawberry Salad with Walnuts
- **Calories:** 400 kcal
- Spinach and strawberries provide Vitamin C and walnuts add zinc, both crucial for immune function.

Dessert: Dark Chocolate with a Handful of Raspberries
- **Calories:** 150 kcal
- Dark chocolate and raspberries, both rich in antioxidants and flavonoids.

Dinner: Garlic Roasted Chicken with Sweet Potatoes
- **Calories:** 490 kcal
- Garlic for its antimicrobial properties and sweet potatoes for a dose of Vitamin A, enhancing immune defense.

Daily Total: 1400 kcal

Day 15: Healthy Aging Day

Breakfast: Avocado and Tomato Toast with Flaxseeds
- **Calories:** 300 kcal
- A source of healthy fats and lycopene, topped with flaxseeds for lignans that promote longevity.

Snack: Greek Yogurt with Sliced Peaches
- **Calories:** 200 kcal
- Calcium-rich yogurt and peaches providing vitamins necessary for bone health.

Lunch: Quinoa and Kale Salad with Pomegranate Seeds
- **Calories:** 450 kcal
- Quinoa for protein, kale for phytonutrients, and pomegranate for antioxidants.

Dessert: Baked Cinnamon Apples
- **Calories:** 150 kcal
- Apples are great for fiber and cinnamon helps control blood sugar levels.

Dinner: Grilled Trout with Asparagus
- **Calories:** 400 kcal
- Trout for omega-3 fatty acids and asparagus for folate, both important for heart health and cognitive function.

Daily Total: 1500 kcal

Day 16: Stress Reduction Day

Breakfast: Berry Spinach Smoothie Bowl
- **Calories:** 300 kcal
- A smoothie bowl filled with antioxidants from berries and iron from spinach to combat oxidative stress.

Snack: Pumpkin Seeds and Sunflower Seeds
- **Calories:** 150 kcal
- Seeds are rich in magnesium, which helps reduce stress and anxiety.

Lunch: Turkey Breast Sandwich on Whole Grain Bread with Avocado
- **Calories:** 450 kcal
- Turkey contains tryptophan which aids in the production of serotonin, a mood stabilizer; avocado provides heart-healthy fats.

Dessert: Greek Yogurt with Honey and Lavender
- **Calories:** 200 kcal
- Greek yogurt for protein and probiotics; honey and lavender are known for their calming effects.

Dinner: Baked Cod with Steamed Broccoli and Sweet Potatoes
- **Calories:** 500 kcal
- Cod is a low-fat protein source, and sweet potatoes are high in fiber and vitamins, supporting overall calm and well-being.

Daily Total: 1600 kcal

Day 17: Metabolic Boost Day

Breakfast: Green Tea and Lemon Detox Water
- **Calories:** 0 kcal
- Green tea boosts metabolism and lemon helps with detoxification.

Snack: Spicy Roasted Chickpeas
- **Calories:** 150 kcal
- Chickpeas are high in protein and the spices can increase metabolic rate.

Lunch: Grilled Chicken Salad with Chili Dressing
- **Calories:** 400 kcal
- Protein-rich chicken and chili to fire up the metabolism.

Dessert: Fresh Pineapple
- **Calories:** 100 kcal
- Bromelain in pineapple aids digestion and boosts metabolic rate.

Dinner: Stir-Fried Tofu with Vegetables in Garlic Sauce
- **Calories:** 450 kcal
- Tofu for protein; garlic and vegetables for their thermogenic properties.

Daily Total: 1100 kcal

Day 18: Physical Endurance Day

Breakfast: Oatmeal with Sliced Bananas and Almond Butter
- **Calories:** 400 kcal
- Slow-releasing carbohydrates from oatmeal and bananas provide sustained energy, while almond butter adds healthy fats.

Snack: Beetroot Juice
- **Calories:** 100 kcal
- Beetroot naturally boosts blood flow and enhances oxygen delivery to muscles.

Lunch: Quinoa and Black Bean Bowl with Mixed Vegetables
- **Calories:** 500 kcal
- Quinoa and black beans are excellent for sustained energy and muscle repair.

Dessert: Dark Chocolate
- **Calories:** 100 kcal
- Dark chocolate for antioxidants and a small caffeine boost.

Dinner: Grilled Salmon with Wild Rice and Kale
- **Calories:** 500 kcal
- Omega-3 fatty acids in salmon enhance muscle recovery; wild rice and kale provide essential minerals and vitamins.

Daily Total: 1600 kcal

Day 19: Mental Health Focus Day

Breakfast: Avocado Toast on Whole Grain Bread with a Poached Egg
- **Calories:** 350 kcal
- The healthy fats in avocado and the choline in eggs support brain function and mood stabilization.

Snack: Mixed Nuts
- **Calories:** 200 kcal
- Nuts provide omega-3 fatty acids and antioxidants, which are crucial for mental health.

Lunch: Spinach Salad with Grilled Chicken, Blueberries, and Walnuts
- **Calories:** 450 kcal
- This meal is rich in folate, protein, and natural antioxidants, all known to boost mood and cognitive function.

Dessert: Dark Chocolate
- **Calories:** 100 kcal
- A small serving of dark chocolate can boost serotonin levels, improving mood and relieving stress.

Dinner: Baked Salmon with Quinoa and Steamed Asparagus
- **Calories:** 500 kcal
- Omega-3 fatty acids from salmon and fiber from quinoa and asparagus help maintain a balanced diet conducive to good mental health.

Daily Total: 1600 kcal

Day 20: Sleep Enhancement Day

Breakfast: Banana and Almond Smoothie
- **Calories:** 300 kcal
- Bananas enhance serotonin and melatonin production, aiding sleep, while almonds add a dose of muscle-relaxing magnesium.

Snack: Chamomile Tea with Honey
- **Calories:** 50 kcal
- Chamomile is known for its natural sedative effects, and honey can slightly spike insulin levels to help regulate sleep hormones.

Lunch: Turkey and Spinach Wrap
- **Calories:** 400 kcal
- Turkey is a good source of tryptophan, which is a precursor to serotonin and melatonin, the hormones that improve sleep quality.

Dessert: Kiwi
- **Calories:** 90 kcal
- Kiwi is rich in serotonin and antioxidants, known to aid sleep onset and duration.

Dinner: Grilled Chicken with Sweet Potatoes and Mixed Greens
- **Calories:** 460 kcal
- Sweet potatoes provide complex carbs that can aid in the production of sleep-inducing melatonin and serotonin.

Daily Total: 1300 kcal

Day 21: Healthy Skin Day

Breakfast: Greek Yogurt with Sliced Strawberries and a Drizzle of Honey
- **Calories:** 300 kcal
- Greek yogurt for protein and probiotics, strawberries for Vitamin C, which is vital for collagen production, and honey for its antibacterial properties.

Snack: Carrot and Celery Sticks with Hummus
- **Calories:** 150 kcal
- Carrots are high in beta-carotene, an antioxidant that prevents skin aging; celery adds hydration; hummus provides healthy fats.

Lunch: Spinach and Avocado Salad with Pumpkin Seeds
- **Calories:** 400 kcal
- This salad is loaded with Vitamin E from pumpkin seeds and healthy fats from avocado, both essential for vibrant skin.

Dessert: Mango
- **Calories:** 100 kcal
- Mangoes are rich in vitamins A and C, which are crucial for skin repair and maintenance.

Dinner: Grilled Trout with a Side of Broccoli and Almonds
- **Calories:** 550 kcal
- Trout is rich in omega-3 fatty acids, and broccoli is a powerhouse of antioxidants and vitamins that support skin health.

Daily Total: 1500 kcal

Day 22: Immune Support Day

Breakfast: Kiwi and Strawberry Smoothie
- **Calories:** 250 kcal
- Kiwis and strawberries are rich in Vitamin C, which is essential for boosting the immune system.

Snack: Brazil Nuts and Dried Apricots
- **Calories:** 200 kcal
- Brazil nuts are a great source of selenium, a key nutrient for immune health, while dried apricots offer a quick energy boost.

Lunch: Chicken Soup with Vegetables
- **Calories:** 350 kcal
- A comforting bowl of chicken soup loaded with a variety of vegetables, providing nutrients and hydration to support immune function.

Dessert: Orange Slices
- **Calories:** 80 kcal
- Fresh orange slices for a vitamin C boost and a sweet, refreshing treat.

Dinner: Baked Cod with a Side of Sautéed Spinach and Garlic
- **Calories:** 450 kcal
- Cod provides lean protein and omega-3 fatty acids, while spinach and garlic both have properties that support immune health.

Daily Total: 1330 kcal

Day 23: High Fiber Focus Day

Breakfast: Oatmeal with Chia Seeds and Blueberries
- **Calories:** 300 kcal
- Oats and chia seeds provide a high-fiber start to the day, while blueberries add antioxidants.

Snack: Almonds and Pear
- **Calories:** 150 kcal
- A snack pairing that offers both fiber and healthy fats to keep you satisfied until lunch.

Lunch: Quinoa Salad with Black Beans and Avocado
- **Calories:** 400 kcal
- Quinoa and black beans are both high in fiber, which aids in digestive health; avocado adds healthy fats.

Dessert: Baked Apple with Cinnamon
- **Calories:** 120 kcal
- A warm, fiber-rich dessert that's also comforting and sweet.

Dinner: Stir-Fried Tofu with Broccoli and Carrots
- **Calories:** 430 kcal
- A dinner rich in dietary fiber and plant-based protein, perfect for rounding out a high-fiber day.

Daily Total: 1400 kcal

Day 24: Hormonal Balance Day

Breakfast: Greek Yogurt with Flaxseed and Pumpkin Seeds
- **Calories:** 300 kcal
- Greek yogurt for probiotics, with flaxseed and pumpkin seeds which are known for their hormone-regulating properties.

Snack: Cottage Cheese with Sliced Cucumber
- **Calories:** 150 kcal
- Cottage cheese provides calcium and protein, while cucumber adds freshness and hydration.

Lunch: Salmon Salad with Leafy Greens and Olive Oil Dressing
- **Calories:** 400 kcal
- Salmon is rich in omega-3 fatty acids, essential for hormonal health; leafy greens provide essential minerals.

Dessert: Dark Chocolate Square
- **Calories:** 100 kcal
- A small portion of dark chocolate can help to regulate mood and satisfy cravings without a sugar overload.

Dinner: Grilled Turkey Breast with Sweet Potato and Asparagus
- **Calories:** 500 kcal
- Lean turkey for protein, sweet potatoes for complex carbs, and asparagus for fiber and folate, all supporting overall hormonal balance.

Daily Total: 1450 kcal

Day 25: Athletic Performance Day

Breakfast: Peanut Butter Banana Smoothie
- **Calories:** 350 kcal
- A protein-packed smoothie with banana for energy and peanut butter for sustained release of nutrients, ideal for pre-workout.

Snack: Beetroot Juice
- **Calories:** 100 kcal
- Beetroot juice is known for increasing nitric oxide levels, which can enhance blood flow and improve exercise performance.

Lunch: Grilled Chicken Breast with Quinoa and Steamed Kale
- **Calories:** 450 kcal
- Lean chicken for protein, quinoa for carbs, and kale for its high micronutrient content, perfect for post-workout recovery.

Dessert: Greek Yogurt with Honey and Almonds
- **Calories:** 200 kcal
- Greek yogurt for muscle repair, honey for a quick energy boost, and almonds for healthy fats.

Dinner: Salmon with Sweet Potato Mash and Green Beans
- **Calories:** 550 kcal
- Omega-3 fatty acids in salmon help reduce inflammation caused by intense workouts, paired with sweet potato for restoring glycogen levels.

Daily Total: 1650 kcal

Day 26: Healthy Aging Day

Breakfast: Oatmeal with Walnuts and Berries
- **Calories:** 300 kcal
- Oatmeal for heart health, walnuts for brain health, and berries for antioxidants.

Snack: Avocado Toast
- **Calories:** 250 kcal
- Avocado for healthy fats and fiber, served on whole grain toast for added B vitamins.

Lunch: Tomato Soup with Whole Grain Roll
- **Calories:** 350 kcal
- Tomato for lycopene, a powerful antioxidant, and a whole grain roll for maintaining healthy digestion.

Dessert: Baked Pear with Cinnamon
- **Calories:** 150 kcal
- Pears and cinnamon both have anti-inflammatory properties, important for aging bodies.

Dinner: Grilled Trout with Asparagus and Mixed Salad
- **Calories:** 450 kcal
- Trout for omega-3s, asparagus for folate, and a salad packed with various nutrients to support overall health.

Daily Total: 1500 kcal

Day 27: Sleep Enhancement Day

Breakfast: Scrambled Eggs with Spinach
- **Calories:** 250 kcal
- Eggs provide tryptophan, and spinach is rich in magnesium, both promoting better sleep.

Snack: Cherry Juice
- **Calories:** 120 kcal
- Cherries are one of the few natural sources of melatonin, which regulates sleep.

Lunch: Turkey and Avocado Wrap
- **Calories:** 400 kcal
- Turkey is another great source of tryptophan, and avocado adds beneficial fats.

Dessert: Vanilla Yogurt with Sliced Almonds
- **Calories:** 180 kcal
- Yogurt for calcium and almonds for a dose of magnesium, both helping in muscle relaxation and better sleep.

Dinner: Baked Cod with Roasted Brussels Sprouts and Quinoa
- **Calories:** 500 kcal
- Cod for protein with a low calorie count, Brussels sprouts, and quinoa for a light yet nutritious meal that won't disrupt sleep.

Daily Total: 1450 kcal

Day 28: Skin Health Day

Breakfast: Smoothie Bowl with Kiwi, Pineapple, and Coconut
- **Calories:** 300 kcal
- Kiwi and pineapple are rich in vitamin C for collagen production, topped with coconut for hydrating healthy fats.

Snack: Carrot and Celery Sticks with Almond Butter
- **Calories:** 200 kcal
- Carrots are high in beta-carotene, and celery provides hydration, both of which are excellent for skin health. Almond butter adds vitamin E, a vital antioxidant for the skin.

Lunch: Spinach Salad with Salmon, Avocado, and Walnuts
- **Calories:** 500 kcal
- Salmon for omega-3 fatty acids, avocado for healthy fats, and walnuts for antioxidants, all nourishing the skin from within.

Dessert: Greek Yogurt with Honey and Mixed Berries
- **Calories:** 200 kcal
- Greek yogurt provides probiotics for gut health which is linked to clear skin, berries for antioxidants, and honey for its antibacterial properties.

Dinner: Sweet Potato and Red Pepper Soup
- **Calories:** 400 kcal
- Sweet potatoes are rich in vitamins A and C, which are crucial for skin health, and red peppers are high in antioxidants.

Daily Total: 1600 kcal

Day 29: Cognitive Function Day

Breakfast: Eggs Benedict with Spinach on Whole-Grain Muffin
- **Calories:** 350 kcal
- Eggs provide choline for brain health, spinach is rich in folate, and whole-grain muffins supply complex carbs for sustained energy.

Snack: Blueberries and Greek Yogurt
- **Calories:** 150 kcal
- Blueberries are often termed 'brain berries' for their high levels of antioxidants, and Greek yogurt provides protein.

Lunch: Tuna Salad on Mixed Greens with Olive Oil Dressing
- **Calories:** 400 kcal
- Tuna is rich in omega-3 fatty acids, crucial for brain function, served over greens which provide essential nutrients.

Dessert: Dark Chocolate
- **Calories:** 100 kcal
- Dark chocolate contains flavonoids, caffeine, and theobromine, which help improve focus and concentration.

Dinner: Grilled Chicken with Quinoa and Steamed Broccoli
- **Calories:** 500 kcal
- Chicken provides lean protein, quinoa offers a full profile of amino acids, and broccoli is a great source of vitamin K, which is known to enhance cognitive function.

Daily Total: 1500 kcal

Day 30: General Wellness Day

Breakfast: Oatmeal with Chopped Nuts and Sliced Bananas

- **Calories:** 300 kcal
- Oatmeal for fiber, nuts for healthy fats and protein, and bananas for natural sweetness and potassium.

Snack: Matcha Green Tea Latte

- **Calories:** 100 kcal
- Matcha is high in antioxidants and provides a gentle caffeine boost for energy without the jitters.

Lunch: Roasted Vegetable and Hummus Wrap

- **Calories:** 400 kcal
- A variety of roasted vegetables provide vitamins and minerals, while hummus adds protein and fiber.

Dessert: Baked Cinnamon Apples

- **Calories:** 150 kcal
- Apples and cinnamon both have anti-inflammatory properties and provide a naturally sweet treat.

Dinner: Baked Halibut with a Side of Asparagus and Brown Rice

- **Calories:** 450 kcal
- Halibut for high-quality protein and omega-3 fatty acids, asparagus for fiber, and brown rice for complex carbohydrates.

Daily Total: 1400 kcal

Part IV: Additional Resources

Part IV of the book serves as a comprehensive supplement to the main content, providing readers with additional tools and references to further their understanding and application of the nutritional and wellness principles discussed throughout the book. This section aims to equip readers with practical resources that can enhance their journey towards a healthier lifestyle.

1. Comprehensive Shopping List for the Healing Kitchen

This resource provides a detailed shopping list that includes all the necessary ingredients to stock a healing kitchen. The list is categorized by food types such as proteins, whole grains, healthy fats, and a variety of fruits and vegetables. It also highlights superfoods and organic options, guiding readers on what to buy to prepare the recipes and meal plans provided in the book.

- **Key Features:**
    - Organized by pantry staples, refrigerated items, and fresh produce.
    - Suggestions for selecting high-quality ingredients.
    - Tips on seasonal purchases to maximize freshness and cost-effectiveness.

2. Weekly Shopping Lists Aligned with the 30-Day Meal Plan

To simplify the meal preparation process, this section offers pre-made weekly shopping lists that correspond with the 30-day meal plan. Each list ensures that readers have all the ingredients they need for a week's worth of meals, helping to minimize food waste and streamline shopping routines.

- **Key Features:**
    - Breakdown of quantities needed to prevent over-purchasing.
    - Alternatives for seasonal or hard-to-find ingredients.
    - Budget-friendly options to help manage food expenses.

3. Techniques for Preserving Nutrients in Foods

Understanding how to properly store and prepare food can significantly impact the nutritional quality of meals. This resource offers techniques for preserving the integrity of nutrients during food preparation and storage, including methods of cooking that retain vitamins and minerals, and tips for storing produce to maintain freshness.

- **Key Features:**
    - Cooking methods like steaming, roasting, and blanching that optimize nutrient retention.
    - Instructions on proper vegetable washing and handling to prevent nutrient loss.
    - Advice on the best storage practices for different types of perishable foods.

4. Safe and Effective Detoxification Practices

This section provides a guide to safe and effective detox methods that can help rid the body of toxins without compromising health. It emphasizes natural detoxification support through diet, supplements, and lifestyle adjustments, providing a cautious approach to popular detox trends.

- **Key Features:**
    - Daily and weekly detox plans incorporating hydrating fluids, dietary fibers, and detoxifying foods.
    - Warnings about common detox myths and potentially harmful practices.
    - Recommendations for natural supplements that support liver and kidney function.

Comprehensive Shopping List for the Healing Kitchen

This comprehensive shopping list is designed to equip readers with all the essential ingredients needed to prepare nutritious meals that align with the teachings of the book. The list is organized into categories to simplify the shopping experience, ensuring that the kitchen is well-stocked with a variety of health-promoting foods.

1. Fresh Produce

- **Vegetables:** Kale, spinach, broccoli, cauliflower, carrots, bell peppers, sweet potatoes, onions, garlic, ginger, mushrooms.
- **Fruits:** Apples, bananas, berries (strawberries, blueberries, raspberries), oranges, lemons, avocados, pineapples, mangoes.

2. Proteins

- **Animal-based:** Free-range eggs, organic chicken breast, wild-caught salmon, turkey, lean cuts of grass-fed beef.
- **Plant-based:** Lentils, chickpeas, black beans, quinoa, tofu, tempeh, edamame.

3. Whole Grains

- **Essentials:** Brown rice, whole grain pasta, quinoa, oatmeal, barley, millet.
- **Specialty grains:** Amaranth, bulgur, farro, teff (ideal for gluten-free diets).

4. Nuts and Seeds

- **Nuts:** Almonds, walnuts, cashews, Brazil nuts.
- **Seeds:** Chia seeds, flaxseeds, pumpkin seeds, sunflower seeds, hemp seeds.

5. Healthy Fats

- **Oils:** Extra virgin olive oil, coconut oil, avocado oil.
- **Others:** Avocados, olives, coconut milk, almond butter.

6. Dairy and Dairy Alternatives

- **Dairy:** Organic Greek yogurt, kefir, grass-fed butter, cottage cheese.
- **Plant-based alternatives:** Almond milk, coconut yogurt, oat milk, cashew cheese.

7. Condiments and Spices

- **Herbs and spices:** Basil, cilantro, parsley, turmeric, cinnamon, black pepper, sea salt, cayenne pepper, rosemary.
- **Condiments:** Apple cider vinegar, balsamic vinegar, raw honey, maple syrup, mustard, tahini.

8. Beverages

- **Teas:** Green tea, herbal teas (peppermint, chamomile, ginger).
- **Others:** Coffee, mineral water.

9. Superfoods

- **Powders:** Spirulina, cacao, maca, matcha.
- **Berries:** Goji berries, acai berries.
- **Others:** Bee pollen, wheatgrass.

10. Snacks

- **Healthy snacks:** Dried seaweed, kale chips, dark chocolate (70% cocoa or higher), fruit bars (no added sugar), roasted chickpeas.

Tips for Using This List

- **Prioritize Fresh and Organic:** Whenever possible, choose fresh, organic produce to reduce exposure to pesticides and chemicals.
- **Seasonal Shopping:** Buy seasonal fruits and vegetables to ensure freshness and cost-effectiveness. This also supports local farming.
- **Bulk Buying:** Purchase items like grains, nuts, and seeds in bulk to save money and reduce packaging waste.
- **Check Labels:** Always read labels on packaged foods to avoid added sugars, unhealthy fats, and unnecessary additives.
- **Plan Ahead:** Plan your meals for the week ahead to ensure you buy only what you need, which helps reduce food waste.

This shopping list serves as a foundation for building a healing kitchen that supports a healthy diet. By stocking these essentials, you'll be well-equipped to prepare a wide array of nutritious meals that promote overall wellness and align with the principles of the book.

Weekly Shopping Lists Aligned with the 30-Day Meal Plan

To ensure a seamless and efficient meal preparation process, these weekly shopping lists are tailored to correspond precisely with the recipes and meal structures outlined in the 30-Day Meal Plan. By organizing shopping this way, readers can minimize food waste, maintain freshness, and ensure they have all necessary ingredients each week.

Week 1 Shopping List

This list covers all the ingredients needed for the first week of the meal plan, ensuring a variety of meals that provide balanced nutrition.

- **Vegetables:**
  - Spinach (1 large bag)
  - Kale (1 bunch)
  - Sweet potatoes (4 medium)
  - Broccoli (2 heads)
  - Avocado (3)
  - Carrots (1 bag)
  - Garlic (1 bulb)
  - Onions (2 medium)
  - Bell peppers (2)
  - Mushrooms (1 pack)
- **Fruits:**
  - Bananas (6)
  - Apples (4)
  - Berries (2 cups, mixed or single type)
  - Lemons (3)
  - Oranges (2)
- **Proteins:**
  - Chicken breasts (4)
  - Salmon fillets (2)
  - Eggs (1 dozen)
  - Canned black beans (2 cans)
  - Tofu (1 block)
  - Greek yogurt (2 containers)
- **Whole Grains:**

- Quinoa (1 bag)
- Brown rice (1 bag)
- Whole grain bread (1 loaf)
- Oatmeal (1 box)

- **Nuts, Seeds, and Healthy Fats:**
  - Almond butter (1 jar)
  - Chia seeds (1 bag)
  - Walnuts (1 bag)
  - Extra virgin olive oil (1 bottle)

- **Dairy and Alternatives:**
  - Almond milk (1 carton)
  - Cheese (optional, for salads or sandwiches)

- **Condiments and Spices:**
  - Sea salt (1 container)
  - Black pepper (1 container)
  - Cinnamon (1 bottle)
  - Turmeric (1 bottle)

- **Beverages:**
  - Green tea (1 box)

Week 2 Shopping List

This list ensures diversity by introducing different ingredients to avoid monotony and sustain excitement in meal preparation.

- **Vegetables:**
  - Asparagus (1 bunch)
  - Zucchini (2 large)
  - Red onions (2)
  - Cherry tomatoes (1 pack)
  - Red bell peppers (2)
  - Cucumber (1)

- **Fruits:**
  - Pineapple (1)

- Mango (1)

- Pears (3)

- Kiwi (4)

- **Proteins:**

    - Lean beef (1 pound, for stir-fry or salads)

    - Turkey breast (1 pound)

    - Canned chickpeas (2 cans)

    - Lentils (1 bag)

- **Whole Grains:**

    - Farro (1 bag)

    - Whole grain pasta (1 box)

- **Nuts, Seeds, and Healthy Fats:**

    - Pumpkin seeds (1 bag)

    - Flaxseeds (1 bag)

- **Dairy and Alternatives:**

    - Coconut yogurt (1 container)

    - Cashew cheese (1 pack)

- **Condiments and Spices:**

    - Balsamic vinegar (1 bottle)

    - Mustard (1 bottle)

    - Honey (1 bottle)

- **Beverages:**

    - Herbal teas (1 box, chamomile or peppermint)

Each weekly list is designed to complement the specific meals planned for that week, ensuring that all ingredients are fresh and readily available for cooking. This methodical approach not only simplifies the meal preparation process but also helps to manage budget effectively by buying only what is necessary for the week's meals.

Techniques for Preserving Nutrients in Foods

Preserving the nutritional value of food is essential for maximizing health benefits from the diet. This section outlines various techniques that can be employed in the kitchen to maintain and even enhance the nutrient content of foods, focusing on preparation, cooking, and storage methods.

1. Choosing the Right Cooking Method

Different cooking methods can have a significant impact on the nutrients in your food. Here's how you can preserve more nutrients during cooking:

- **Steaming:** This is one of the best methods for preserving vitamins and minerals when cooking vegetables, fish, or poultry. Steaming is gentle on the food and doesn't leach nutrients as boiling can.

- **Blanching:** Quickly boiling vegetables and then plunging them into ice water can help preserve their color, texture, and nutrients. This is ideal for vegetables that you may want to freeze or use in salads.

- **Sautéing:** Quick, high-heat cooking like sautéing can preserve flavors and nutrients. Use healthy oils like olive or avocado oil to enhance absorption of fat-soluble vitamins.

- **Roasting:** Cooking vegetables at high temperatures can enhance certain nutrients like lycopene in tomatoes and beta-carotene in carrots. Roasting can also concentrate flavors without significant nutrient loss.

2. Minimizing Nutrient Loss in Preparation

How you prepare foods can also affect their nutritional content:

- **Washing:** Wash fruits and vegetables just before use, not immediately after bringing them home. Prolonged exposure to water can cause water-soluble vitamins like vitamin C and B vitamins to leach out.

- **Peeling:** Many nutrients are found in the outer layers of fruits and vegetables. Whenever possible, use vegetables and fruits with their skins to maximize fiber and nutrients intake.

- **Cutting:** Expose less surface area to air to prevent oxidation of nutrients. Cut fruits and vegetables close to cooking or eating time, and use sharp knives to reduce damage to the cells.

3. Proper Storage Techniques

Storing foods properly can greatly affect their nutritional quality:

- **Refrigeration:** Keep perishable produce in the refrigerator to slow down the decay process and nutrient degradation. Most vegetables and fruits benefit from refrigeration, except for a few like tomatoes and potatoes.

- **Airtight Containers:** Store grains, nuts, and seeds in airtight containers to protect them from oxidation and preserve their nutrient content.

- **Freezing:** Freezing is one of the best ways to preserve nutrients in foods for longer periods. It halts the loss of sensitive vitamins and enzymes, particularly in fruits and vegetables.

4. Using Antioxidants

Adding antioxidants can help preserve foods naturally:

- **Lemon Juice:** Applying lemon juice to cut fruits and vegetables can prevent oxidation of vitamin C and color degradation.

- **Vitamin C Powder:** A sprinkle of vitamin C powder on cut fruits and vegetables not only enhances nutrient content but also preserves their freshness.

5. Cooking with the Lid On

Cooking with the lid on can help to trap steam and heat, cooking the food more gently and preserving heat-sensitive vitamins such as vitamin C and many B vitamins.

Safe and Effective Detoxification Practices

Detoxification practices can be beneficial for cleansing the body of toxins and improving overall health when performed correctly and safely. This section of the book outlines a series of safe and effective methods to support the body's natural detoxification processes without compromising health.

1. Hydration

Hydration is fundamental to detoxification. Water helps to flush toxins from the body through the kidneys and supports optimal function of the lymphatic system, an integral part of the immune system.

- **Daily Water Intake:** Aim for at least 8-10 glasses of water per day. You can enhance detoxification by starting your day with a glass of warm lemon water to stimulate digestion and liver function.

- **Herbal Teas:** Incorporate herbal teas such as dandelion, milk thistle, or green tea, which contain compounds that support detoxification and liver health.

2. Dietary Fiber

Fiber plays a crucial role in removing waste and toxins from your body via the digestive tract.

- **Increase Fiber Intake:** Include plenty of fiber-rich foods in your diet, such as fruits, vegetables, whole grains, and legumes.

- **Diverse Sources:** Vary your fiber sources to benefit from different types of dietary fiber, such as soluble and insoluble, each supporting detoxification in different ways.

3. Nutrient-Rich Diet

Eating a nutrient-rich diet helps support the liver and other detoxifying organs. Focus on foods rich in antioxidants, vitamins, and minerals that promote detoxification.

- **Antioxidant-Rich Foods:** Incorporate berries, nuts, seeds, green tea, and leafy greens, which are high in antioxidants like vitamin C and E.

- **Cruciferous Vegetables:** Broccoli, cauliflower, and Brussels sprouts enhance liver detoxification enzymes and provide fiber.

4. Regular Exercise

Physical activity increases blood flow, improves digestion, and accelerates the removal of toxins through sweat.

- **Consistent Exercise Routine:** Engage in regular aerobic exercise such as walking, cycling, or swimming for at least 30 minutes a day.

- **Include Sweating:** Activities like using a sauna can help eliminate toxins through perspiration. Ensure you are well-hydrated and listen to your body to avoid dehydration.

5. Limit Exposure to Toxins

Reducing your exposure to external toxins is just as important as removing toxins from your body.

- **Household Chemicals:** Opt for natural cleaning products.

- **Personal Care Products:** Choose beauty and personal care products that are free from harmful chemicals such as parabens, sulfates, and phthalates.

- **Food Contaminants:** Buy organic produce where possible to avoid pesticide residues. Wash fruits and vegetables thoroughly, or peel them.

6. Mindful Practices

Stress can impede the body's natural detoxification by affecting the liver and other organs.

- **Mindfulness and Meditation:** Regular practice can reduce stress and support body functions.

- **Adequate Sleep:** Ensure 7-9 hours of quality sleep per night to support the body's regenerative processes.

7. Detox with Professional Guidance

For those considering a more rigorous detox plan, such as a detox diet or fast:

- **Consult Healthcare Providers:** Always consult with a healthcare professional before starting any new detox plan, especially if you have underlying health conditions or are taking medication.

- **Guided Detox Programs:** Consider participating in detox programs that offer professional supervision and support.

Conversion charts

Length

US (inches)	UK (centimeters)
1 inch	2.54 cm
12 inches (1 foot)	30.48 cm

Volume

US	UK Equivalent
1 teaspoon	4.93 ml
1 tablespoon	14.79 ml
1 fluid ounce	29.57 ml
1 cup	236.59 ml
1 pint (16 fl oz)	473.18 ml
1 quart (32 fl oz)	946.35 ml
1 gallon (128 fl oz)	3.785 L

Weight

US	UK Equivalent
1 ounce	28.35 grams
1 pound	453.59 grams
1 stone	6.35 kg

Cooking Temperature

Fahrenheit (°F)	Celsius (°C)
32°F (freezing point of water)	0°C
212°F (boiling point of water)	100°C
250°F	120°C
275°F	135°C
300°F	150°C
325°F	160°C
350°F	175°C
375°F	190°C
400°F	200°C
425°F	220°C
450°F	230°C
475°F	245°C

Thank you so much for purchasing my book! I'm thrilled to have you as part of my reading family.

If you could take a moment to scan the QR code below and leave your honest review on Amazon, I would be deeply grateful.

If you are reading the ebook version, please click on this link:

https://www.amazon.com/review/create-review?&ASIN=B0CWMCM7BK

Your feedback is incredibly important to me—it helps me grow as a writer and makes our community stronger. I genuinely love hearing from you and value your thoughts immensely!

HERE IS YOU FREE GIFT!

👇 SCAN HERE TO DOWNLOAD IT

🎁 **Over 10 hours of exclusive Dr. Barbara O'Neill's videos.**

🎁 **15 Transformative Juice Blends for Detox, Energy, and Immunity, which elevate your health to its peak with nature-inspired beverages.**